RESEARCH METHODS

A Framework for Evidence-Based Clinical Practice

Wendy L. Hurley, PhD, ATC, CSCS
Associate Professor of Motor Behavior
Kinesiology Department
State University of New York College at Cortland
Cortland, New York

Craig R. Denegar, PhD, PT, ATC, FNATA
Department of Physical Therapy
University of Connecticut
Neag School of Education
Storrs, Connecticut

Jay Hertel, PhD, ATC, FACSM, FNATA
Associate Professor of Kinesiology and
Physical Medicine & Rehabilitation
University of Virginia
Charlottesville, Virginia

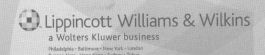 Lippincott Williams & Wilkins
a Wolters Kluwer business
Philadelphia · Baltimore · New York · London
Buenos Aires · Hong Kong · Sydney · Tokyo

Acquisitions Editor: Emily Lupash
Product Managers: Meredith Brittain/John Larkin
Marketing Manager: Allison Powell
Designer: Doug Smock
Compositor: MPS Limited, A Macmillan Company

First Edition

Printed in China

Library of Congress Cataloging-in-Publication Data

Hurley, Wendy L.
Research methods : a framework for evidence-based clinical practice / Wendy L. Hurley, Craig R. Denegar, Jay Hertel. — 1st ed.
　　p. ; cm.
　　Includes bibliographical references and index.
　　Summary: "This research methods textbook distinguishes itself from other textbooks by providing a unique framework and perspective for users/students to establish the relevancy of research in their clinical practice. Many, if not most, students in professional preparation allied health care programs view the research methods/statistics course requirement of the curriculum as an obstacle to be overcome, or at best, as a necessary evil. Most research methods textbooks promote these notions because of the way they are presented. Of course, most times they are written by researchers or statisticians and are absolutely correct in presenting the theoretical underpinnings and mechanistic applications of the scientific method. They correctly present explanations as to why one type of methodology requires a certain type of statistical analysis based on the characteristics of the study population, the type of data collected, or the underlying assumptions pertinent to a specific statistical model. So, while technically beyond reproach, their failure is in establishing how and why research activity and understanding is integral to a professional practice"—Provided by publisher.
　　ISBN 978-0-7817-9768-9 (alk. paper)
　　1. Medicine—Research—Methodology. 2. Evidence-based medicine. I. Denegar, Craig R. II. Hertel, Jay. III. Title.
　　[DNLM: 1. Biomedical Research—methods. 2. Evidence-Based Medicine—methods.
　　3. Research Design. W 20.5]
　　R850.H87 2011
　　610.72—dc22
　　　　　　　　　　　　　　　　　　　　　　　　　　　　　　　　2010026652

To purchase additional copies of this book, call our customer service department at **(800) 638-3030** or fax orders to **(301) 223-2320**. International customers should call **(301) 223-2300**.

Visit Lippincott Williams & Wilkins on the Internet: http://www.lww.com. Lippincott Williams & Wilkins customer service representatives are available from 8:30 am to 6:00 pm, EST.

9　8　7　6　5　4　3　2　1

RRS1007

To Gram—When I was a child, you read to me as I sat on your lap, you encouraged my curiosity, you allowed me to ask questions, you supported my dreams and imagination, and you always showed me love and acceptance. I miss you. To Dr. Bruce W. Young, Mr. David J. Tomasi, Dr. Lori A. Michener, Dr. Bradley D. Hatfield, Dr. W.E. Buckley, Dr. Craig R. Denegar, and Dr. Karl M. Newell—My beloved teachers, respected mentors, and trusted professional role models. Your lessons continue to provide guidance and direction as I hear your words in my mind's ear and see your examples in my mind's eye. This book would never have been possible without your belief in me, and your lasting influences on me both personally and professionally. It is my greatest privilege to remain your humble and loyal student. I honor you with my gratitude, love, and devotion. To my students—We learn together, and I grow as you teach me what I need to do to become better at helping you learn how to learn. I am fortunate to share my academic passions and my favorite sagacious musings from the philosophies of Zen, Buddhism, and Taoism with you. To Brent—You understand me, and I love you. And, to Luka—Always.

WLH

To Sue, Charlie, and Cody for their love, support, and daily inspiration.

CRD

To my parents, Jim and Kay Hertel, for providing the opportunity for me to pursue a career in athletic training and sports medicine research, and to all of the students I've had the opportunity to work with over the past 15 years. If I manage to teach others half of what you have taught me, I'll be satisfied.

JH

FOREWORD

This research methods textbook distinguishes itself from other textbooks by providing a unique framework and perspective for users/students to establish the relevancy of research in their clinical practice. Many, if not most, students in professional preparation allied health care programs view the research methods/statistics course requirement of the curriculum as an obstacle to be overcome, or at best, as a necessary evil. Most research methods textbooks promote these notions because of the way they are presented. Of course, most times they are written by researchers or statisticians and are absolutely correct in presenting the theoretical underpinnings and mechanistic applications of the scientific method. They correctly present explanations as to why one type of methodology requires a certain type of statistical analysis based on the characteristics of the study population, the type of data collected, or the underlying assumptions pertinent to a specific statistical model. So, while technically beyond reproach, their failure is in establishing how and why research activity and understanding is integral to a professional practice.

In this textbook, the authors appreciate professional realities that have relevancy to professional preparation and the role of research within that preparation. First, they promote that understanding research is a *required competency* in allied health care preparation. That is, most allied health care professionals are going to be consumers of research literature for the duration of their professional lives. This is often enforced by continuing education requirements that reflect the understanding that medical and allied medical bodies of knowledge are ever expanding and/or being refined and must be communicated to clinicians. Thus, at a minimum, professional preparation programs must provide the opportunity for the student to establish competencies in reading, critically evaluating, and synthesizing research into their clinical practice.

The reality is that most medical and allied medical professions have accepted that their disciplines need to follow an evidence-based best practice approach to clinical practice and professional preparation in order to be effective today. Most of their professional organizations actively promote through funding and dissemination vehicles this research paradigm. This is not at the exclusion of other valuable research paradigms, but rather as an emphasis commensurate with current disciplinary interest.

The authors have taken these realities and developed the research elements of this textbook to be professionally relevant to clinical movement practitioners (e.g., physical therapists and certified athletic trainers). They use a commonsense-style presentation of the conceptual and theoretical bases for the clinical research enterprise and provide clear examples of application, evaluation, and integration into clinical practice.

Part I introduces the reader to the basic tenets of the research enterprise as it relates to clinical practice. A wonderful chapter is presented on how to read and evaluate research articles. This is a very pragmatic chapter that highlights the elements of an article so the reader can critically appraise the quality of the article. The history of evidence-based clinical practice is presented along with a chapter about how research can be used to establish best practices. The last chapter in this section provides an overlay of ethical principles that need to be operative in research and clinical practice enterprises.

Part II has seven chapters that effectively make the case that the conceptual, elemental parts of research have a role in the reader's effort to establish an evidence-based practice. This is accomplished by describing how a reader could have a clinical question and that the question is what dictates the research methodology and analysis. One chapter provides the reader with a way to find resources on clinical practice topics and evaluate the quality of the resources. Another establishes that there is a hierarchy of evidence and the reader needs to know what level or quality of evidence is important for them to use in their clinical practice. Several chapters are nicely presented that introduce the most common types of scientific inquiry and statistical analysis related to evidence-based practice.

Part III carries this utilitarian presentation approach to the research enterprise even further. The chapters are organized into clinical categories rather than research method categories. That is, Chapter 13 presents what clinical research methodology and analysis is appropriate when the reader is trying to find out about the evaluation and diagnosis of orthopaedic conditions. Chapter 14 is about screening and prevention of illnesses and injuries and what kinds of clinical research and analysis are appropriate. Chapter 15 presents the research options that clinical movement practitioners can use to develop evidence about the efficacy of treatment/intervention options they may want to use. Chapter 16 further develops the concepts of treatment outcomes and broadens the focus to present common methods and relevant data analysis techniques. The last two chapters in this part focus on how to extend research results to a clinical practice and how to organize many research results into a usable body of clinical evidence.

Parts IV and V provide sections that are unique to this text. But, again, the utilitarian approach is taken. These sections are "how-to's" for a clinical movement practitioner to appreciate how clinical research results are disseminated. As a research consumer, this is important for them to know. Also, the authors provide some guidance on how to effectively write a funding proposal for a research project. Again, many students in professional preparation programs begin to favor the research element of their discipline and want to become actively involved in developing and answering their own clinical questions. Finally, the authors provide insight into how clinical evidence can be used in clinical learning and teaching.

The genius of this text is that it is written for clinical professionals to understand and appreciate research elements that are going to positively affect their clinical practice. All the research methodology and analysis contained herein is within the context of improving clinical outcomes. In other words, the authors illustrate how clinical practice should drive the research enterprise rather than the converse. In this way, the information becomes relevant to something clinical professionals value and are therefore willing to accept and incorporate research competencies in their clinical practice.

W.E. Buckley, PhD, MBA, ATC
Professor of Exercise and Sport Science, and Health Education
Department of Kinesiology
The Pennsylvania State University

PREFACE

*Process transforms any
journey into a series of small
steps, taken one by one, to reach
any goal. Process transcends
time, teaches patience, rests
on a solid foundation of careful
preparation, and embodies trust
in our unfolding potential.*

*~Dan Millman (Millman D.
The Laws of Spirit: Simple,
Powerful Truths for Making
Life Work. Tiburon, CA:
H J Kramer Inc; 1995.)*

PURPOSE AND AUDIENCE

The purpose of this book is to provide a theoretical framework that will enable students and practitioners to interpret and apply research into an evidence-based best practice model. This book will serve as a primary course textbook in upper-level undergraduate and graduate allied health programs for clinical movement practitioners in both athletic training education programs and physical therapy programs. The focus of this book is research methods, with emphasis on application to evidence-based best practice for clinical allied health programs.

This book is intended to fill the void that exists in medical professions for a textbook on research methods for evidence-based clinical practice for movement practitioners. We've been teaching research methods for a combined 30 years to both undergraduate and graduate students in allied health programs that emphasize evidence-based clinical practice, and throughout this time, there has continued to be a void in existing research methods textbooks to address the specific needs of disciplines and educational programs that follow an evidence-based best practice approach to clinical practice and clinical education. As a result, we've been left to use our own personal notes on research methods supplemented by research methods textbooks designed and intended for nonclinical programs such as Physical Education, or nonmovement practitioners such as nurses.

Existing materials currently do not provide the breadth and depth of discipline-appropriate informational substance necessary for application to evidence-based clinical practice for movement practitioners in the professional practices of physical therapy and athletic training. The approach to research methods is often dry and theoretical. If examples are provided, they tend to be methodological and scientific rather than practical. As a result, the texts are often uninteresting and read like instruction manuals. All too often, the unfortunate outcome has been that students reject their research methods text or put it aside because they feel as though they cannot connect with the material and the manner in which it is presented.

While the procedural methods of empirical research are consistent across disciplines, the examples and connections to clinical programs are left the responsibility of the professor. Often this has resulted in feedback from students who complain about the expense of buying a textbook that they don't like and don't use because they prefer to use our lecture notes and examples rather than purchase the course textbook. It has been our experience that with the lack of targeted information in the textbook, students struggle to make application to their core curriculum and all too often the result is that students disengage from the learning process and often draw the erroneous conclusions that research is not for them or their future profession. After years of students asking us why we didn't write our own textbook on this subject matter, we feel that it is time to offer a discipline-appropriate course textbook in research methods for movement practitioners in evidence-based clinical practice.

While the concept of evidence-based clinical practice is still relatively new, the body of literature on this topic has grown considerably over the last 5 years. It seems that perhaps this notion has been slow to catch on in the United States, but internationally it has seemed to be more widely recognized as a hot topic. As grant monies become more available nationally to focus on this area in medicine and clinical practice, it is likely that the concept will become more widespread throughout colleges and universities in the United States. (To this point, we felt it important to include a chapter that specifically addresses the issue of grant writing and provides helpful guidelines, examples, and suggestions for writing funding proposals.) This text references much of this current literature and contemporary material with the sole purpose of targeting this untapped audience of allied health professionals and clinical movement practitioners (i.e., physical therapists and certified athletic trainers).

APPROACH

The focal point of our approach to research methods is to provide guidance and direction for students, instructors, and practitioners on how to acquire, read, interpret, assess, and apply research as evidence in clinical practice has not been provided in traditional research methods textbooks. We tend to view statistical analysis as the flip side of research methodology, or two sides of the same coin.

We approach the subject matter conceptually and practically. Using a common-sense style, conceptual and theoretical frameworks are introduced and discussed with clear application and integration to evidence-based clinical research. While much research methodology is known this information will be restated in a clear, detailed manner targeting practitioners in evidence-based clinical care and students in professional preparation allied health care programs. Discipline-specific vocabulary, examples, and case studies will be used to help the target audience better understand the role and process of research in evidence-based clinical practice.

CHAPTER FEATURES

Each chapter of *Research Methods* provides the following elements to enhance the usability of the text and offers a fresh approach to research methods for clinical movement practitioners and students interested in learning about evidence-based clinical practice:

- Key terms and concepts are bolded throughout the chapter to help the reader focus their attention on scientific nomenclature and vocabulary essential to a basic understanding of the chapter content and context.
- Chapter objectives detail what the reader will learn in the chapter and highlight important pedagogical outcomes while also serving as a three-fold self-assessment for readers (What are some important reasons for me to read this chapter? How does this knowledge help me prepare to read it? And, after reading this chapter, can I satisfy this list of learning outcomes?). Readers are encouraged to make use of the chapter objectives to help guide their reading and assess their level of reading comprehension.
- Concept checks reinforce important chapter content and purposefully reiterate noteworthy theory and viewpoints.
- Examples throughout chapters make concepts easier to grasp and apply to real-life research and clinical decision-making situations.
- A chapter summary at the end of each chapter provides a comprehensive review of the chapter and provides a take-home message for the readers.
- A list of key points further elucidates concepts, theories, and viewpoints presented and elaborated throughout the chapter as both foundation to the current chapter and groundwork to subsequent chapters, thus presenting a full-circle approach by reinforcing the importance of key terms, chapter objectives, concept checks, examples, and the chapter summary within the textbook.
- Chapter references and suggested readings are provided to aid the reader with supplemental materials for breadth and depth of knowledge, and demonstrate appropriate use and formal citation of original sources in empirical research.
- Figures and tables offer illustrations to provide the reader with visual examples that help support important information detailed in the text.

- End-of-chapter critical thinking questions and thought-provoking discussion-based problem-solving questions serve as necessary opportunities for discussion, review, assessment, and critical appraisal to help organize and guide readers' thought processes as we lead them through the thought-structured progression of problem-solving, which is a foundational requirement for learning to apply research methodology and follow an evidence-based model of clinical practice.

By providing consistent features in each chapter, this approach guides the reader as they encounter new vocabulary and learn to interpret and apply content knowledge in a way that makes sense to them. In this manner, the text is both a learning tool and an informational resource for research methods.

ORGANIZATION

The book is organized into five parts. Part I (Chapters 1 to 5) is structured as an opening presentation of underlying conceptual frameworks and theoretical underpinnings in clinical research and evidence-based practice, and an introduction to the skills for critiquing and analyzing research is introduced. Chapter 1 covers the concept of empirical research and the basic tenants of research methodology as a collective paradigm. Chapter 2 provides a guide for how to read research and offers a framework for evaluating research articles. Chapter 3 introduces the notion of evidence-based clinical practice and explains how to distinguish best practices. Chapter 4 addresses the historical perspective of evidence-based medicine to provide lead into the necessity of ethics in research and practice (covered in Chapter 5).

Part II (Chapters 6 to 12) is organized around the research process in terms of statistical analyses and the idea of research as evidence. More specifically, this section addresses how the question drives the methods when seeking answers to clinical questions, because we are of the pedagogical and theoretical perspectives that it is difficult to "teach" research methods without simultaneously addressing statistics. Chapter 6 covers informational sources, search strategies, and critical appraisal of research as evidence. Chapter 7 addresses the issue of hierarchy of evidence. Chapter 8 deals with qualitative inquiry, while Chapter 9 begins to sort out quantitative inquiry. Chapters 10 and 11 describe research designs and data analysis while introducing the statistical perspective of research methods. Chapter 10 discusses the fundamentals of statistical analysis, focusing on validity and reliability of measures. Chapter 11 covers tests of comparison. Chapter 12 highlights measures of association.

The concepts that are introduced in Parts I and II and then developed and elaborated in Part III focuse on clinical research diagnosis, prevention, and treatment. In this way, Part III (Chapters 13 to 18) is ordered to describe research designs and data analysis for each type of study, and then provide some examples to illustrate its application. Our goal is to address and apply concepts of research methods into prevention, diagnostics, and intervention outcomes. We are of the perspective that these are the issues at the heart of evidence-based medicine—why disease and injury occur (epidemiology) and what can I, as a clinician, do to prevent the condition in the patient in my office (clinical epidemiology), etc. Chapter 13 addresses evaluation and diagnosis from the perspective of research methods and data analysis. Chapter 14 looks at screening and prevention of illness and injuries, again from the perspective of research methods and data analysis. Chapter 15 explores the notion of treatment outcomes across the disablement spectrum. Chapter 16 expands on this and looks at treatment outcomes from the perspective of research methods and data analysis. Chapter 17 covers the topics of clinical prediction rules and practice guidelines. And, Chapter 18 explores the application and usefulness of systematic review and meta-analysis in evidence-based clinical practice.

Parts IV and V are unique to our book on several levels. The topics covered in these chapters are uncommon in most traditional textbooks and are even rarely mentioned in a book on research methods. Part IV (Chapters 19 and 20) is concentrated on the dissemination of research. Specifically, Chapter 19 offers guidelines and suggestions for presenting research findings; and, Chapter 20 offers a detailed guide with examples for writing the funding proposal. Part V (Chapters 21 and 22) covers the integration of evidence-based medicine into the education experience. Chapter 21 explores the notion of evidence in learning and teaching. Chapter 22 wraps up the discussion and comes full circle to revisit the topic of evidence in the context of the clinical experience.

ADDITIONAL RESOURCES

Research Methods includes additional resources for both instructors and students that are available on the book's companion website at http://thePoint.lww.com/ Hurley.

Instructor Resources

Approved adopting instructors will be given access to the following additional resources:

- Answers to the critical thinking problems found in each chapter
- One to two example assignments for each chapter
- A chapter assignment template—with accompanying guidelines, directions, and suggestions—that can be used by instructors to create their own chapter assignments
- PowerPoint slides for each chapter
- An image bank of all the figures and tables in the book

Student Resources

All purchasers of the textbook can access the searchable Full Text On-line by going to the *Research Methods* website at http://thePoint.lww.com/Hurley. See the inside front cover of this textbook for more details, including the passcode you will need to gain access to the website.

ACKNOWLEDGMENTS

No book is the result of any one person's efforts, yet we accept any mistakes as ours alone. We would like to thank the following people whose efforts were essential to this project:

- Our product manager, Meredith Brittain, and her editorial staff for their talents, continued hard work, patience, and assistance in bringing this vision to fruition.
- Our reviewers, for their time, feedback, and suggestions for improvement.
- Our contributing authors for their time, expertise, and generous participation. These include the coauthors of Chapter 20, Amy Henderson-Harr (Assistant Vice President, Research and Sponsored Programs, State University of New York College at Cortland) and Allan Shang (Assistant Professor of Anesthesiology, Duke University School of Medicine, and Senior Research Scientist, The Fitzpatrick Institute for Photonics, Duke University Pratt School of Engineering).
- We would also like to acknowledge the following individuals who contributed suggestions for the text: Timothy J. Bryant (Lecturer III, Kinesiology Department, State University of New York College at Cortland), for his help with Chapters 5 and 8; Brent Thomas Wilson (Assistant Professor, Communication Disorders and Sciences Department, State University of New York College at Cortland), for his help with Chapters 5 and 8; and, Amy Henderson-Harr, for her help with Chapter 5.
- Our students and patients, past and present. We offer special acknowledgment to the following students for their assistance in this project: Caitlin Latham, Lauren Lenney, Patrick Sullivan.
- Our contemporaries in education, research, and medicine.
- The many past generations of teachers, clinical researchers, and medical practitioners who came before us. We have benefited from your countless, sometimes unrecognized, sacrifices, and your successes and failures paved the way for evidence-based practice.

We would also like to thank our families and friends for their understanding and support throughout the many hours during which our work keeps us away from those most precious parts of our lives: the persons, the times, and the occasions that we cannot recover after they are missed or gone.

CONTENTS

PART III
CLINICAL RESEARCH: DIAGNOSIS, PREVENTION, AND TREATMENT   213

Reviewers

Diane P. Brown, PhD, OTR
Associate Clinical Professor
School of Occupational Therapy
Texas Woman's University
Denton, TX

Allyn Byars, PhD, CSCS, *D
Associate Professor
Department of Kinesiology
Angelo State University
San Angelo, TX

Mary Ellen Camire, PhD
Professor
Food Science and Human Nutrition
University of Maine
Orono, ME

D. Scott Davis, PT, MS, EdD, OCS
Associate Professor
Department of Human Performance and Exercise Science
West Virginia University
Morgantown, WV

Dawn M. Hankins, PhD, ATC, LAT
Associate Professor and Curriculum Director for Athletic Training
Athletic Training, School of Nursing and Health Professions
McKendree University
Lebanon, IL

Patti Kalvelage, MS, OTR/L
Senior Lecturer, MOT Program
Department of Human Health and Services
Governors State University
University Park, IL

Suh-Jen Lin, PT, PhD
Associate Professor
School of Physical Therapy
Texas Woman's University
Dallas, TX

Elizabeth Rink, PhD
Assistant Professor
Health and Human Development
Montana State University
Bozeman, MT

Barbara Sanders, PT, PhD, SCS
Professor and Chair, Department of Physical Therapy
Associate Dean, College of Health Professions
Texas State University
San Marcos, TX

Hal Strough, PhD, ATR, ATC
Department Chair/Assistant Professor
Athletic Training
The College of St. Scholastica
Duluth, MN

Laura K. Vogtle, PhD, OTR/L
Professor and Director, Postprofessional Master's Program
Department of Occupational Therapy
University of Alabama at Birmingham
Birmingham, AL

Bruce Watkins, PhD
Associate Professor
Sport Management
University of Michigan
Ann Arbor, MI

Barbara Prudhomme White, PhD, OTR/L
Associate Professor
Occupational Therapy, College of Health and Human Services
University of New Hampshire
Durham, NH

INTRODUCTION TO CLINICAL RESEARCH

CHAPTER 1

RESEARCH: AN OVERVIEW

Just as treasures are uncovered from the earth, so virtue appears from good deeds, and wisdom appears from a pure and peaceful mind. To walk safely through the maze of human life, one needs the light of wisdom and the guidance of virtue.

Buddha (as quoted in Baird, 2000, p. 331)

CHAPTER OBJECTIVES

After reading this chapter, you will:

- Know what research is and what research is not.
- Understand the role of theory in research.
- Know the appropriate steps to follow during the research process.
- Learn how to identify a topic and be aware of the ways in which to search and review the literature.
- Be able to explain how to define a topic.
- Understand the importance of an operational definition when defining a topic and how to correctly phrase an operationally defined hypothesis.
- Know how to plan methods and to gather and interpret data in an attempt to test the hypothesis.
- Understand the role that research methods play in evidence-based clinical practice.

KEY TERMS

anecdotal	evidence-based practice	theoretical research hypothesis
data	independent variable	theory
dependent variable	paradigm	validity
empirical research	reliability	variables

INTRODUCTION

For many of us, the notion of research can seem daunting, ambiguous, or even conceptually intangible. Some of the more imaginative among us may envision the scientific research process as "brainiac," dangerous, secretive, or even science fiction-like. For others, the results of research may have an unrecognized yet assumed impact on multiple levels of everyday living. We may presume the decisions and decision processes inherent in medicine and healthcare are not only necessary but also valid and reliable. But what about the false assumptions that we make regarding research and/or how it is used to "protect" us?

Many of us might be as truly unaware of the extent of research in our lives as we are uninformed about the pitfalls of quackery that expose us to worthless or even harmful products that are legally marketed. Sometimes it might seem hard to keep up with the latest reports of clinical studies and medical guidelines. At times it might even seem as though one news report contradicts another, and it could be a challenge to determine which information is trustworthy. How do we differentiate credible research and determine what is the right and most appropriate answer to the questions we ask? If we seek to apply research, how do we weigh research with instinct-honed professional expertise and personal preference? These are among the issues that are central to clinicians who seek to become practitioners of evidence-based medicine. For example, how can clinicians use the most directly relevant research (evidence) to help guide them when facing diagnosis and treatment decisions for individual patients (**evidence-based practice** [EBP])? Similarly, how can clinicians learn to access, evaluate, and interpret research literature as they seek to apply the principles of clinical epidemiology to day-to-day clinical practice (Bulpitt, 1987; Godfrey, 1985; Haynes et al., 1986; Sackett et al., 1991)?

Research can at times feel overwhelming, especially to those not formally trained in research methodology. The goal of this chapter is to provide common-sense style guidance and direction in the methods of research. The intent is to help bridge the gap between clinical practice and research. This chapter will provide a theoretical framework that will enable students and practitioners to become informed consumers of research as they learn to evaluate, interpret, and apply research into an evidence-based "best" practice model.

WHAT RESEARCH IS AND WHAT RESEARCH IS NOT

Some may consider research an affliction of the seriously curious-minded individuals who constantly question why and spend countless hours pondering cause and effect. It is true that scientists sometimes devote their entire careers to the pursuit of knowledge in a quest for answers to questions stemming from personal and/or professional interest to them. Aside from cartoon-like illustrations and

Hollywood depictions, research is more than the mission of a scientist gone mad with an all-consuming passion for truth.

What Is Research?

Research is a careful, logical, and systematic process of investigation. **Empirical research** is a methodological approach to problem solving in which decisions are based on findings and conclusions established as a result of analyzing collected **data about variables** and the relationships that connect them. Data are collected through observation and/or experimentation, and later scrutinized through a series of statistical analyses to determine results. The results of research often lead to more questions and more areas of investigation.

Further investigation requires future research. Thus, like an expanding puzzle, knowledge is pieced together as research begets research. This complex, sequential method of inquiry is usually based on tentative explanation and discussion of facts, findings, and **theory**. For itself, theory is central to the research process. While the goal of research may be to originate theory, an existing theory can be replaced only by a new theory that has been empirically tested and supported by data. This is the cyclic nature of research.

In the continuum of research, applied research offers direct clinical applicability while basic research may have little direct clinical application. In between these two types of research lies the debate of ecologic **validity**. It has been suggested that levels of relevance for finding solutions to practical problems might incorporate some degree of basic and applied research, depending on the setting and primary objective of the research (Christina, 1989).

Basic research tends to take place in carefully monitored and controlled laboratory settings. The goal of basic research is to addresses theoretical issues or underlying explanations to questions in basic science (e.g., biology). Applied research can take place in laboratory and nonlaboratory settings. In either circumstance, the settings are carefully designed to approximate authentic and functioning environments (e.g., clinical or sport environments). Applied research can provide and contribute to theory-based knowledge, but also aims to provide direct solutions to practical problems.

What Research Is Not?

There are limits to research. If we consider research to be a purposeful method of problem solving and investigation, then we must recognize that answers to research questions are only as good as the questions that are asked. Likewise, data collected through observation and experimentation are only as accurate as the methods and tools used to collect them. Consequently, the results of the research process are only as accurate as the statistical analyses that are used to test it. And so on. Research is a complex system of reasoning. By its very nature, the process of research is limited by (and dependent on) the accuracy, validity, and **reliability** of each step of the process.

Research is not a method of "proof." In other words, research does not "prove" anything. Rather, it lends supportive evidence for or against the existence or nature of relationships among or between variables of interest. It is a process of investigation that provides perspective on how (or if) one variable or group of variables affects or influences another variable or group of variables.

Research is not haphazard. It is planned and procedural. Research is a time-consuming and, at times, tedious process of examination and investigation. It is a careful, unhurried, deliberate series of steps that are completed in an exact order. The steps are designed to confirm precise measurement.

The outcome of research is not predetermined. Research is not conducted to justify results; it is done to determine results. In the same respect, research reports results that were found. It does not report results that were expected or hoped to be found. Sometimes, finding nothing at all is as important and profound as finding something as a result of the research process.

Research is not unrepeatable. By its very nature, research is subject to and intended for replication. The results of research must be repeatable in order to be reliable and valid.

✔ CONCEPT CHECK

Research lends supportive evidence for or against the existence or nature of relationships among or between variables of interest. It is a process of investigation that provides perspective on how (or if) one variable or group of variables affects or influences another variable or group of variables. Research is not a method of "proof."

Why Study Research?

While you may not aspire to become a scientist or to establish a career in academe, it could be argued that every college student or practitioner should have an overview of research methods. An appreciation for the methods of research will help you understand how to find possible answers to a question, and why the actual steps in answering the question are important. This scientific method of research provides a framework for the process of acquiring knowledge through problem solving. By examining this framework, you will learn how to apply research methods in realistic circumstances. More specifically, you will learn how to follow an evidence-based approach to problem solving by using methodological criteria to systematically access, evaluate, interpret, and apply evidence. Such methodological review of existing evidence is fundamental to the process of acquiring knowledge, problem solving, and making well-informed decisions in clinical practice.

There is growing agreement among practitioners that research is the distinct element that distinguishes a profession from a trade (Knight & Ingersoll, 1998; Thomas & Nelson, 2001). Much of clinical practice is upheld as an "art," yet evidence-based medicine has provided justification for the value of sharing and learning from the experience of others in the evolution of evidence-based clinical practice. Research methods provide a plan for asking and answering questions, and the dissemination of research findings provides the means for the sharing of information. In the current era of EBP, students and practitioners need to be able to efficiently access the literature, analyze the strength of evidences, conduct article appraisal, and understand basic research designs. Understanding research methods is a logical and necessary first step to EBP.

THE ROLE OF THEORY IN RESEARCH

While the topic of theory and theoretical foundations in research will be discussed in more detail in chapter 3, it is important to provide a brief explanation at this point of what is meant by the term. The role of theory in research is that of a frame of reference, a "school of thought," or a **paradigm** of science. Theory can be a goal or a guide to research. In this way, empirical research can be thought of as a process or set of ideas used for asking and answering questions. Research gives us a way to find answers to questions, and make decisions based on those answers. The answers that result from research are formulated into theory, a tentative explanation for the facts and findings that evolve from the research process. In this manner, scientific theory is consistent with, and accounts for, the results of empirical research. Similarly, theory is used to guide and direct further investigation and collection of empirical data to determine how things are, and why.

✔ CONCEPT CHECK

The role of theory in research is that of a frame of reference, a "school of thought," or a paradigm of science. Theory can be a goal or a guide to research.

THE RESEARCH PROCESS

The step-by-step process of empirical research is intended to find out determinably unbiased answers to specific questions and to report those answers in a manner that does not lead to deceptive or ambiguous interpretation. The research process is a dynamic and purposeful method of problem solving and investigation into the questions of why and what will happen in a relationship between or among variables of interest. Research gives us the best answers that we have, for now, and it provides us with a widening and deepening knowledge base that we can use to find better answers, as we learn more. Research produces new data, and adds to what is already known.

Stages of the Scientific Research Process

The stages of the scientific research process are the same, regardless of the problem or question being addressed. Each stage serves as a necessary step in the process. The steps can be thought of as individual points in a blueprint for detailed inquiry and examination into some particular topic of interest. Collectively, the steps frame a method of problem solving.

The stages of the process are:
1. Identifying a topic
2. Searching and reviewing the literature
3. Defining a topic
4. Stating a general question or a problem
5. Phrasing an operationally defined hypothesis
6. Planning the methods to test the hypothesis
7. Collecting data
8. Analyzing data and interpreting results
9. Writing about the findings

The focus of this text is on the stages of the scientific research process; nonetheless, it is noteworthy at this point to mention chapter sequence in the formal written proposal or thesis.

Stage 1: Identifying a Topic

Getting started with the first step can seem frustrating and uncertain because of the difficulty of how to choose a topic, or deciding what would be a "good" topic. A helpful rule of thumb is to select a general subject or issue that is of interest, either personally or professionally (or both). You may or may not already know something about the topic, but you must like it enough to want to learn more about it. Without genuine appeal and curiosity, any topic can quickly become uninteresting. Keep in mind that the research process is lengthy and extensive, and enormous time can be spent considering the topic in question. Tremendous focus and energy can be exhausted during the investigation process. If you don't really like the topic you're studying, then you'll probably hate it by the end of the research process. Many graduate students can attest to losing interest in their research projects, or even disliking them by the end of their work.

It is usually recommended to start with a general topic until you've had a chance to explore the existing literature on the subject and begin to narrow down your topic in a more specific context. For example, a general topic of "knee injury" would be an appropriate starting point. The topic is broad, but until you've explored and reviewed the literature, you may not appreciate the various approaches and avenues of research on the topic. Perhaps, after beginning to search the literature on this topic, you discover that your interest lies more within the context of "anterior cruciate ligament (ACL) injury." However, this is still a broad category, and it will require more searching and reviewing of the literature.

A common mistake is to "become infatuated with" with a topic before it has been thoroughly searched and reviewed in the literature. Stated differently, at the beginning stage of the research process, the topic is still evolving as a work in progress and it is important to stay open-minded to possibilities perhaps not yet considered. Most likely, the topic will change or become modified to some extent. A broad, general topic can become clarified, focused, and refined; however, an overly specific, narrow topic can be so limited that it leaves little room for exploration.

✔ CONCEPT CHECK

When choosing a research topic, we suggest you begin by selecting a general subject or issue that is of interest to you either personally or professionally (or both).

Stage 2: Searching and Reviewing the Literature

Before exploring a specific question, it is important to become knowledgeable about the subject matter and existing literature connected to the vastness of that topic. In other words, it is necessary to learn the current status of the topic by searching and reviewing the available literature connected to it. The purpose is to carry out a careful and thorough examination of the body of published work concerned with a particular subject in order to find and familiarize you with the information that exists on that topic. Initially, the search will be purposefully broad and general before it becomes restricted or limited in scope or extent. As the search becomes more narrowed, the topic will begin to take shape and become more defined.

Continuing with the previous examples of the topics of "knee injury" and "ACL injury," the next step would be to search the literature on ACL and ACL injury. This might include locating and examining the research on anatomy and physiology of the ACL, joint mechanics and clinical biomechanics of the tibiofemoral joint, etiology and epidemiology of ACL injury, common mechanisms of injury to the ACL, contemporary surgical procedures and rehabilitation protocols for ACL injury, etc. This process allows for developing an acquired and learned appreciation for the breadth of the "big picture" topic, and also provides opportunity to pinpoint a more defined, more manageable issue or question associated with the more global "big picture" topic. Consistent with the notion of EBP, guidelines will be introduced in Chapters 2 and 3 of Part I, and detailed throughout Chapters 6-18 of Part II and Part III to help you learn to access the literature efficiently, analyze the strength of evidences, conduct article appraisal, and understand basic research designs.

Stage 3: Defining a Topic

After doing a primary literature search, the goal is to decide on a particular and detailed issue or question while avoiding vagueness and indefinite scope. It is at this point that the topic is more clearly defined and stated. As the topic is clarified and defined, the explicit intention or purpose of the inquiry into the topic must also be made clear. This is also referred to as the statement of the problem.

Stage 4: Stating a General Question or a Problem

The problem statement is a deliberate and understandable explanation that expresses the question or issue of interest in definite terms. The statement is usually one sentence in length. The statement not only defines the topic, but also formally announces the intention or reason for the investigation. The purpose statement sets the stage for the study as it will be developed and expanded later using existing literature to justify or rationalize the idea. More simply, the problem statement clearly states the main topic and the point of the study. It is a concise explanation and description that briefly notes what the study will be about and why the study or experiment will be done. For example, if you are interested in studying the effects of perceived stress and pain on ACL rehabilitation, then you might state your problem as follows: "The purpose of the study is to understand the effects of pain and psychological distress on adherence to scheduled rehabilitation following ACL reconstruction."

The task of defining the topic and then stating the problem in one clear sentence is more challenging than it might initially seem. The following helpful rule of thumb was shared by a fellow colleague: if the purpose cannot be plainly articulated in 30 seconds or less, then the topic and problem statement have not been clearly defined.

Stage 5: Phrasing an Operationally Defined Hypothesis

The operationally defined research hypothesis is logically connected to the topic, and links directly to the statement of the problem. The operationally defined hypothesis is a theoretical hypothesis. It is not the same as a mathematical or statistical hypothesis that will be tested as a null hypothesis.

The **theoretical research hypothesis** implies directionality among the variables of interest, and states the probable or theorized connection between or among those variables. It describes the relationship expected to be found, and under what conditions. The research hypothesis is considered "operationally defined" because it must follow operational definitions stated for words or phrases that might be used differently from their usual or explicit meanings.

The operational definitions make obvious how the words will be used and what their meanings are in the context of the current study. Accordingly, the research hypothesis must be consistent with the connotations, explanations, and descriptions of operationally defined terms. The terminology would have to be coherent and consistent with precise meanings, distinctive labels, or details unique to the variables of interest as defined in the current study. Operational definitions may or may not be consistent among existing research. Stated simply, the meaning of words may vary from study to study.

For example, the word "injury" may have contradictory definitions and classifications in different studies. The criteria used to distinguish what constitutes an "injury" in one study may be different from the criteria used in another study. The operational definitions of "injury" will state what is meant by this variable and explain how it will be used for the purposes of each study.

As previously explained, the purpose of the research hypothesis is to depict the expected connection among or between variables of interest. The variables of interest are the things or stuff being questioned or measured in the study. A well-written research hypothesis clearly states how it is anticipated that the **independent variable** of interest will influence or cause change in the **dependent variable** of interest. By definition, variables must have two or more categories of distinguishing qualities or distinctive characteristics, a range of values, parameters, or quantifiers. The identification of independent and dependent variables is important, and often confused. The independent variable is something that is manipulated by the researcher, and the dependent variable is something that is measured by the researcher. The research hypothesis describes how expected changes in the dependent variable depend on the independent variable as a result of the study.

Following along with the example of studying the effects of perceived stress and pain on ACL rehabilitation, the hypothesis might incorporate the information that pain is measured by subjective pain ratings, as well as indicate the measures of psychological distress. Bearing in mind that such ratings of stress and pain would depend on patient perception throughout the ACL rehabilitation process, these measurements would be considered as dependent variables while patient perception would be considered an independent variable. Furthermore, "pain" might need to be operationally defined, and copies of rating scales used to measure subjective pain might need to be provided as a supplement for clarification in an appendix.

Stage 6: Planning the Methods to Test the Hypothesis

After the research hypothesis has been operationally defined, the most appropriate methods to test the hypothesis have to be decided. A research question or problem can often be addressed from more than one perspective, using more than one type of methodology. Searching and reviewing the existing literature can provide perspective on how similar questions or problems have been examined in the past. Additionally, reviewing the discussions, limitations, and suggestions for future research directions from relevant earlier studies can be helpful in planning the methods to test the hypothesis of the current study.

When planning the methods and procedures, it is important that what is being measured in the study is clearly connected to the hypothesis and the statement of the problem. The methods must focus on the variables of interest and how these variables will be measured or evaluated so as to best answer the research question. The methods are like a detailed recipe or formula. They explain the step-by-step directions describing what variables will be measured or tested, and how. The methods must be accurately followed and must be able to be replicated. Simply stated, if someone else were to follow the methods of a study exactly, then they should be able to come to the same results as the original researchers. It is important to keep in mind that the research questions drive the research methods, and that methods need to be flexible, broad, and available for clinical use (e.g., practical).

✔ CONCEPT CHECK

The methods must focus on the variables of interest, and how these variables will be measured or evaluated so as to best answer the research question.

Stage 7: Collecting Data

In the data collection stage, information about the variables of interest is carefully gathered and documented. The methods and procedures planned how to collect the data, and it is during this stage that these methods and procedures are executed. As the data collection is so closely associated with the methods and procedures, this will be discussed in detail in later chapters on qualitative and quantitative research (Chapters 8 and 9).

Stage 8: Analyzing Data and Interpreting Results

Once the data has been collected, it must be analyzed and interpreted. In order to determine which statistical tests are most appropriate to analyze the data collected, the researcher must keep in mind what general question was being asked or what problem was being addressed in the study or experiment. It is important to remember that the research problem and the research question(s) drive both the research methods and the data analysis. It is difficult to separate research methods from data analysis because these are like two sides of the same coin.

Students should recognize that statistics are not simply a tool that is used *after* the data has been collected. In evidence-based approaches, it is particularly important to *simultaneously* merge research methods and data analysis at every level of the research process in order to help generate more meaningful research questions that are both clinically meaningful and methodologically sound. This notion will be further discussed and elaborated in Part III of this book. Part III will take a "big picture" look at the application and integration of data analysis and statistical methods in diagnosis, prevention, and treatment in clinical research. Research designs and data analysis will be discussed for each type of study introduced, and examples will be provided to illustrate application.

While you might not need to know the details of statistical analysis, research methodology will be presented in detail, because you might become researchers or professors in academic and clinical settings in the future. Introduction to "basic statistics," or common statistical tools traditionally covered in an entry-level statistics course, usually precedes a course in research methods. Whether or not you may have had formal training in statistics, statistical concepts must be applied in a research methods course as part of the research process—particularly when approached from an EBP perspective. Rather than separating the concepts of research methods and statistics, coverage of statistics is thematically linked and woven throughout chapters in Parts II and III of this book, including clinical interpretation of statistical results and application to real-world examples.

Stage 9: Writing about the Findings

After the data have been analyzed and interpreted, the results of the study must be reported. If something of interest was measured, what was the outcome? How did one variable influence or change another? Regardless of the results, it is important to stick to the facts and report what was found even if what was found differs from what was expected. To some extent, how the results are written up depends on the nature of the report. Will the results be presented in a journal article? Will the results be presented as a pilot study for a grant application? Or will the results be presented at a conference? More specific guidelines for writing and reporting findings will be discussed in detail in Part IV.

Another possibility is that the results will be written up as a formal written project proposal or thesis, which is a culminating scholarly activity that students are sometimes required to prepare. At the graduate school level, a thesis can be thought to reflect and demonstrate a natural outgrowth of the students' intellectual, scientific, and philosophical ideas associated with their particular academic experiences. By comparison, an undergraduate project proposal can be considered as a much smaller scale opportunity to review the existing literature on a topic of interest and demonstrate the ability to carry out investigative processes in problem solving and critical writing under faculty supervision.

While the standards and politics of subjective expectations associated with quantity and quality of content may vary (Pyrczak, 2000), the sequence of chapters in a formal written thesis or proposal is traditionally presented as follows: Chapter 1 (topic introduction), Chapter 2 (literature review), Chapter 3 (methods), Chapter 4 (results), and Chapter 5 (discussion). The project proposal typically consists of only the first three chapters, and is written in future verb tense because the project has not yet been done. The classic thesis is distinguishable as having all five chapters, and is written in past tense because the study would have been completed. A common end goal of the thesis process is publication. According to the Pennsylvania State University Graduate School (2006), "after the student has graduated and the thesis is published, it serves as a contribution to human knowledge, useful to other scholars and perhaps even to a more general audience" (p. 2). Dissemination of research will be covered in Part IV of this book.

RESEARCH AND THE CLINICAL PRACTITIONER

An important part of any research study or clinical practice is to find a common language with which to talk about certain topics or problems of interest. Clinicians and researchers alike may have various backgrounds and expertise seemingly different and distinct from a topic that may be of mutual interest. Accordingly, the same problem may be addressed from different perspectives and discussed in different contexts. The same words may hold very different meanings depending on background and expertise of the individuals using those words. With that in mind, the following section will describe and explain how the phrase "evidence-based best practice" will be used in this chapter.

What Is Evidence-Based Practice?

EBP implies a process of deductive reasoning. In other words, it is the process by which decisions about clinical practice are guided from evidence in research based on scientific models and theoretical paradigms. This approach is in contrast to the strategy of inductive reasoning where scientific explanation is retrospectively considered in attempt to understand clinical outcomes. As noted in the beginning of this chapter, EBP can be thought of as a framework to help with evaluation and interpretation of research (evidence) when applied to clinical practice.

The phrase "evidence-based practice" is used in reference to the notion of establishing performance procedures and techniques supported by and derived from empirical research rather than clinical customs and traditions based on **anecdotal** "proof" of effectiveness. In this process of systematic development, findings from empirical research are interpreted, applied, and integrated (or translated) into clinical practice. Rather than following perhaps changeable subjectively judged remedies and coincidental treatments, empirical evidence is based on reliable objective measurements following formal comparative procedures. In this manner, EBP applies the science of research to the artful skill of clinical practice. In other words, EBP translates science into practice. This method provides an interdisciplinary framework for clinicians to access, interpret, evaluate, and apply contemporary theory and research into an evidence-based clinical practice model. The notion of evidence-based clinical practice will be discussed in detail in Chapter 2, and applied throughout the remainder of this book.

CHAPTER SUMMARY

Research is a formal process of questioning and exploring particular relationships among or between variables of interest. The research process can be explained in nine steps: (i) identifying a topic, (ii) searching and reviewing the literature, (iii) defining a topic, (iv) stating a general question or a problem, (v) phrasing an operationally defined hypothesis, (vi) planning the methods to test the hypothesis, (vii) collecting data, (viii) analyzing data and interpreting results, and (ix) writing about the findings. Although the various steps may be explained with minor dissimilarity, together they are commonly recognized as research methods.

During the research process, ideas are tested but not proven. The information yielded from research can be used to generate a more complex series of ideas or theories. Research findings can be translated into clinical practice so that treatment protocols and evaluative techniques are the result of careful scientific study. Consequently, evidence-based clinical practices are developed from a systematically organized body of knowledge about a specific subject or problem. As such, evidence-based clinical practices are carried out according to methods that are grounded in theory and science, and then balanced with clinical expertise and practical experience. By considering research methods as a type of decision-making framework, clinicians can interpret and apply scientific findings to an evidence-based clinical practice model.

KEY POINTS

- Empirical research is a problem-solving method for decision making.
- Evidence-based clinical practices are based on tested relationships and logical, deductive reasoning.
- Research lends supportive evidence for already existing relationships between variables.
- Research does not prove anything.
- Research results must be repeatable in order for the research to be reliable.
- Problem statements should formally announce the intention of the research question.

The researcher manipulates the independent variable(s).

 The dependent variable is what the researcher measures.

 Evidence-based practice is the process by which decisions about clinical practice are supported from research using scientific models and theoretical paradigms.

Critical Thinking Questions

1. Why is research not meant to prove something?
2. Evidence-based clinical practice is preferred for what reason?
3. Are theories proved through experiments and investigations?
4. How can evidence-based best practice be used to translate research findings to the clinical professions?
5. What is the role of theory in research?

Applying Concepts

For the following problem-solving exercises, visit the MEDLINE and PubMed websites and search a variety of topics that you think are interesting to you. Then attempt to narrow down your search and select a specific topic. Bring three articles pertaining to your specific topic to class with you.

1. Consider the clinical implications of a research article in which the results do not match the conclusion(s) and an article that manipulates the findings of the study to justify a desired clinical effect or outcome.

2. Explain and describe why the topic you selected is important to you either personally or professionally, and consider why it might be a potentially interesting research topic.

REFERENCES

Baird D. *A Thousand Paths to Wisdom*. Naperville, IL: Sourcebooks, Inc.; 2000.

Bulpitt CJ. Confidence intervals. *Lancet*. 1987;1(8531):494–497.

Christina RW. Whatever happened to applied research in motor learning? In: Skinner JS, Corbin CB, Landers DM, et al., eds. *Future Directions in Exercise and Sport Science Research*. Champaign, IL: Human Kinetics; 1989:411–422.

Godfrey K. Simple linear regression in medical research. *N Engl J Med*. 1985;313(26): 1629–1636.

Haynes RB, McKibbon KA, Fitzgerald D, et al. How to keep up with the medical literature: V. Access by personal computer to the medical literature. *Ann Intern Med.* 1986;105(5):810–816.

Knight KL, Ingersoll CD. Developing scholarship in athletic training. *J Athl Train.* 1998;33:271–274.

Pyrczak F, ed. *Completing Your Thesis or Dissertation: Professors Share Their Techniques and Strategies.* Los Angeles, CA: Pyrczak Publishing; 2000.

Sackett DL, Haynes RB, Guyatt GH, et al. *Clinical Epidemiology, a Basic Science for Clinical Medicine.* 2nd ed. Boston, MA: Little Brown & Co Inc; 1991:218.

The Pennsylvania State University Graduate School. Thesis Guide. Available at: http://www.gradsch.psu.edu/current/thesis.html. Accessed November 2006.

Thomas JR, Nelson JK. *Research Methods in Physical Activity.* 4th ed. Champaign, IL: Human Kinetics; 2001.

SUGGESTED READING

1. Kuhn TS. *The Structure of Scientific Revolutions.* Chicago, IL: University of Chicago Press; 1970.
2. Popper KR. *The Logic of Scientific Discovery.* London: Hutchinson; 1968.

CHAPTER 2

HOW TO READ RESEARCH: EVALUATING RESEARCH ARTICLES

By Three Methods We May Learn Wisdom: First, By Reflection, Which Is Noblest; Second, By Imitation, Which Is Easiest; and Third, By Experience, Which Is Bitterest.

~Confucius (551 BC–479 BC, as cited in *Cole's Quotables* on *The Quotations Page*, http://www.quotationspage.com)

CHAPTER OBJECTIVES

After reading this chapter, you will:

- Know some basic tips for reading research.
- Understand why most research is read.
- Know the appropriate steps to follow when learning to read research.
- Learn how to identify various sections of a research article.
- Be able to explain what to expect in each section of a scientific article.
- Understand common difficulties in reading research.
- Know how to plan an effective and efficient reading strategy.
- Understand the role and benefit of self-assessment in determining your level of reading comprehension.

KEY TERMS

appraisal	plan	scientific writing
critical analysis	preparation	self-assessment
interpretation	reading comprehension	strategy

INTRODUCTION

When first learning to read research, many students and practitioners alike complain of feeling overwhelmed by variations in formal layout, writing styles, and technical terminology from journal to journal. A common complaint is a resounding expression of frustration at "not being able to see the forest for the trees" when attempting to read formal, scientific reports of research. The purpose of this chapter is to provide tips for reading research. Our goal is to provide a mini guidebook to help you keep away from the pitfalls of what is sometimes considered a shadowy and mazelike journey through the minutiae of **scientific writing**.

As a brief overview of the general ideas of this chapter, you will learn the following points about reading and evaluating research: The purpose should be clearly stated in the introduction—that the methods permit achieving the purpose, that the data are tied to the central question or questions, that the results make sense, given the data, and justify the conclusion, and finally authors are open regarding the limitations of the study and thus the strength of the conclusions (Figure 2-1). Our goal is to weave this theme as a thread throughout this chapter and guide you through the elements of scientific writing.

For explanation purposes, we use the example of reading a map to illustrate likenesses to reading research. Similarly, we submit that research should be viewed as a respectful and purposeful process of appreciation and discovery,

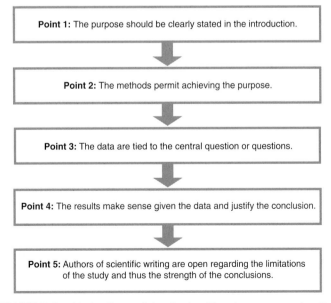

FIGURE 2-1   Navigation points of a health science research article.

similar to backcountry hiking or orienteering. Analogous to "Leave No Trace" outdoor ethics, the first rule of reading and conducting research is to **plan** ahead and prepare.

✔ **CONCEPT CHECK**

Some common difficulties when reading research include feeling overwhelmed by variations in formal layout, writing styles, and technical terminology from journal to journal.

WHEREABOUTS

Before you begin your travels, it could be argued that it would be helpful to have in mind either a destination or an objective. In other words, what is the reason or purpose for your intended travel? For example, are you traveling to get somewhere? Or, are you traveling to leave somewhere? We suggest that it is practical to take into account four initial aspects before you set out:

1. The point from which you are starting
2. The point to which you are going
3. The purpose for your venture
4. Even if you have no deliberate stopover or purpose for your excursion, the plausible time limit for this particular trip

Consider the following question: Would you prepare differently if you were planning to trek along a public walkway versus in a national park? How might you prepare if you were planning a multistate hike of the 2175-mile footpath known as the Appalachian Trail that follows the crest of the Appalachian Mountain ridgelines from Georgia to Maine? By comparison, what might you plan differently if you intended to stroll leisurely on a jaunt through the local city park during your 30-minute lunch break? Your purpose will largely influence and determine your **strategy**.

Just as there are obvious advantages to planning ahead and preparing a travel strategy before embarking on a demanding outdoor adventure trip, it can be to your advantage to plan ahead and prepare a reading strategy before you delve into evaluation and **appraisal** of a challenging scientific article. The essential crux of your reading strategy requires that you clearly establish your intention or reason for reading the specific article. For example, are you reading for pleasure? Or, are you reading for evidence discovery because you seek accurate and reliable answers to a specific clinical question? Here again, your purpose will largely influence and determine your strategy.

If you explore an unfamiliar location with the express purpose of sighting a rare genus of flora or fauna, then would it not be helpful to be familiar with its appearance? Usually if you know what you're looking for and have a fairly good idea as to where you might find it, then the overall search strategy can be much more efficient and effective. The same holds true when reading research. As described in the preceding example of a sighting trip, most research is read for the like purpose of finding something out (i.e., observing, finding, or revealing certain information).

We suggest that students consider the following questions in **preparation** for reading scientific writing: who, what, where, when, how, and why? The answers to these questions can help frame the approach you take to planning ahead and preparing, thus improving your likelihood for successfully reaching your goal(s): *Who* were the participants in the study? *What* was the purpose of the experiment? *Where* did the study and data collection occur? *When* did the study take place? *How* were data collected? *Why* should you care about the results—why are the findings important? Reading with these questions in mind can be helpful in developing an uncomplicated albeit unsophisticated preparatory routine or system for navigating scientific writing. Refer to Box 2.1.

Additionally, these simple questions can serve as a final checklist to help you gauge the extent to which you were able to comprehend the basic details of any research article. If after having finished reading an article an answer to any one or

---

BOX 2.1 | **Questions to Ask in Preparation for Reading Scientific Writing**

READ WITH THE FOLLOWING QUESTIONS IN MIND

Who were the participants in the study?
What was the purpose of the experiment?
What were the variables of interest?
Where did the study and data collection occur?
When did the study take place?
How was the data collected?
Why should we care about the results?
Why are the findings important?

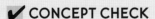 **CONCEPT CHECK**

We suggest that our students consider the following questions in preparation for reading scientific writing: who, what, where, when, how, and why?

more of these questions is not clear, then we recommend rereading the relevant section(s) to find out the answer(s). The redundancy of this rudimentary system is deliberate so as to help students and practitioners become skillful at planning ahead and preparing to read scientific writing, as well as to learn to self-assess their level of **reading comprehension** when attempting **critical analysis** of a research article.

NAVIGATING SCIENTIFIC WRITING

Although referencing style and heading organization may vary slightly from journal to journal, the basic structure of scientific writing is reflective of easily recognizable commonalities. It is our suggestion that you focus on familiarizing yourself with these commonalities so that you can become more confident and efficient at navigating your way through the landscape of scientific writing.

The commonalities in the body of a scientific article can be used as a type of navigation tool, like a compass, to provide basic guidance and directional information when trying to find your way through a research article. Similar to using a compass or reading a map, trial and error learning can be effective; however, many a lost hiker or student might argue that a few instructions given at the beginning could make the learning process less painful. In response to such requests, we will attempt to provide a type of guided discovery tour to scientific writing in hopes that these instructions might minimize panicked cries for help in the middle of the night when the underprepared or overconfident novices begin to realize that they are lost.

When acquainting yourself with scientific writing, it can be helpful to keep in mind that the abstract serves as a type of map legend and emphasizes noteworthy informational bits or common points of interest located within the article. The challenge for the research novice is to figure out how to make the necessary connections from point to point of diverse and often unfamiliar prose so as to logically locate and link the introduction and purpose to the conclusion and discussion sections of a scientific article. The challenge for an orienteering novice is to figure out how to navigate from point to point of diverse and often unfamiliar terrain so as to logically locate and link control points using a map and compass. Once more, it is helpful to plan ahead and prepare.

The section headings of a scientific article are analogous to the contour lines of a topographic map. The contour lines provide insights into land surface by using quantitative representations to depict terrain and ground elevation. To persons skilled at using a map and compass to navigate unfamiliar terrain, the topographic map provides important and detailed information about the type of terrain to expect in various geographic regions between these contour lines. By comparison, to persons untrained in navigational skills, a topographic map may appear overly detailed and confusing if the contour lines offer no meaning.

To persons skilled at interpreting and using research articles, the headings of a scientific article indicate the type of information to expect in the various sections of a research article. The section headings provide structural organization and designate the location of distinctive information, thus informing the trained reader about what to expect in each section of the article. To an untrained reader of research, the section headings are of no use because they hold no consistent meaning. The point of this comparison is that the contour lines of a topographic map and the section headings of a research article are only helpful to persons trained and skillful at reading, recognizing, and interpreting the information they provide.

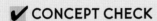 **CONCEPT CHECK**

The headings of a scientific article indicate the type of information to expect in the various sections of a research article.

Where to Start

Although there are certainly many different approaches and anecdotal tips for how to read research, we offer the following steps as a soft, flexible framework rather than a rigid, uncompromising progression. As you become more adept at reading scientific writing, you will undoubtedly discover your own preferred steps. We suggest the steps suggested in Table 2-1.

TABLE 2-1   Suggestions for reading scientific writing

A FLEXIBLE FRAMEWORK: HOW TO READ RESEARCH

1. Begin by reading the title:	Does it make sense to you?
2. Next, read the abstract:	Does it make sense to you?
3. Consider the key terms:	Are you familiar with the terminology?
4. Read the introduction:	Do you have a good understanding of the general topic?
5. Read the body of the article methods, results, and discussion:	Do you get a sense of how one section transitions to the next?
6. Scan the tables and figures:	Do they make sense to you?
7. Consider the references:	Are they current, have you read any of them?

If you can answer "NO" to any one of the questions 1 to 6 from Table 2.1, then we urge you to reevaluate the appropriateness of your article selection, as you may not yet be ready for the level of complexity or difficulty of the article at this point. If the article was assigned to you rather than selected by you, then we strongly encourage you to carefully repeat the suggested steps while keeping a notepad nearby. List and look up any unfamiliar words. Use the notepad to list any remaining questions you have after reading the article section by section at least two times in its entirety. The list of questions will be helpful when you later discuss your confusions with a professor or colleague. Lastly, we suggest that you consider reading some of the supportive articles listed as references. The references can often provide important background information and prerequisite knowledge about the topic or relevant points of discussion made by the authors of the current article.

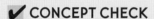

✔ CONCEPT CHECK

We suggest that you consider reading some of the supportive articles listed as references.

Section Headings: What to Expect

Sections and section headings provide order and enhance the transitions through the path of the manuscript. Following the analogy of orienteering, it is important to consider the points in Figure 2.1 as a series of sequential global positioning satellite (GPS) coordinates that will guide you like the needle on a compass to your final destination. Keeping these points in mind will serve as your handbook to help direct you through the manuscript.

The Title

The title should be highly descriptive and provide direct insight into the topic of the article; however, the title is merely a starting point and cannot fully represent the scope and content of the article. Regardless of the length of the title, it is important to remember that the title alone usually lacks the necessary details upon which you will need to determine the relevancy and readability of the article. In most cases when conducting a search of the literature, it is necessary to read the abstract as well as the title before determining if an article is germane to your investigation.

The Abstract

Abstracts are typically limited in length and many journals have abstract word limits as low as 150. The abstract provides a snapshot view of the article and highlights the author(s)' perception of the rudimentary yet fundamental information detailed in the body of the article.

The Body

Just as nonmilitary GPS receivers are accurate to within 10 feet, there may be some variation in the structure of a research article; however, you can comfortably expect for published research in health science to organize the body of the article using Introduction, Methods, Results, and Discussion sections.

The Introduction Section   The Introduction section should identify a problem or a question in need of study. Readers should expect an appropriate yet brief review of the most important and pertinent literature on the topic. The introduction sections should conclude with a clear statement of purpose for the current research.

> ✔ **CONCEPT CHECK**
>
> The purpose should be clearly stated in the introduction.

The Methods Section   The Methods section of an article should permit the reader to replicate the study completely. The reader should expect the Methods section to accurately describe *how*, *when*, and *where* data were acquired. Likewise, the methods should provide sufficient detail to replicate the data analysis. It is not uncommon to see the use of subheadings in a Methods section.

> ✔ **CONCEPT CHECK**
>
> The methods permit achieving the purpose; and, the data are tied to the central question or questions.

The Results Section   The Results section should provide answers to the question or questions posed in the introduction. The reader should expect the reports of statistics, as well as tables and figures to complete and enhance the presentation of the findings. The reader should expect the most important results to be reported first.

> ✔ **CONCEPT CHECK**
>
> The results make sense, given the data, and justify the conclusion.

The Discussion Section   The Discussion section should put the results in scientific and, where appropriate, clinical perspective and offer one or more conclusions. The reader should expect the discussion of the results to logically connect the results of the current study with previous literature as well as formulate recommendations and ideas for future research. The limitations of the study should be addressed by the authors.

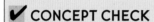

CONCEPT CHECK

Authors of scientific writing are open regarding the limitations of the study and thus the strength of the conclusions.

CHAPTER SUMMARY

The objective of this chapter was to provide basic guidance and direction for reading research. We offered suggestions and insights to help the reader progress from section to section of a scientific article. Although we noted the benefits of planning and preparation, we feel it is necessary to stress the significance of patience and diligence when reading scientific writing. Checklists and helpful tips are only as useful as the time you commit to using them; becoming skillful at reading research takes time and repetition. The more familiar you become with the research literature, the more skillful you will become at reading research, and vice versa. Eventually, students of research methods realize that they must immerse themselves in the research literature if they are to fully understand the research process. A hasty review of the literature or a superficial grasp of the research is difficult to hide from others more experienced and/or knowledgeable. There are no shortcuts to reading or conducting research, and accurate **interpretation** of research is key to a successful evidence-based approach.

KEY POINTS

- The essential crux of your reading strategy requires that you clearly establish your intention or reason for reading the specific article.
- Most research is read for the like purpose of finding something out (i.e., observing, finding, or revealing certain information).
- Sections and section headings provide order and enhance the transitions through the path of the manuscript.
- The title is merely a starting point and cannot fully represent the scope and content of the article.
- Abstracts are typically limited in length with a 150 word limit being common.
- The Introduction section should identify a problem or a question in need of study.
- The Methods section of an article should permit the reader to replicate the study completely.

- The Results section should provide answers to the question or questions posed in the introduction.
- The Discussion section should put the results in perspective and offer one or more conclusions.

 ## Critical Thinking Questions

1. What is the first rule of thumb of reading and conducting research?
2. What is the primary challenge for the research novice trying to read a scientific article?
3. Why should you consider reading some of the supportive articles listed as references?

 ## Applying Concepts

For the following problem-solving exercises, visit the MEDLINE and PubMed Web sites and search a variety of topics that you think are interesting to you. Then attempt to narrow down your search and select a specific topic. Bring three articles pertaining to your specific topic to class with you. You may use the same topic as the three articles previously attained for the problem-solving exercises in Chapter 1, but you may *not* use the same three articles.

1. Complete the questions listed in Box 2.1 for each of the three articles you selected. Be prepared to lead discussion and verbally summarize these articles using the answers to the questions in Box 2.1 as your guide. Keep in mind that you are required to recap the articles using your own words to explain and describe the answers to questions in Box 2.1. Your summary cannot be a replica of the authors' abstract. Explain and describe; do not plagiarize (i.e., do not copy illegally, lift, bootleg, or reproduce published words or creative work to which you do not own copyright).

2. Explain and describe why the results of the study you selected are important to you either personally or professionally, and consider how this study might be potentially expanded or further explored as a research topic.

SUGGESTED READING

1. For more information on "Leave No Trace" outdoor ethics, visit http://www.lnt.org.

CHAPTER 3

EVIDENCE-BASED CLINICAL PRACTICE: DISTINGUISHING BEST PRACTICES

Great spirits have always found violent opposition from mediocrities. The latter cannot understand it when a man does not thoughtlessly submit to hereditary prejudices but honestly and courageously uses his intelligence.

Albert Einstein (1879–1955) (as quoted in the *New York Times*, March 19, 1940)

CHAPTER OBJECTIVES

After reading this chapter, you will:

- Understand what is meant by evidence-based clinical practice.
- Be able to explain and discuss the issues at the heart of evidence-based medicine.
- Recognize the roles of theory and models in research.
- Recognize the roles of theory and models in evidence-based clinical practice.
- Learn how to follow an evidence-based practice approach.
- Understand the difference between a systematic review and a traditional review.
- Be able to describe and explain the role of evidence in defining and advancing clinical practice.
- Recognize the role and limits of research in evidence-based practice.
- Understand the steps in the systematic inquiry process.
- Be able to describe and explain the cyclic nature of accessing the best information available for evidence-based practice.

KEY TERMS

clinical epidemiology	epidemiology	paradigm shift
critical appraisal	evidence	prevention
diagnostics	exhaustive search	theoretical model
disablement model	outcomes	

INTRODUCTION

Perhaps the greatest challenge for many practitioners who wish to engage in evidence-based clinical practice is to distinguish how to address research into **prevention**, **diagnostics**, and intervention **outcomes**. The issues at the heart of evidence-based medicine (EBM) reflect this quandary of how to apply the clinical research literature and attend to the important underlying matters of concern: why disease and injury occur, understanding how widespread the conditions are (epidemiology); and, what can we do to prevent the condition in the patients in our offices (**clinical epidemiology**). Clinical epidemiology should encompass diagnosis, treatment, and prognosis of conditions in patients in addition to prevention. Diagnostics is an obvious issue because of the fact that without identification the next piece (treatment) is meaningless. The other issue is cost containment.

The research methods and thus the data analysis are markedly different for prevention and diagnostic studies thus requiring separate approaches. The same can be said for treatment outcomes, particularly with a **disablement model**. Students and practitioners alike may fumble with these issues along with the questions of what constitutes **evidence** and how the strength of evidence can be weighed, interpreted, and applied. These issues will be covered in detail in Chapter 15, which explores the concept of "evidence" as it applies to the advancement of health care practice and patient care, but before we get ahead of ourselves let us first consider the role of evidence in defining and advancing clinical practice.

In the era of evidence-based practice (EBP), there is growing expectation for students and practitioners to be able to access the research literature efficiently, analyze the strength of evidence, conduct article appraisal, and understand basic research designs. While it might not be necessary to know the details of statistical analysis, undergraduate and postprofessional doctoral students will need to know the research methodology in detail because they will be researchers or professors in academic and clinical settings in the future. Acquiring skills in research and **critical appraisal** is fundamental in learning to assess and regard the significance of efficiently accessing and effectively determining the applicability, reliability, and validity of published research in order to distinguish best clinical practices. The goal of this chapter is to guide you through academic theory and research methods to practical applications of EBP in patient care and clinical advancement.

✔ CONCEPT CHECK

Acquiring skills in research and critical appraisal is fundamental in learning to assess and regard the significance of efficiently accessing and effectively determining the applicability, reliability, and validity of published research in order to distinguish best clinical practices.

WHAT IS EVIDENCE-BASED PRACTICE?

Modern health care has demonstrated a trend that seems now to require clinicians not only to develop individual medical skills, but also to become skillful at navigating within an evidence-based, technology-driven information cycle. As stated in Chapter 1, EBP refers to the process by which decisions about clinical practice are supported from research using scientific models and theoretical paradigms. In this process, clinicians use the best, up-to-date clinical care research evidence to help in the diagnosis and treatment of individual patients.

The progression of "evidence-based" clinical practice necessitates that clinicians be able to access, evaluate, interpret, and apply the medical literature by following methodological criteria used to systematically determine the validity of the clinical evidence. You can think of evidence-based clinical practice as a three-pronged approach to patient care: (i) valid research findings grounded in theory and science; (ii) clinical expertise and practical experience; and (iii) the medical needs, psychosocial interests, and ethical and religious values of the individual patient.

Fundamentally, EBP can be viewed as a systematic inquiry process through which students and/or practitioners assess, ask, acquire, appraise, and apply evidence to answer clinical problems. The Center for Health Evidence (CHE), part of the University of Alberta, designed a **theoretical model** that illustrates the process of practicing EBM. This model is known as Hayward's evidence-based information cycle (Figure 3-1). It shows the cyclic nature of accessing the best information on the effectiveness of each intervention. Following this notion, EBP can be explained as simply an approach to medical practice in which clinicians endeavor to apply research evidence in decision-making processes underlying best practices in patient care.

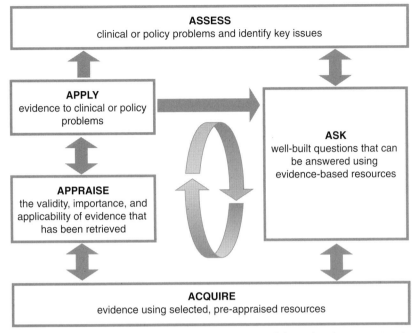

FIGURE 3-1 Evidence-based information cycle. (Adapted with permission from http://www.cche.net/info.asp. Framework developed by Dr. Robert Hayward, Director of Centre for Health Evidence. Accessed October 21, 2009.)

✔ **CONCEPT CHECK**

Fundamentally, EBP can be viewed as a systematic inquiry process through which students and/or practitioners (i) assess, (ii) ask, (iii) acquire, (iv) appraise, and (v) apply evidence to answer clinical problems.

Evolution of the Evidence-Based Clinical Practice Paradigm

The development of EBM appears to have a relatively recent timeline, being first introduced in the early to mid-1990s (Claridge & Fabian, 2005; Sehon & Stanley, 2003). Whether or not EBM constitutes a true "**paradigm shift**" (Guyatt et al., 2002; Sehone & Stanley, 2003) conforming to the philosophical definition introduced by Thomas Kuhn (1970), it has nonetheless gained considerable attention and debate as an importantly different medical approach. EBM has not advanced equally across all medical specialties; consequently, it has not been adopted uniformly. With this in mind, it seems plausible that such general disparity in acceptance and implementation has conceivably added to the debate and confusion over the development of evidence-based clinical practice.

While the notion of applying evidence to clinical practice is not novel, the more historical customs of following traditional dogma and anecdotal accounts as "evidence" of alternative treatment approaches have generated misapprehension about today's judicious and systematic attempts to establish clinical practices that are consistent with the best research evidence. Recognizing that valid evidence and sound data from high quality, ethical clinical research does not immediately translate into EBP, students and practitioners must be trained to independently and skillfully appraise the research evidence (Claridge & Fabian, 2005; Guyatt et al., 2000). Those same skills necessary to provide an evidence-based solution to a clinical dilemma can be recognized as a series of actions and principles that symbolize the evolution of the evidence-based clinical practice paradigm itself: identify and define the problem, plan and carry out a well-organized search to find the best evidence, critically appraise the evidence/literature, and carefully weigh the "evidence and its implications" with regard to patient values and belief system (Guyatt et al., 2000; Haynes et al., 2002; Sackett et al., 2000). With regard to the evolution of the (evidence-based clinical practice) paradigm, the distinguishing characteristic of EBP is the hierarchy it assigns to specific categories of evidence (Sehon & Stanley, 2003).

Fact versus Fallacy

Now that we have provided some conceptual clarification as to what is meant by EBM and evidence-based clinical practice, let us separate fact from fallacy and make clear what EBP is not. EBP is not an attempt to replace clinician judgment with scientific research. Similarly, EBP is not a safeguard to confirm or manage practitioners' clinical judgment. It is not a standardized treatment approach determined and dictated by science. And, EBP is not agenda driven by administrators or policy makers with the single objective to reduce medical expenses for more costly conditions by eliminating patient treatment options. EBP is not an authoritarian or repressive approach to clinical interventions and patient care (i.e., treatment, diagnosis, and prevention). While EBP does acknowledge and has appreciation for rational boundaries inherent in practitioner intuition, practical clinical experience, and knowledge and interpretation of pathology and human physiology, it does not denounce these more traditional means to clinical knowledge.

THE ROLE OF THEORY: DEFINITION AND BASIC TENETS

Theory is often considered to be abstract, or expressing something that can only be appreciated intellectually. Theory is based on general principles rather than specific instances. It can be explained as a set of facts, propositions, or principles analyzed in their relation to one another and used, especially in science, to explain phenomena. Theory connects and lends explanation to a set of circumstances, principles, ideas, or techniques that, when seen as distinct from actual practice, can be applied to a particular subject. The focus of theory is on internal structure and form, emphasizing how concepts or ideas interrelate with one another. Theory provides a conceptual description that gives the main points of something: a plan, organization, or structured set of ideas that has been reduced so that only its most basic and necessary elements are still functioning. Theory can be likened to an ideological skeleton, an internal notional framework upon which connecting ideas or practices are developed and drafted so that they can be tested in conjunction with one another.

Theory in Clinical Practice

Theory serves to guide and support clinical practice decisions. In other words, theory serves as a type of conceptual framework for a set of ideas, principles, or guidelines that can provide a contextual outline for students and practitioners in the process of coming to a conclusion or determination about a clinical situation. Theory can offer a hypothetical template that provides a general background or context to particular clinical decisions. Theory can be thought of as the ideologic glue with which applied clinical practice strategies and techniques are built and connected; theory provides support and rationale for *why* and *how* clinical practices work in relation to one another, and at their most basic level. Theory provides the conceptual framework upon which clinical problems are scrutinized and clinical decisions (i.e., causation, prognosis, diagnostic tests, and treatment strategy) are made in an attempt to provide optimal patient care.

✔ CONCEPT CHECK

The role of theory in evidence-based clinical practice is a type of conceptual framework for a set of ideas, principles, or guidelines that can provide a contextual outline for students and practitioners in the process of coming to a conclusion or determination about a clinical situation.

Theory in Research

As discussed in Chapter 1, theory provides both a goal and a guide to empirical research. The term "theory" can refer to a set of hypothetical circumstances or principles used to systematically examine complex concepts. It can also be used to provide the underlying explanation for particular areas of speculative knowledge concentrated on causality or phenomenological existence in the basic sciences. Stated more simply, theory represents a frame of reference, school of thought, or paradigm of science.

In scientific research, theory is introduced and based on a set of testable hypotheses or a conjectured relation between independent and dependent variables. While scientific theory is similar to scientific law, the primary difference is that, by its very essence, a scientific theory is much more complex and dynamic than a scientific law. More precisely, while a scientific law provides explanation for a specific single occurrence, a scientific theory refers to an entire group of related phenomena.

The law of gravity and Einstein's theory of relativity provide examples for differentiating between these terms in a research context. According to Newton's Law of Gravity, a force of attraction exists between all objects that have mass. This law can be expressed mathematically in a single equation and scientific research can be and has been done to test the effects of gravity (following the argument that this law is true). Einstein later proposed his General Theory of Relativity based on Newton's Universal Law of Gravitation as supporting evidence for his argument. In this example, the law of gravity remains the central premise and the theory of relativity expands upon gravitational phenomena to examine the complex concepts of space and time. A classic definition of theory in science follows:

> Theory is a system of logically interrelated, specifically non-contradictory, statements, ideas, and concepts relating to an area of reality, formulated in such a way that testable hypotheses can be derived from them (deGroot, 1969, p. 40).

Theoretical Frameworks and Models

Theoretical frameworks and models are used to represent a type of physical analogy (e.g., the brain is like a computer). More formally, a theoretical model can also be a type of strict statement of relations that can be put into equation (e.g., Theory of Relativity). As offered by Horak (1991), theoretical frameworks and models can potentially provide opportunity for clinicians in physical therapy and athletic training to move from "skilled hands *technology*" toward evolution into "a *profession* of problem solvers." For a review of the stages of the scientific research process and theoretical paradigms, please look at the detailed descriptions provided in Chapter 1.

The Role of Theory in EBP

As described in the preceding sections, theory serves important roles in both clinical practice and research. Viewed or regarded together, the dual functions of theory are inherently preserved in EBP as a result of applying research evidence to clinical practice. Similarly, if EBP is reflective of a paradigm shift in clinical practice then it could be reasoned that the theoretical underpinnings of EBP could be elaborated and explained using theoretical models and frameworks for distinguishing best clinical practices.

THE ROLE OF RESEARCH IN EBP

Research is a process of scientific, methodological investigation designed to acquire knowledge about particular clinical issues or support or revise theory in clinical practice based on the knowledge discovered. In evidence-based clinical practice, the information made known through research is interpreted and applied by clinicians to help guide and support practice decisions. In other words, research results can offer evidence that provides empirical support and validation for clinical decisions (i.e., causation, prognosis, diagnostic tests, and treatment strategy) made in an attempt to provide optimal patient care. Research findings are carefully interpreted and weighed with clinical experience, clinical expertise, and clinical instincts, and applied to the patient problem with sensitivity to the patient's emotional needs and personal value system.

There is no substitute for clinical experience; thus, the role of research in EBM is that of a complement to clinical experience and patient preference. It is necessary that practitioners and students identify clinical problems and ask good questions. Clinical questions serve to drive the research methods and the data analysis; similarly, identification of clinical problems gives focus to a systematic review of medical and clinical literature. From a more global perspective, the role of research in EBM is to provide the basic guidelines for conducting, interpreting, and applying empirical research to clinical practice. In this context, it could be reasoned that the role of research in EBM is to drive the clinical profession forward and advance the clinical profession.

✔ **CONCEPT CHECK**

In evidence-based clinical practice, the information made known through research is interpreted and applied by clinicians to help guide and support practice decisions.

HOW DOES THE CLINICAL PRACTITIONER USE RESEARCH AND EBP?

Students enrolled in curricula that implement principles of EBM are taught how to make patient care decisions based on current, valid, and germane empirical and theoretical evidence. Similarly, through didactic and clinically integrated activities they learn skills necessary to assess, ask, acquire, appraise, and apply evidence to answer clinical problems and communicate new knowledge in clinical decision-making (Guyatt et al., 2000; Haynes et al., 2002; Khan & Coomarasamy, 2006; Sackett et al., 2000). By comparison, clinical practitioners not involved with or concerned about educational practices may wish to implement EBM into their clinical practice simply to update themselves and stay current with the latest medical literature.

The clinical practitioner may seek to incorporate holistic perspectives and include EBM principles in their practice by asking clear and answerable questions about specific clinical problems, systematically searching and obtaining relevant research literature, appraising the research evidence for quality and appropriateness, carefully interpreting and weighing the evidence with their own clinical expertise and experiences, and then deciding if or how best to apply the evidence with regard to the patient's personal values and belief systems (Gronseth, 2004; Khan & Coomarasamy, 2006; Sackett et al., 1996). Although students are taught the process of EBM, the process may seem overwhelming and intimidating to the clinical practitioner faced with day-to-day practice issues of economics and time constraints. The goal of the following sections is to empower clinicians with EBM techniques for finding, identifying, and using the best evidence help bridge the gap between research and clinical practice.

Basic "How-to" Guidelines: Finding, Evaluating, and Applying Evidence

Essentially, EBP is about recognizing clinical problems, asking good clinical questions, finding, critically evaluating, analyzing, and synthesizing the evidence, and applying the best, most relevant evidence to clinical decisions and patient care recommendations. Suggested step-by-step procedures may vary slightly with the addition or omission of minor steps in the procedure but all emphasize the same basic progression. We suggest the following as a fundamental ladder of "how to" steps for the EBP process.

How to Define a Question or Problem: Assess and Ask

The EBP process begins with a clinical question or a clinical problem. The problem and question must be specific, clear, and answerable. Stated another way, clinical questions must be distinctive (i.e., prognostic, diagnostic, or therapeutic) and clearly based on the nature of the clinical problem (i.e., causation, prognosis, diagnostic tests, and treatment strategy). Therefore, step one involves considering population, intervention, and outcome issues as foundation for the question. This is done through *assessment* whereby you identify key issues and then *ask* good answerable questions. Thorough assessment yields important information about these basics which, taken together, provide necessary context to conceptualize the present clinical problem or question.

Consider it in this manner: before you can ask a good question you first need to have an unambiguous concept as to what it is you are asking about. In other words, you have to at least know a little bit about something before you can ask a clear, answerable question about it. In EBP, it is imperative that clinicians identify the clinical problem and formulate a good, clear, answerable clinical question because the question actually guides the search strategies for finding the evidence, determining the relevance of the evidence, and evaluating the quality of the evidence. The answers will only be as good as the questions asked. Assessment yields information; and, informed questions yield informed answers. Good information generates more good information.

How to Access Research Literature Efficiently and Gather Evidence: Acquire and Appraise

Once you have articulated a good, clear, answerable question, then you need to find current, valid, high-quality evidence that provides answers to your question. As stated in the previous section, your question will guide your search strategies for finding the evidence, determining the relevance of the evidence, and evaluating the quality of the evidence. A systematic review of the literature will enable you to access theoretical and research literature efficiently so as to carry out a comprehensive, unbiased search of the evidence that is connected to your question or problem.

In accordance with empirical research methodology, you must maintain meticulous record of all electronic databases and search terms that you use to acquire your evidence. The steps you follow in your search must be accurate and correct in all details so that your search strategies are obvious and can be reproduced. The goal of your search is to collect all the available, relevant literature connected to the patient(s), intervention, and outcomes identified in your assessment. You want to find out everything you can about the specific clinical problem or clinical question of interest.

The search to acquire and appraise relevant literature is commonly considered an **"exhaustive" search**, figuratively and literally. For this reason alone, it is especially important that your question is clear and answerable; otherwise, the results of your search will not be well focused and will not bear clearly upon an answer to your question or a solution to your problem. Your search results should produce appropriate quality and quantity of evidence. If the information generated by your search is not well focused or of sufficient magnitude, then subsequent appraisal of the information will not be efficient or comprehensive and may not be effective in providing enough high-quality evidence from which to synthesize well-supported clinical decisions.

At this point it may be helpful to review the suggestions on identifying a topic and beginning a search as described in Chapter 1. Even if you are not writing a formal thesis proposal or planning to conduct an empirical study, the stages of the scientific research process still apply to the steps of a systematic review. As noted in Chapter 1, the stages of the scientific research process are the same, regardless of the problem or question being addressed. The steps can be thought of as individual points in a blueprint for a detailed inquiry and examination into some particular topic of interest. Each stage serves as a necessary step in the process; and, collectively, the steps frame a method of problem solving. Systematic review is a method of investigative problem solving used in EBP. Accordingly, it is important to keep in mind that EBP is a framework for applying research evidence to clinical practice.

How to Analyze the Strength of Evidence: Appraise

As you acquire and amass relevant literature, you need to know how to critically appraise and analyze the strength of the evidence as you review it for appropriateness and usefulness. A vital part of the appraisal process is recognizing the quality or level of evidence. Hierarchy largely determines the level of evidence. Detailed discussion and direction for ascertaining the hierarchy of evidence are provided in Chapter 7. At that point, you will learn what constitutes evidence and how the strength of evidence can be weighed, interpreted, and applied. For now, we will focus on understanding basic research designs. At this point, you need only to be aware that there are different strengths of evidence and that the hierarchy of strength of evidence is one component of the article appraisal process. If your interest in research methodology has developed into an obsession and you cannot wait to swathe yourself in the knowledge contained between the pages of Chapter 7, then you may peek ahead.

It is important to understand that in an ideal world, all research evidence would be consistent and of high quality. Ours is not an ideal world. To account for this fact, you must perform a systematic review in order to build consensus as you synthesize the information gained from your examination and evaluation of the literature. You would like to find consistent results from one study to another, a low risk of bias, and general conclusions that demonstrate clear-cut and uncomplicated relevance to the clinical question. For a plethora of reasons, such is not often the case. Therefore, it is imperative that students and clinicians know how to conduct critical appraisals based on evaluating the strength of the research evidence and how it connects to the clinical problem, and draw highly plausible, evidence-based conclusions.

How to Conduct Article Appraisal

In the context of this text, we use the phrase "article appraisal" to refer to appraisal of evidence discussed relative to quality. For the purposes of this text, we will consider quality with regard to statistical and methodological issues of bias, power, and generalizability of results.

Various critical appraisal tools have been developed and can be downloaded and used to assess the applicability, reliability, and validity of published research.

Specialized critical appraisal tools range from systematic reviews to randomized controlled trials (RTCs) to qualitative research to cohort studies.

Critical Appraisal Skills Programme (CASP, 2006) provides suggestions for general guidelines for critical appraisal. Included in these suggestions are three key questions: (i) Is the study valid? (ii) What are the results? (iii) Will the results help my patients?

Additionally, CASP (2006) suggests consideration of rigor, credibility, and relevance during article appraisal. Rigor refers to methodological rigor and addresses the appropriateness of the research methods in the study. Credibility refers to the credibility of the research findings and addresses the presentation and meaningfulness of the results. Relevance refers to the clinical importance of the study and addresses the usefulness and applicability of the results to treating patients.

The themes of critical appraisal include consistent valuation or litmus tests to rate precision, exactness, significance, consequence, and validity and reliability of the scientific and statistical methods used in the study, as well as the results obtained from the study.

How to Understand Basic Research Designs

Understanding basic research designs is central to critical appraisal. Discussion of basic research designs will be covered in detail in subsequent chapters. Part II of this text focuses on seeking answers and how the question drives the methods. Part III of this text focuses on issues methodological and statistical application to clinical research dealing with diagnosis, prevention, and treatment.

How to Use the Evidence to Help Yourself and Your Patients/Population: Apply

After the literature has been critically appraised and the appropriateness of the findings has been established, the student or clinician must next determine how best to apply the knowledge obtained from the research evidence. The goal at this point is to summarize the findings and determine how or if the evidence conclusively connects to the clinical problem so as to provide a clear consensus and answer to the clinical issue in question. The challenge is to establish conclusions directly supported by the evidence and apply those findings to the question, while minimizing bias and reducing random error. A meta-analysis, while not accounting for bias and not always the most appropriate approach, offers a statistical method for combining studies to reduce error and estimating the effect of the intervention on the outcome (Gronseth, 2004; Petitti, 1994). Detailed explanation and discussion of systematic review and meta-analysis will be provided in Chapter 18.

> ✔ **CONCEPT CHECK**
>
> Essentially, EBP is about recognizing clinical problems, asking good clinical questions, finding, critically evaluating, analyzing, and synthesizing the evidence, and applying the best, most relevant evidence to clinical decisions and patient care recommendations.

CHAPTER SUMMARY

In evidence-based clinical practice, research findings are applied to clinical practice in the form of clinical recommendations. Clinical recommendations are suggested or approved by the practitioner as the best course of action based on conclusions drawn from the evidence that was summarized and interpreted during a careful systematic review of the existing research literature. The research evidence is weighed with clinical insights and expertise to determine optimal patient care.

The systematic review process is guided and directed based on the clinical question. The more skilled the clinician or student is at precisely defining a patient problem, and what information is required to resolve the problem (assessing), the better the clinical question will be (ask). A better clinical question leads to a more efficient search of the literature (acquire); better selection of relevant studies and better application of the rules of evidence leads to determination of the validity of the evidence (appraise); better evaluation of the evidence leads to better application of evidence to the patient problem (apply). This process of literature review and evaluation is known as the "critical appraisal" of evidence; and, critical appraisal is the crux of evidence-based clinical practice and deciding best practices.

KEY POINTS

- The distinguishing characteristic of EBP is the hierarchy it assigns to specific categories of evidence.
- Evidence-based practice is not an attempt to replace clinician judgment with scientific research.
- Theory is based on general principles rather than specific instances.
- In scientific research, theory is introduced and based on a set of testable hypotheses or a conjectured relation between independent and dependent variables.
- Rigor refers to methodological soundness and addresses the appropriateness of the research methods in the study.
- Credibility refers to the integrity of the research findings and addresses the presentation and meaningfulness of the results.

- Relevance refers to the clinical importance of the study and addresses the usefulness and applicability of the results to the clinician and patient.
- There is no substitute for clinical experience; thus, the role of research in EBM is that of a complement to clinical experience and patient preference.
- The stages of the scientific research process are the same, regardless of the problem or question being addressed.
- The systematic review process is guided and directed based on the clinical question.

Critical Thinking Questions

1. What is the greatest challenge for many practitioners who wish to engage in evidence-based clinical practice?
2. What three key questions are included in the suggestions offered by CASP (2006) as general guidelines for critical appraisal?
3. How should students and clinicians conduct critical appraisals of the research literature?

Applying Concepts

1. Form small discussion groups of three to five people. Consider the progression of "evidence-based" clinical practice. Talk about why it is important that clinicians be able to access, evaluate, interpret, and apply the medical literature by following methodological criteria used to systematically determine the validity of the clinical evidence. Provide an example based on a clinical scenario and identify applicable prevention, diagnostics, and intervention outcomes.
2. Provide examples of theory and law as they connect to clinical practice search topic.

REFERENCES

CASP. The CASP elearning resource: An Introduction to Evidence-Based Practice. (http://www.caspinternational.org/ebp) This website was developed by the Critical Appraisal Skills Programme (CASP) and the Department of Knowledge and Information Science, part of the Public Health Resource Unit, Oxford, UK; 2006.

Claridge JA, Fabian TC. History and development of evidence-based medicine. *World J Surg.* 2005;29(5):547–553.

deGroot A. *Adrianus de Groot's Methodology: Foundations of Inference and Research in the Behavioral Sciences, Psychological Studies 6*. The Hague: Mouton; 1969:40.

Gronseth G. From evidence to practice. *NeuroRx: The Journal of the American Society for Experimental NeuroTherapeutics*. 2004;1:331–340.

Guyatt GH, Meade MO, Jaeschke RZ, et al. Practitioners of evidence based care. *Br Med J*. 2000;320:954–959.

Guyatt GH, Haynes B, Jaeschke R, et al. Introduction: the philosophy of evidence-based medicine. In: Guyatt G, Rennie D, eds. *Users' Guides to the Medical Literature: A Manual for Evidence-Based Clinical Practice*. Chicago: AMA Press; 2002:3–12.

Haynes RB, Devereaux PJ, Guyatt GH. Physicians' and patients' choices in evidence based practice. *Br Med J*. 2002;324:1350.

Horak F. Assumptions underlying motor control for neurologic rehabilitation. In: Contemporary Management of Motor Control Problems, Proceedings, 11 Step Conference, Foundation for Physical Therapy. New York: 1991.

Khan KS, Coomarasamy A. A hierarchy of effective teaching and learning to acquire competence in evidence-based medicine. *BMC Med Educ*. 2006;6:59.

Kuhn TS. *The Structure of Scientific Revolutions*. 2nd ed. Chicago: University of Chicago Press; 1970:xii, 210.

Petitti DB. Statistical methods in meta-analysis. In: Petitti DB, ed. *Meta-Analysis, Decision Analysis and Cost-Effectiveness Analysis*. New York: Oxford University Press; 1994:90–114.

Sackett DL, Rosenberg WM, Gray JA, et al. Evidence based medicine: what it is and what it isn't. *Br Med J*. 1996;312(7024):71–72.

Sackett DL, Straus SE, Richardson WS, et al. *Evidence-Based Medicine: How to Practice and Teach EBM*. 2nd ed. Edinburgh: Churchill Livingstone; 2000.

Sehon SR, Stanley DE. A philosophical analysis of evidence-based medicine debate. *BMC Health Ser Res*. 2003;3:14. Available at: http://www.biomedcentral.com/1472-6963/3/14.

SUGGESTED READING

1. Couto JS. Evidence-based medicine: a Kuhnian perspective of a transvestite non-theory. *J Eval Clin Pract*. 1998;4:267–275.

2. Guyatt GH, Rennie D. *Users' Guide to the Medical Literature: A Manual for Evidence-Based Clinical Practice*. Chicago: AMA Press; 2002.

3. Miles A, Bentey P, Polychronis A, et al. Evidence-based medicine: why all the fuss? This is why. *J Eval Clin Pract*. 1997;3:83–86.

4. Russell Keeps Post by Vote of 11 to 7; Court Fight Begun: Leaders in the Russell Controversy, Times Wide World Photos. *New York Times* (1857–current file). New York: March 19, 1940:p. 1 (2pp.).

CHAPTER 4

EBM: A HISTORICAL PERSPECTIVE

In the beginner's mind there are many possibilities. In the expert's mind there are few.

Shunryu Suzuk (as quoted in The Quotations Page, www.quotationspage.com)

CHAPTER OBJECTIVES

After reading this chapter, you will:

- Have an appreciation for the role of clinical epidemiology in evidence-based medicine.
- Understand why the practice of evidence-based health care requires the continued pursuit of clinical research and the dissemination of that research to the provider.
- Know that the research-consuming clinician must be able to appraise the research literature in order to apply the best available evidence to their clinical decision making.
- Learn how and why evidence-based medicine is central to the advancement of medicine.
- Be able to explain the differences between basic research, field research, and translational research.
- Know that clinical research asks questions about the usefulness of diagnostic tools and the effectiveness of prevention and treatment efforts.
- Understand the general goals of clinical research and evidence-based practice.
- Appreciate how the study of cost analysis will bring additional evidence to the decision-making process once a level of proficiency is developed in consuming and critically appraising research related to screening, diagnosis, prevention, and treatment.

KEY TERMS

art of medicine	clinical judgment	paradigm
bench research	Cochrane collaboration	randomized clinical trials
biomedical research	information technology	translational research
clinical epidemiology	interventions	

INTRODUCTION

Perhaps the most remarkable aspect of the "history" of evidence-based medicine (EBM) is that it is not very long. In 2005, Dr. David Eddy acknowledged that since 1990 EBM has become increasingly more accepted and established in the field of medicine. He continued by stating that the term "evidence-based medicine" first appeared in print in papers authored by Dr. Gordon Guyatt in 1991 and 1992 (Evidence-Based Medicine Working Group, 1992). Given the long history of efforts to treat conditions of the body and mind, EBM is in its relative infancy.

As with many new concepts, the development of what has been described as the dominant new **paradigm** in medicine has origins dating back before the label was attached. Many have labored and written to develop the central concepts of EBM, but most new, large endeavors can be traced to a few pioneers. The work of Chalmers I. Archie Cochrane (1909 to 1988), known as Archie and after whom the **Cochrane collaboration** is named, has been identified as the springboard for the development of EBM (2006). While even a short biography on Archie Cochrane (Chalmers, 2006) is fascinating, his efforts to promote the use of **randomized clinical trials** to collect data to inform clinical practice certainly were important to the development of the paradigm of EBM.

Drs. David Sackett, Gordon Guyatt, and colleagues have also had a vast impact on the promotion and teaching of EBM as well as the methods of identifying best evidence. These authors also coined the term **clinical epidemiology**, which is really the vehicle through which evidence-based health care is practiced.

While medicine was the original focus of the EBM, the paradigm has spread throughout health care. The concepts and principles apply to nonphysician providers including physical therapists, occupational therapists, and certified athletic trainers. In today's complex health system, an understanding of EBM and clinical epidemiology is important to all providers striving to improve patient care by employing the best diagnostic strategies, and most effective prevention and treatment intervention.

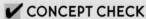 **CONCEPT CHECK**

Clinical epidemiology can be described as the vehicle through which evidence-based health care is practiced.

HISTORY AND DIRECTION OF CLINICAL FIELDS

EBM did not simply emerge as a new way of doing things. In order to place the paradigm of evidence-based medicine in the context of modern health care, it is important to consider medical practice of the mid -20th century. According to Eddy (2005), approximately 40 years ago, medical decisions were based on underlying supposition. Physicians would deduce right thoughts and right actions through the "**art of medicine**" or "**clinical judgment.**" Physicians synthesized information to determine the best course of action. Medical decision making as a field of study did not exist.

The flaws in the assumption that the preparation and practice of physicians consistently result in optimal care are revealed (i) when research fails to demonstrate the efficacy of **interventions** and the effectiveness of care and (ii) when the management of patients with similar conditions varies widely between providers, care facilities, and regions (Eddy, 2005).

Consider for a moment the similarities between the education and practice of physicians and that of nonphysician health care providers including physical therapists, certified athletic trainers, and occupational therapists. Take, for example, the once common practice of administering corticosteroid medications via iontophoresis in the treatment of tendinopathy. Although this treatment persists, the bulk of the research literature fails to confirm benefit and many providers no longer consider iontophoresis as a treatment option.

If you dare, consult with several providers regarding their treatment of conditions such as nonspecific low back pain, patellofemoral pain syndrome, lateral epicondylalgia, or a host of other musculoskeletal complaints. Recommended interventions are likely to vary, sometimes considerably between those whom you consult. It can be safely assumed that each clinician would be providing his or her best opinion based on their personal training and experiences. Similarly, each clinician can likely recall and discuss similar cases where the patient reported substantial improvement and great satisfaction with their care. Could it be that each of the recommended plans of care is of equal benefit? Probably not!

Thus, the traditional educational and clinical preparation of nonphysician health care providers to make the decisions that result in optimal care suffers from the same deficiencies as that of physicians. The paradigm of evidence-based practice has emerged so that the best clinical research is applied to the treatment decisions made on similar patients across disciplines, facilities, and regions. The practice of evidence-based health care requires the continued pursuit of clinical research and the dissemination of that research to the provider. The integration of the best available research into clinical decision making directly targets concerns that practice is inconsistent with the research evidence. Moreover, since the best evidence is now more available to care providers everywhere because of the advances in **information technology** practice patterns, when based on the best evidence, plans of care will likely become more similar.

The universal practice of evidence-based health care is a lofty goal. Over time, advances in information technology and clinical research are changing health care practices, improving the outcomes of care, and in some cases, reducing the costs of care by eliminating unnecessary diagnostic procedures and ineffective interventions. Much of this book is devoted to research methods and data analysis, not because we strive to prepare clinical researchers but because the research-consuming clinician must be able to appraise the research literature in order to apply the best available evidence to their clinical decision making.

✔ CONCEPT CHECK

The paradigm of evidence-based practice has emerged so that the best clinical research is applied to the treatment decisions made on similar patients across disciplines, facilities, and regions. The best evidence is now more available to care providers everywhere because of the advances in information technology practice patterns.

RESEARCH IN MEDICINE

Research is without a doubt central to the advancement of medicine. **Biomedical research** is a vast and diverse field where questions related to the functions of the body, disease, responses to medications, injury mechanisms, and disease and injury patterns are but a few that are addressed. Biomedical research is much like a spiderweb, with strands representing areas of study that are often intricately connected to address complex problems.

Take, for example, the challenge of preventing anterior cruciate ligament (ACL) tears. In the last 50 years, much has been learned regarding the anatomy and histology of the ligament. Biomechanists have explored normal and pathologic loading. Epidemiologists have identified those most at risk of injury, and factors contributing to risk have been identified. Each research effort has expanded the understanding of ligament structure, injury, and treatment. With greater understanding, efforts at prevention of ACL injuries have included rule changes, bracing, and exercise programs. These efforts have been based on existing knowledge and are well intended. Sound reasoning and good intentions, however, do not necessarily lead to effective interventions.

Archie Cochrane championed randomized-controlled clinical trials as the best means of determining which interventions are truly effective in preventing and treating illnesses and injuries. The need for and methods of such research are presented in detail in subsequent chapters. However, the importance of "clinical research" or investigations where the effectiveness of diagnostic strategies, prevention efforts, and therapeutic interventions in patients or at-risk populations in informing health care practice cannot be understated, and separates the practice behaviors described by Eddy and the practice of evidence-based health care.

✔ CONCEPT CHECK

Biomedical research is a vast and diverse field where questions related to the functions of the body, disease, responses to medications, injury mechanisms, and disease and injury patterns are but a few that are addressed. Biomedical research is much like a spiderweb, with strands representing areas of study that are often intricately connected to address complex problems.

CLINICAL RESEARCH

Medical research, like research in other fields, is not of singular design or purpose. The diversity in how and where research is conducted has lead to components of the large research picture being labeled. Basic science or **bench research** is often thought of as being conducted in a laboratory environment under tightly controlled conditions. Field research is conducted away from the laboratory, often in a natural setting. **Translational research** is a more recent term used to describe investigations that apply the results from basic science to the care of patients. Sometimes referred to as "bench-to-bedside," translational research seeks to speed the development of more effective patient care strategies. The completion of the translation of research findings to patient care requires what is perhaps best labeled clinical research.

✔ CONCEPT CHECK

Basic science or bench research is often thought of as being conducted in a laboratory environment under tightly controlled conditions. Field research is conducted away from the laboratory, often in a natural setting. Translational research is a more recent term used to describe investigations that apply the results from basic science to the care of patients.

Clinical research asks questions about the usefulness of diagnostic tools and the effectiveness of prevention and treatment efforts by enrolling patients and at-risk individuals. Consider the discussion of ACL injuries in the previous sections. It makes sense that exercise regimens that train athletes to land in ways that reduce loading of the ACL would decrease the incidence of injury, especially in populations shown to be at higher risk. However, this assumption warrants testing before investing resources in such training initiative and perhaps failing to pursue effective alternatives. Such clinical research completes the translation from basic science to patient applications and lies at the heart of EBM.

✔ CONCEPT CHECK

Clinical research asks questions about the usefulness of diagnostic tools and the effectiveness of prevention and treatment efforts by enrolling patients and at-risk individuals.

CLINICAL RESEARCH AND EVIDENCE-BASED PRACTICE

Clinical epidemiology has been described as the use of data collected from the study of samples drawn from populations to make decisions about the care of individual patients. This clinical research addresses issues across a spectrum of patient care from screening and diagnostic accuracy to prognosis to the effectiveness of prevention and treatment strategies. This research also includes cost analyses.

The design of research to investigate questions in each area, and the factors that are considered when assessing methodological quality, vary with the type of research being conducted. Many of the methodological considerations and strategies for data analysis are presented in Part II of this book. From this work comes the data to guide decisions regarding the utility of diagnostic tests and screening examinations in specific populations. Certainly, clinicians seek tests and procedures that will identify problems when they exist (specificity) but rarely lead to false-positive findings (sensitivity). Clinicians also want to recommend prevention efforts that are generally effective and pose a low risk of adverse events. The same is true of treatment efforts.

✔ CONCEPT CHECK

Certainly a general goal of clinical research and EBM is to seek tests and procedures that will identify problems when they exist (specificity) but rarely lead to false-positive findings (sensitivity). Clinicians also want to recommend prevention efforts that are generally effective and pose a low risk of adverse events.

Prognosis is a complex concept. Studies of prognosis can assist in identifying treatments that are most likely to lead to a favorable outcome or avoid the use of interventions that have little effect on achieving long-term treatment goals. Cost analyses require a unique set of research skills and are not addressed in depth in this book. It is important to grasp the concepts related to the other aspects of clinical epidemiology before tackling this important topic. Health care is very costly, yet some very expensive diagnostic and treatment procedures have limited impact on the overall quality of care provided. Once a level of proficiency is developed in consuming and critically appraising research related to screening, diagnosis, prevention, and treatment, the study of cost analysis will bring additional evidence to the decision-making process. This information is increasingly of interest to patients and consumers bearing an increased responsibility for paying for the services they receive.

✔ CONCEPT CHECK

Once a level of proficiency is developed in consuming and critically appraising research related to screening, diagnosis, prevention, and treatment, the study of cost analysis will bring additional evidence to the decision-making process.

CHAPTER SUMMARY

The paradigm of evidence-based health care is neither old nor fully established. The past few decades have witnessed tremendous changes in health care. The health care system continues to change, and new discoveries and technologies offer hope of better treatment of a host of diseases and medical conditions. Greater emphasis on translational research seeks to speed the use of new information and technology to patient care. Unfortunately, not all new procedures and treatments truly improve the outcomes of health care, and sometimes there are adverse unanticipated events. Thus, clinical research is essential to informing the practices of individual providers. The volume of clinical research continues to increase rapidly. Advances in information technology also permit clinicians greater and more rapid access to the medical literature than at any time in history. It is essential that practicing clinicians and, more importantly, tomorrow's clinicians are prepared to access, read, critically appraise, and lastly apply research findings to the clinical decisions and recommendation made in the care of each patient.

According to David Katz (2001):

> Evidence has securely claimed its place among the dominant concepts in modern medical practice. To the extent possible, clinicians are expected to base their decisions (or recommendations) on the best available evidence. Physicians may see this as one possible silver lining in the dark cloud of managed care.

Despite the challenges of working within the health care system, this is an exciting time in the history of health care. The practice of health care has changed, and while the decisions of providers are often questioned, more tools are available to develop best practice than ever. Ultimately, learning how to practice evidence-based health care is not about the provider but about the improved care delivered to the patient, and we are all patients many times in our lives.

KEY POINTS

- The term "evidence-based medicine" first appeared in print in papers authored by Dr. Gordon Guyatt in 1991 and 1992.
- The efforts of Archie Cochrane to promote the use of randomized clinical trials to collect data to inform clinical practice were important to the development of the paradigm of EBM.
- The paradigm of evidence-based health care is neither old nor fully established.
- Greater emphasis on translational research seeks to speed the use of new information and technology to patient care.
- Clinical research is essential to informing the practices of individual providers.
- Advances in information technology also permit clinicians greater and more rapid access to the medical literature than at any time in history.
- It is essential that practicing clinicians and, more importantly, tomorrow's clinicians are prepared to access, read, critically appraise, and lastly apply research findings to the clinical decisions and recommendation made in the care of each patient.
- Ultimately, learning how to practice evidence-based health care is not about the provider but about the improved care delivered to the patient, and we are all patients many times in our lives.

 Critical Thinking Questions

1. Who is credited with having coined the term *clinical epidemiology*?
2. Why do the concepts and principles of EBM apply to both physicians and nonphysician providers including physical therapists, occupational therapists, and certified athletic trainers?
3. What elements are essential for the continued practice and integration of EBM?

(continued)

4. What is clinical epidemiology?

5. What role do studies of prognosis have in EBM?

 Applying Concepts

1. Consider the role of clinical epidemiology in EBM. Would it have been plausible for EBM to have developed without the study of clinical epidemiology? Is it possible to practice EBM without considering, interpreting, or applying clinical epidemiology? Explain and provide rationale as to *why or why not.*

2. Consider the roles and influences of randomized clinical trials (RTC) and clinical epidemiology in the practice of EMB.

REFERENCES

1. Chalmers I. Archie Cochrane (1909–1988). In: *The Lind Library*; 2006. Available at: www.jameslindlibrary.org. Accessed August 19, 2008.

2. Eddy DM. Evidence-based medicine: a unified approach. *Health Aff.* 2005;24:9–17.

3. Evidence-Based Medicine Working Group. Evidence-based medicine: a new approach to teaching the practice of medicine. *JAMA.* 1992;268(17):2420–2425.

4. Guyatt GH. Evidence-based medicine. *ACP J Club.* 1991;114(2):A-16.

5. Katz D. *Clinical Epidemiology and Evidence-based Medicine.* Thousand Oaks, CA: Sage Publications; 2001.

CHAPTER 5

ETHICS AND RESPONSIBLE CONDUCT IN RESEARCH AND CLINICAL PRACTICE

We do not act rightly because we have virtue or excellence, but we rather have those because we have acted rightly. We are what we repeatedly do…

Aristotle, as quoted in BrainyQuote
(http://www.brainyquote.com/quotes/quotes/a/
aristotle408592.html)

CHAPTER OBJECTIVES

After reading this chapter, you will:

- Understand what role culture takes on in the advancement of medical care.
- Know how the Belmont Report supports the clients/patients' right to know the procedures that they will be exposed to or the extent to which they will be involved in as participants.
- Be aware of how ethical procedures transcend the boundaries of the United States via international agreements on health, medicine, and medical research.
- Realize how the federal government can intercede to make ethical guidelines clear and aid in the advancement of medical practices.

KEY TERMS

Belmont Report	confidentiality	human participants
beneficence	disclosure	
clinical practice	ethical issues	

INTRODUCTION

The question of ethics goes beyond the notion of shaping "right" from "wrong." It could be reasoned that the majority of ethical considerations and moral standards in research and **clinical practice** have evolved from two basic tenets. Arguably, these tenets are both ideological and philosophical in nature.

The first tenet can be summarized as follows: It is essential to think about all probable risks and/or potential harm regarding the use of humans as participants. This first guideline is reassuring and honorable; however, not necessarily plausible as we cannot logically foresee and prevent all possible harms. Nevertheless, the prevailing theme (intended to reflect our ethical values in the research community) is that our first obligation is to protect the participant from physical and psychological injury. This principle is similar to the modern translation of the Hippocratic oath, "First do no harm." (Hippocratic oath, *OrkoV*, attributed to Hippocrates of Cos [460–370 BC] taken from the Latin phrase, *Primum non nocere*, translated by Francis Adams as quoted in the Internet Classic Archive: http://classics.mit.edu/Hippocrates/hippooath.html)

The second tenet is an associated line of reasoning: the benefit (to the participant) of participation in the research must outweigh any potential risk (to the participant) associated with participation. Yet again, this second guideline is not always attainable. There may be occasions when participation in research poses only negligible risk (to the participant), yet participants derive no obvious benefit from their participation.

The goal of this chapter is to provide an overview of historical context and justification for the theoretical and practical application of ethics, responsible conduct, and ethical decision-making in medicine, research, and clinical practice. Determination of rationale and intention will be suggested as keys to help recognize high-standard, transparent ethics and responsible conduct, and as tools to help students and clinicians draw more parallels to clinical practice and identify some definite ethics breaches. A big-picture objective will be to reinforce the notion of evidence-based practice (EBP) and its interconnectedness with ethical codes of conduct in both research and clinical practice.

It is important to note that this chapter will promote the integration of ethical and professional conduct at the highest standards across culturally diverse patient populations, as well as translational and interdisciplinary research necessary for advancement in the medical community. Ethical guidelines, however, are not exempt from the changes and updates develop from research that identifies best practices or conflicting ethical values. We take the approach that ethical and responsible conduct in research and clinical practice is crucial for both establishing and promoting excellence, as well as public trust, in medicine. As this chapter will provide a relatively brief synopsis on this vast subject, we strongly encourage students and practitioners, alike, to take a course on Ethics, Medical Ethics, or Biomedical Ethics.

GENERAL BACKGROUND

As stated in Chapter 1, research is a process of scientific, methodological investigation designed to acquire knowledge about particular clinical issues or support or revise theory in clinical practice based on the knowledge discovered. Ethics and responsible conduct guide the research process. In establishing ethical guidelines, as in evidence-based clinical practice, the information made known through research is interpreted and applied to help guide and support practice decisions and advance ethical and responsible conduct.

In other words, research results can offer evidence that provides empirical support and validation for clinical decisions (i.e., causation, prognosis, diagnostic tests, and treatment strategy), as well as provide a stimulus for federal regulatory requirements and institutional policies made in an attempt to provide ethical guidelines for responsible and professional conduct and optimal patient care. For example, beginning January 4, 2010, all institutions that apply for financial assistance from the National Science Foundation (NSF) were required to provide, as part of their grant proposal, certification of training and oversight in the responsible and ethical conduct of research for all researchers who participate in NSF funded projects (NSF-10, January 2010; AAG Section IV B). Similarly, all researchers who apply for financial assistance from the National Institutes of Health (NIH) must complete online training education for ethical and responsible conduct in research with **human participants** (NIH Human Participant Protections Education for Research Teams at http://cme.cancer.gov/c01/nih_intro_02.htm).

Ethical codes do not exist in a vacuum or in isolation from mainstream society, as a whole. Ethical codes in the healthcare profession are developed and established to protect the patient or client legally and provide a procedural conduct approach for the practitioner. The degree of importance of having such codes in the healthcare profession has resulted in many ethical standards of practice that have been legislated into state and federal laws. While such codes of conduct are passed into law, the origin, practice, and interpretation of them are left to those in the specific profession where they are applied at a variety of institutional levels.

The issues of ethics and responsible behavior in research and healthcare have not always been reflective of clear-cut, contemporary convention. Ethics in medical research and clinical practice have evolved over centuries of unscripted human interaction, religious dogma, war, and government report. Today, ethics have developed into a three-pronged Buddhist-like approach to determining and demonstrating right thought, right word, and right action. Yet, the distinction between right and wrong is not always evident or easily predictable. Often, what is more easily recognizable and agreed upon is the apparent discrepancy between that which is deemed "wrong" versus "right." More than judgments of "wrong" versus "right" actions or "bad" versus "good" decisions, **ethical issues** contrast appropriate and inappropriate behaviors, and are based on personal, moral, professional (i.e., cultural), and societal views of accepted, principled criteria and guidelines for responsible conduct (Bourdieu, 1995). These levels influence one another in a nonlinear and give-and-take fashion, yet do have hierarchical order with societal norms serving as the supervisory rank (Baudrillard, 1990).

Currently, many institutionalized professions have adopted an explicit code of ethical procedures or conduct to reduce misinterpretations and encourage proper behavior in the workplace while reducing confusion on how to act properly. Since the medical profession maintains a strong and stable stance on acceptable practices, the only way the standard or paradigm of clinical practice is changed is through the advances of legitimized research (Kuhn, 1970). When well-respected medical professionals conduct research on new clinical procedures, diagnostic or treatment techniques (and find benefit from their use), then these new practices become more legitimized. This is important to understand for the practitioner when dealing with the general public because if there is doubt in the treatment they are to receive, patients will want to confirm that the recommended treatment is a normal and highly successful procedure.

✔ CONCEPT CHECK

Often a code of ethics is learned through experience and implicitly understood by all members of the group, and these norms are often unwritten.

MODEL OF INTERPRETATIVE PRACTICE

This brings us back to the concept of EBP and its connection with ethical codes of conduct. When examining EBP for the practitioner, the break from previous practices should be evident and responsive to both the caregiver and the patient. It is important to remember that EBP takes into account the perspective that the consideration and experience of the clinician, the most current research/literature available, and the patient themselves must all be weighed in determining the "best" or "most suitable" clinical practice. Each one of these three parts needs to be examined with respect to their role in this model of practice.

✔ CONCEPT CHECK

It is important to remember that EBP takes the perspective that the consideration and experience of the clinician, the most current research/literature available, and the patient themselves must all be weighed in determining the "best" or "most suitable" clinical practice.

The Clinician

When clinicians are considered as to their roles or status it may vary based on the designated role, professional experiences, and the period when they received their education. For instance, the type of clinician may vary from certified athletic trainers to physical therapists to doctors (general practitioner/GP). These three allied professions and their knowledge of injury diagnosis and treatment can either vary greatly or be on an equal level. The reasons for this similarity or disparity have to do with the level and frequency of experience that a clinician has with the problem the patient is experiencing, the quality and extent of their own education (formal, learned experiences, and self-taught), as well as their knowledge and understanding of relevant, current research on the problem. It is important for the patient to understand and be aware of the parity of knowledge that exists within the diagnosis and treatment of injuries in the medical community.

Research/Literature of the Field

The second part of the EBP model, research/literature of the field, is critical to the practice of delivery of care to the patient. This area requires the clinician to review two important aspects of practice within this framework. One is keeping up with the current literature and advances in procedures/techniques and second is the ability to interpret the literature as it is presented or reported in the journals. In an age where any professional can be overwhelmed by the new information being produced in their field, it is important to be able to devote time to staying up to date. Likewise, as studies are published the clinician needs to keep a critical eye on interpretation and application of the literature being published and how it applies to the way they treat people.

> EXAMPLE

Focus on Results and Methodology

For example, let's consider a physical therapist working with individuals recovering from strokes. Such individuals should maintain an interest in the literature on the benefits of aerobic exercise for cognitive and neuromuscular improvements. Their interpretation and critical assessment skills of such studies should focus on not only the results of such studies but also on the methodology of how those results were achieved. For example, studies that downplay the use of treatments that in themselves are dynamic to coordination and human movement may need further examination as to their utility and application with patients. Such a study may not have lasted long enough (overall duration) or the protocol of duration or progression may not have been fully implemented long enough to determine whether positive results could be manipulated or achieved.

Upon careful review of studies dealing with benefits or lack of benefits from various treatments including therapeutic exercise, one can detect problems or design flaws in the research protocol that affect the results. For example, if there are conflicting studies in the literature that state that aerobic exercise was of little effect in older individuals with regard to cognitive function and mental effect, this might cause alarm with conventional wisdom of what we know about exercise and its effects. Upon closer examination of such studies that downplay the use of aerobic exercise, one can find in the protocol that the time and duration of the aerobic exercise could be minimal in comparison to what other data had found to work with improving health conditions for older populations.

The Patient

The patient is the third part of the EBP model and must be viewed as an individual. Similarly, it must be understood that (based on the medical problem they may have) patients also bring with them a variety of emotions, skills, education, religious beliefs (culture), and personal history when they seek treatment. To direct a patient to the most productive and successful treatment, each aspect of their background should be considered. The decision to guide an individual to a proper treatment should entail finding out what other treatments they have received in the past and how successful were those treatments. It also helps to find out the religious background of a patient. Without that knowledge, a clinician can run into a number of problems such as recommending someone for a treatment that violates their belief system. An example of this consistently occurs with those practicing under the tenets of the Christian Science Church that does not traditionally accept medical practices but instead promotes healing of physical and mental illnesses and disorders through prayer.

Another aspect to consider with the patient is educating the patient on the various types of treatments available. The role of the clinician becomes twofold, educator and advocator at the same time. A part of the education process of following proper ethical codes is to allow the patient to be involved in the process of their own treatment.

HISTORICAL CONTEXT

A physical therapist friend of mine once offered the following words of advice to me in terms of patient treatment and learning to gauge how far to push someone as they regain muscular strength, range of motion, and so on: *"… sometimes you have to cross the line in order to establish it."* She was not suggesting blatant disregard for patient perceptions of pain, nor was she suggesting cruelty or mistreatment under the excuse of a Darwinian mindset of species adaptation and survival. She was simply noting that sometimes we learn through trial and error, even when we are acting deliberately and intentionally exercising appropriate precautions. Perhaps, the same approach could be recognized in the development and advancement of ethical and professional standards for conducting research. However, the lessons of history have shown bold denial in the disturbing convictions with which our predecessors repeatedly chose to ignore prudence and benevolence in the name of science.

Disregard of Basic Ethical Principles of Conduct: Failure to Protect Human Participants

The following are selective examples of some of the more horrendous narratives that demonstrate inhumane research and egregious acts of brutality against human participants that have occurred throughout history, both nationally and internationally. These accounts are provided to exemplify historical perspectives and their significant impact on the development of ethical standards governing research using human participants. For a more detailed listing, please refer to Box 5.1. It illustrates a timeline for important historical research perspectives and their significant impact on the development of ethical standards governing research using human participants. For a more detailed account, please refer to McGuire Dunn & Chadwick (1999).

BOX 5.1	Historical Studies and Key Issues in Ethical Research: A Timeline

Part I: Background

- 1946 The Nuremberg Doctors' Trial: Nazi Doctors performed medical experiments; battlefield medicine; injury treatment; and, exposure to chemical warfare agents

- 1963 The "Milgram Study": Yale University social psychology researcher (Stanley Milgram) performed obedience to authority experiment; deception; resulting concerns for psychological stress, social, legal, and economic harm to participants

- 1932–1972 The Tuskegee Syphilis Study: United States Public Health Service (later known as Center for Disease Control); untreated syphilis; knowing violation of participant rights; "scientific opportunity"; resulting in National Research Act including requirements for informed consent and review of research by institutional review boards (IRBs); and creation of the National Commission for the Protection of Human Subjects of Biomedical and Behavioral Research (later wrote the Belmont Report).

- 1963 The Jewish Chronic Disease Hospital Study: New York's Jewish Chronic Disease Hospital; cancer research conducted on senile patients suffering from chronic diseases; consequent review by Board of Regents of the State University of New York resulted in findings of fraud, deceitfulness, and unprofessional conduct.

Part II: The Development of Codes of Research Ethics

- 1947 The Nuremberg Code: Voluntary consent; benefits outweigh risks; ability to withdraw

- 1964 Declaration of Helsinki: Concern for the interest of the participant must prevail

- 1979 Belmont Report: Ethical concepts of respect, beneficence, and justice

Source: McGuire Dunn C., Chadwick G. *Protecting Study Volunteers in Research: A Manual for Investigative Sites.* CenterWatch, Inc., University of Rochester Medical Center; 1999:2 4; Henderson-Harr, A. (2004). *Historical Perspectives and their Significant Impact on the Development of Ethical Standards Governing Research Using Human Participants.* Cortland, NY: State University of New York College at Cortland, Research and Sponsored Programs Office.

EXAMPLE

Tuskegee Syphilis Study

Before detailing this travesty, we would be remiss not to point out that this *"experiment"* was conducted by the U.S. Public Health Service (PHS) and continued from 1932 until 1972. The name of the study is derived from the Tuskegee Institute, the historically black university and its affiliated hospital founded by Booker T. Washington. It is widely held that participants were falsely informed that they were being treated for "bad blood" when in reality they were being studied to determine the effects of tertiary syphilis. Treatment and cure were shamelessly admitted to be of no consequence to those conducting the study. Left untreated in the course of 40 years of study, some of the participants unknowingly infected their wives, and, in turn, some of their children.

Under the believed purpose of contributing to an important study designed to compare the effects of syphilis between white and black men, the Tuskegee Institute was enlisted to help recruit African-American male participants in a study of the prevalence of syphilis. Similarly, plantation owners and black church leaders were solicited to encourage participation. It is said that even the Surgeon General of the United States played a part in persuading the men to go on with the study.

Any participant found to suffer from syphilis remained not only untreated, but also uninformed as to the fact that they were infected with the disease. Even after the PHS started administering penicillin for the treatment of syphilis in 1943, participants in the Tuskegee study remained uniformed, were denied medical treatment, and were prevented from receiving treatment by other agencies such as the U.S. Military. In 1973, the late Senator Edward Kennedy called for congressional subcommittee meetings and ultimately succeeded in a total revision of Health, Education, and Welfare regulations for working with human participants in research. This legislative accomplishment marked an important milestone in setting regulations for the responsible conduct of research involving human participants.

The Nuremberg Doctors Trials

The Nuremberg trials (also known formally as the Trials War Criminals before the Nuremberg Military Tribunals) of World War II occurred from 1945 through 1949. The "Doctors' Trial" was held from December 9, 1946 to August 8, 1947 and focused on heinous Nazi human experimentation that took place at the hands of some 20 German medical doctors performing ongoing testing on concentration camp prisoners. Prisoner participation was forced and torture was an extreme example of coercion tactics used by the German Nazi regime at Auschwitz and other camps, while methods of experimentation often ended in the deaths of the participants. Experiments were explained with the rationale of helping the

(continued)

German military (in particular, the Air Force), eliminating the Jewish race, and "curing" homosexual prisoners of their homosexuality.

These so-called "medical experiments" were performed without consent on detained prisoners of war, as well as unfortunate civilians of occupied countries. Some of the torturous experimentation included poison experiments; freezing experiments; sterilization experiments; twins experiments; incendiary bomb experiments; malaria experiments; high altitude experiments; sea water experiments; sulfonamide experiments; battlefield medicine experiments including treatment of gunshot wounds, burns, traumatic amputations, and chemical and biological agent exposures; and mustard gas experiments. These experiments were later deemed crimes and the doctors who conducted the "experiments" were put on trial at what became known as the Doctors' Trial. Widespread news broadcasts of these beyond-abusive crimes eventually led to trial judgments and a set of standards that we now know as the Nuremberg Code of medical ethics.

The Nuremberg Code (http://ohsr.od.nih.gov/guidelines/nuremberg.html) was actually a list of ethical standards that collectively established a new paradigm shift in morality by which the defendants were judged and their guilt determined. Thus began the "Modern" era of human research protections that originated from the Nuremberg Code.

The Code states that
1. Informed consent of volunteers must be obtained without coercion.
2. Human experiments should be based on prior animal experimentation.
3. Anticipated scientific results should justify the experiment.
4. Only qualified scientists should conduct medical research.
5. Physical and mental suffering and injury should be avoided.
6. There should be no expectation of death or disabling injury from the experiment.

Medical ethics commonly include the following six values that developed out of the Code: (i) autonomy; (ii) **beneficence**; (iii) nonmaleficence; (iv) justice; (v) dignity; and (vi) truthfulness and honesty (informed consent has stemmed from these).

ETHICAL PRINCIPLES AND HUMAN PARTICIPATION PROTECTIONS

Informed Consent

Informed consent is critical for the researcher, but even more important for the research participant. It is the job of the researcher to lay out the protocol of the experiment to the participant/patient/client, and to inform them on the benefits, obligations, and any potential risks they may incur by participating in the research project being presented to them. Consent forms have to be extremely explicit in their language, and must clearly state the roles of the researcher/practitioner and participant/client in the research study. Depending on the nature of the research, the participant must be informed of such matters of **confidentiality**. If participants are going to be referred to by name they need to agree to this within the informed consent. Likewise, due to the nature of most medical research it is clearly laid out in the informed consent that the participant will remain anonymous in the study. However, as mentioned above, there are special cases where approval for identification might be needed as in compiling social histories or in case studies. Either way, it is critical that the language of the consent form makes this point clear to the participant.

For the research practitioner informed consent forms may take on the mantle of just another procedure to go through prior to beginning their research. Nevertheless, the informed consent form is in fact a contract between the participant and the researcher. Another way of viewing this is while the research practitioner should already have the knowledge of ethical procedures such as Helsinki Agreement and the **Belmont Report**, the participant often is not informed of such detailed ethical protocols and procedures. This is where the research practitioner has to take on the role of educator and advocator for their participants/clients in order to protect not only the participants but also themselves. Consent forms are the foundational bridge between researcher and research participant, and part of the necessary procedure to maintain ethical standards while conducting research with human participants.

National and International Practices

The Belmont Report

The Belmont Report (http://www.bop.gov/news/BelmontReport.jsp) originated from the Department of Health, Education and Welfare (HEW), and it concentrates on and lays down the guidelines for the protection of human subjects used in research. It is a requirement that all researchers read this report prior to submitting research requests to the HEW Board if research is to be conducted on HEW facilities. The report covers three areas of ethical principles and conduct of behavior in research: (i) boundaries between practice and research, (ii) basic ethical principles, and (iii) application of these principles to do research. The next sections summarize each of these three areas of the report.

Boundaries between Practice and Research   In a medical setting these two terms are often blended together and thought of as the same. However, they need to be separated and defined as the separate entities they are. The Belmont report makes it clear about how these two are different. Practice is often when the practitioner adjusts or slightly deviates from the standard protocol of treatment to help an individual client or patient (NCPHS, 1979). Research refers to a rigidly designed protocol that needs to be or is being tested, whereby the goal is to develop a hypothesis and to contribute to the body of knowledge in the field (NCPHS, 1979). Additionally, another aim of research is the repeatability of the results across trials and populations.

Basic Ethical Principles   The attempt here is to outline the justifications for applying codes of conduct while proceeding forward with research on human subjects. Much of this is framed in the cultural and societal codes we value. The most relevant ones here relate to respect for persons, beneficence, and justice (NCPHS, 1979).

Respect for persons
The respect for persons/clients recognizes that each individual is just that, an individual, and they should not be pressured into doing something they either feel uncomfortable doing or that violates their own personal belief system. On the most basic of levels this means giving the individual respect and autonomy. In some cases the practitioner may be the sole advocate for the client to be involved in a research study where the outcomes may be of benefit or possibly harm to their client due to reduced autonomy (NCPHS, 1979). These cases may occur when the individual is unable to communicate verbally or in any other cognitive way. Such examples would be in case of a child under the age of 2 years or someone who is in coma, or any other incapacitated form.

Beneficence
Beneficence refers to the ability of the practitioner to secure and stabilize the condition or well-being of the client while they are receiving treatment or are involved in a research project (NCPHS, 1979). Beneficence can also be understood as acts of kindness, charity, or comfort to the individual client that go beyond their normal obligation to the client. The guiding statute here for the practitioner is that the client should be receiving maximum benefit from participation in the study while minimizing their exposure to threat or harm (NCPHS, 1979). Another consideration for beneficence is being able to see when there is a depreciable return of benefits to the client in the face of constant or increased risks to their health over time. In these cases beneficence requires that a client be removed from such involvement.

Justice
This aspect of ethical codes of conduct arises over who should benefit from the findings of the research produced. It is often thought that the benefactors of medical research are those coming from a better social class, ideal health, age or weight, and financial standing. When this does occur an injustice has occurred. The goal is to equalize the playing field by applying the idea of equally distributing knowledge and treatment to correct the problem of injustice.

Applications and Informed Consent under the Belmont Report   Under the Belmont Report guidelines of informed consent consist of **disclosure** to the client of what the research entails. The potential client has the choice to accept or reject participation once all procedures and requirements of participation have been disclosed to them. This also includes understanding of the study by the subject and what will happen to the data collected on them once it has concluded (NCPHS, 1979).

The disclosure of information to clients includes but is not limited to research procedures, the goal or purpose of the study, any potential risks or possible benefits, adaptations to the stated procedures, explicit statements regarding the opportunity for the client to ask questions about the study, and the option to drop out of the study at any time for any reason (NCPHS, 1979). Another consideration is to disclose to the client their individual results and the overall results once the study has been concluded. In the case of researchers conducting interviews, case studies, or other forms of qualitative research, the client should be given a copy of their responses and the opportunity to edit or add to their responses and sign off on a second and final informed consent before concluding the study. Here the overall guiding theme throughout this process is that the standard of care is to be given to the client who is volunteering for the study.

In most cases full disclosure is the norm; however, there are some cases where incomplete disclosure is needed in order to maintain the validity of the study. Such cases arise where if the clients were to have full disclosure of all intentions of the study the results would be manipulated by their own actions (NCPHS, 1979). The ethical rule to follow in such cases is to go back to the well-being of the client/subjects participating in the study, whereby not fully informing them no harm will come to them (NCPHS, 1979). And again the client would be informed of the results and the reason for incomplete disclosure at the completion of the study. What is not acceptable here is when a researcher chooses to give only incomplete disclosure of the study because it is an inconvenience to them or in some cases the researcher fears that they will lose some of their subject pool if they give full disclosure.

With any study the client needs to be fully aware of what is being asked of them. An adequate amount of time must transpire before any client is allowed to participate in a study. This gives the client the opportunity to fully understand their role in the study and ask for clarification of just what is being asked of them. The degree of understanding of what the client is being asked to do is ensured by giving the client a questionnaire regarding the procedure(s) or putting them through a simulation or practice run prior to commencing the studying with the subject (NCPHS, 1979). Another consideration for comprehending the role of the client in a study is when the subject or subject pool have limited cognitive capabilities (e.g., infants, toddlers, and coma patients) and require a third party (often the closest family member) acting in the clients' best interest.

✔ CONCEPT CHECK

Under the Belmont Report guidelines of informed consent consist of disclosure to the client of what the research entails. The potential client has the choice to accept or reject participation once all procedures and requirements of participation have been disclosed to them.

Assessment of Risks and Benefits

While this has already been reviewed to some degree in the previous sections it needs to be restated that any potential benefit or risk to the client needs to be explicitly stated in the informed consent. There are a number of considerations that need to be taken into account so as to not put the client in harm's way during the research process. These considerations are as follows: brutal or inhumane treatment (physical, mental, or emotional); risks should be minimized and if risks are viewed to bring harm to potential clients then human subjects should not be used; review committees need to insist on the justification of human subjects in research work; the type and percent risk must be stated; full disclosure of risks and benefits must be explicitly stated in the informed consent (NCPHS, 1979).

Subject Selection

In the selection of subjects for research studies all of the guidelines already stated apply. The selection process of subjects needs to follow the guidelines of what has been approved by what is considered an expert but yet objective institutional body that is not directly conducting the research. In some cases the idea of randomness satisfies the need of where the pool of subjects can be recruited to participate. However, subject selection must be taken with care so that certain populations are not exploited or repeatedly used for studies (World Medical Association, 2008; NCPHS, 1979). This is what is known as a form of injustice in the selection of subjects for research work. In the past there have been abuses that have warranted the protection of groups or entire social classes of people from being overused and even abused in the name of research. Groups that are the most vulnerable to overselection in human research work include institutionalized groups/individuals, economically disadvantaged groups, minority groups, and the very sick (NCPHS, 1979).

World Medical Association Declaration of Helsinki

The World Medical Association (WMA) is an institutional body that has set procedure, policies, and codes of conduct for doctors and medical researchers to follow on a global level. Such organizations set these procedures in order to provide guidance to developing nations that have less informed or nonexistent national bodies in a given area. Additionally, international bodies such as the WMA aid in furthering medical knowledge in developed nations in an effort to maintain a high standard of ethical treatment of research subjects while not impeding the progress of research in the field of medicine on a global level.

Purpose of WMA

The overall purpose of the WMA is twofold. The first being, "The health of my patient will be my first consideration" (World Medical Association, 2008). The second tenet relates to an ethical code, "A physician shall act only in the patient's interest when providing medical care which might have the effect of weakening the physical and mental condition of the patient" (World Medical Association, 2008). Much of the general practice and procedures in the treatment of subjects/clients by the WMA mirror the standards set by the Belmont Report, which has already been outlined.

Principles for all Medical Research

Where the WMA extends beyond the Belmont Report is as follows. The WMA requires that any medical research involving human subjects be research based (World Medical Association, 2008). This also conforms to the groundwork of the EBP concept proposed in this book. The WMA stresses caution must be used when conducting research not only in regards to human subjects but to the environment or to the welfare of animals (World Medical Association, 2008).

As with any sanctioned research the WMA requires that the experimental protocol goes through an ethical review committee that is independent of the investigator or any other influence (World Medical Association, 2008). It is also requested that updates or monitored reports on the progress of the research is submitted to this independent committee throughout the research process (World Medical Association, 2008). This is of particular importance in the occurrence of any adverse developments during the research process.

While it seems to be a requirement, the WMA is quite clear on the fact that medical research should only be conducted by qualified individuals (World Medical Association, 2008). Also in agreement with the Belmont Report the WMA is clear on any inherent risks to human subjects, provided the subjects are healthy. Here as in the Belmont Report, medical research should be conducted only if the importance of the medical objectives outweighs the risks and hazards to the subject (World Medical Association, 2008).

The WMA is in agreement with the EBP concept and the Belmont Report with regards to informed consent. Here practitioners/doctors/medial researchers must provide full disclosure aims, methods, sources of funding, any possible conflict of interest (cultural, religious, or otherwise), the relationship of the researcher(s) to the institution, and the benefits and the risks of the proposed research to the client/subject (World Medical Association, 2008). Another obligation to be stressed here that falls within the guidelines of the WMA is that when the data go to publication the results are reported accurately, all facets of the research are reported, sources of funding, institutional affiliation, and any possible conflict of interest (World Medical Association, 2008).

✔ CONCEPT CHECK

Also in agreement with the Belmont Report the WMA is clear on any inherent risks to human subjects, provided the subjects are healthy. Here as in the Belmont Report, medical research should be conducted only if the importance of the medical objectives outweighs the risks and hazards to the subject (World Medical Association, 2008).

MEDICAL RESEARCH COMBINED WITH MEDICAL CARE

With regards to medical research there are sometimes cases where research studies and medical care share the same environment and relate to the health status of the individual under the care of a doctor. In such cases these two should only be combined when warranted by the value of the research to aid in the physical well-being of the client (World Medical Association, 2008). Under these circumstances additional standards and rigors of control are placed on the researcher in order to protect the patient. Another consideration is the application of a new protocol for medical use and its application. Here it should only be used after it has been tested against current and most accepted protocol (World Medical Association, 2008).

Another case where problems can result is when a patient/client refuses to take part in a study even if their participation may help them and improve their health. If a client refuses to participate, then the relationship between the doctor and patient or practitioner/client should not change. In other words, there should be no retribution to a patient or change in the professional relationship for electing to not take part in a proposed study (World Medical Association, 2008). For example, once the study has concluded and the protocol under study has found to aid the condition of the patient who refused to take part in the study, then that patient should not be denied the new treatment.

This process of care-related ethical treatment of patients relates to one last statute by the WMA. That relates to the use of unproven medical treatments or protocols that have the potential to save the life of the patient, restore health, or eliminate suffering. The applications of these protocols still can only be administered with the patient's informed consent but then also knowing the method to be used on them is untried (World Medical Association, 2008).

MILITARY AND OTHER SPECIAL INTEREST RESEARCH

The funding of research at the university level can come from a number of different sources. These sources include but are not limited to universities in the form of internal grants, the private sector, the state government, and the federal government. Federal funding particularly from the military comes with a reference to warfare and the destruction of human property and life. To some researchers this type of funding is objectionable due to the very nature of source and how their results will be interpreted by the military. However, research done for the military can take on a variety of purposes and needs that are responses to preserving human life. Fundable research for preservation and protection of life by the military includes but is not limited to extreme environmental stresses placed on the human body, protective gear and body armor, and application of medical treatments in the field. The problem for any individual or group looking for funding from the military often centers around the aspect of the intention to use the research or what is produced by the research toward peaceful means and not as an offensive tool for destruction. The question for many is how will their work be used once it is out of their control.

An example of how military medical research has helped and caused problems for the last seventy years is in the development of a variety of drugs that were introduced during World War II; namely, the development and use of amphetamines and human growth hormone during and after the war. Amphetamines were developed to keep soldiers alert when they put on extended duty on the front lines. Those taking the drugs were put on picket duty; the role of this position is to alert the rest of the company, regiment, and larger segments of the army if an attack is coming. The eventual fallout from the development of amphetamines after the war was the illegal distribution of a strong stimulant that was potentially addictive.

Likewise, human growth hormone was developed for the medial branch of the military occupation forces in Europe to treat children who were malnourished and undersized due to rationing and starvation during the war. The drug was developed to allow these children to reach their physical genetic potential. Ultimately the drug found its way into the hands of international and professional athletes as a means to increase muscle mass and enhance performance.

Government funded research in medical and other fields of science has in the past been a hurdle for researchers to overcome or at least the perception was that it came with roadblocks and a long process to acquire an independent or joint patent of what was developed in the research study. Prior to 1980, universities and other nonprofit organizations were faced with the problem over who had the rights to inventions or medicines when they had been developed with the assistance of federal taxpayers money and who would receive the windfall from these new inventions. Often the process for public distribution of new inventions and medicines was arduous and time consuming when it came to distributing them to the public because of legal and ethical snarls over ownership of the patents and trademarks due to federal funding. In 1980, Senators Robert Dole and Birch Bayh put forth legislation to allow private research firms and universities to retain title to inventions with federal funding which in turn allows these agencies to promote commercial concerns for these inventions (Council on Governmental Relations, 2008). Retaining title to inventions by the institution did not help, but ensured the practice of private institutions or universities being able to accept funding from interested research partners in the future (Council on Governmental Relations, 2008). Further additions to this act were made in 1984 and 1986 to ensure that the products developed from federal funding in private institutions continued to find quicker access to the public for commercial use (Council on Governmental Relations, 2008). Additionally, universities are encouraged by the government to file for patents on inventions they develop with federal grants (Council on Governmental Relations, 2008). The trade-off for the government under the Bayh-Dole Act occurs because they retain the license to practice the patent throughout the world as well as retaining march-rights to the patent (Council on Governmental Relations, 2008).

The Bayh-Dole Act has several provisions that address a number of ethical issues related to the titling of inventions. For instance, universities have to properly manage the invention in the public market when it is distributed for commercial use (Council on Governmental Relations, 2008). Proper managing of these inventions is set and enforced by the related or appropriate federal agency that granted the funding to the research firm or university (Council on Governmental Relations, 2008). While this may appear to be the government interfering with research and development, it is in reality quite the opposite. Agencies such as the National Institutes of Health (NIH) have electronic reporting systems that allow institutions such as universities to enter reports and data directly into database systems that allow the NIH to manage and review the progress of the agency receiving the grant (National Institutes of Health, 2008). Additionally, such measures have not inhibited research but have actually increased the development and distribution of new inventions and medicines tenfold since the passing of the Bayh-Dole Act (Council on Governmental Relations, 2008). Because of the Bay-Dole Act some of the following discoveries have been made possible: developing artificial lung surfactant for use with newborn infants, process for inserting DNA into eucaryotic cells and for producing proteinaceous materials, recombinant DNA technology, central to the biotechnology industry, and TRUSOPT (dorzolamide) ophthalmic drop used for glaucoma (Council on Governmental Relations, 2008).

Besides the upside to liberating research institutions to conduct research, receive funding for it, the Bayh-Dole Act also puts in place a series of ethical checks and balances for proper disbursement of said inventions. This is done as already stated by freeing up the institution to commercially produce the invention but at the same time answer for how they are spending the grant money and how they are proceeding with the development of the new invention for further or expanded use in the open market.

✔ CONCEPT CHECK

The Bayh-Dole Act put in place a series of ethical checks and balances for proper disbursement of said inventions, along with a greater attention to the details to monitor proper protocols and procedures are being followed by agencies receiving grants.

CHAPTER SUMMARY

The role of ethics and responsible conduct in treatment of human participants is a product of protection for the research participant. In short, the researchers pledge two primary assurances to their participants: (i) that they will not be placed in harm's way and (ii) that they will not be denied access to information concerning their well-being. Such ethical guidelines for participant treatment go through a series of checks and balances to ensure proper treatment of the client, whereby the client will be provided with practitioners within the medical field to advocate for them. It is important to understand that the institutions (medical, academic, or otherwise) must establish and uphold guidelines of ethical practice for uniform treatment of research participants.

While all professionals should adhere to written and formally agreed upon ethical standards sometimes their ability to deliver services within those parameters might be different due to their educational background, professional position, world-view, and age. In other words, although style and technique of application may vary, all professionals within a given institution have ethical guidelines to keep them within a common code or practice for how they treat and interact with clients. Ethical treatment includes, but is not limited to, the methods of selection of research participants and patients who agree to participate in experimental studies or treatment protocols.

While the interaction with the ethical treatment of patients for medical research or returning them to health is the goal of healthcare professionals, there are other matters of importance that require ethical consideration within the healthcare field. As noted previously, legislation has helped in reducing the problems of who has the rights to medical developments and other products that would benefit clients. The solution of the Bayh-Dole Act helped to bridge that gap. The institution funding the development of a new product and the institution producing the product from outside funding can have equitable common ground. This shared role in the delivery of the product without getting entangled in territorial snares and differences of ethical choices allows both parties to adhere to the same practice and to speed the delivery of the product to clients.

KEY POINTS

- The role of ethical treatment of clients is a product of protection for the client.
- Ethical guidelines for client treatment go through a series of check and balances to ensure proper treatment of the client.
- Institutions, medical or otherwise, must establish and uphold guidelines of ethical practice for uniform treatment of clients.
- Ethical treatment includes but is not limited to the methods of selection of clients for research or aiding them in regaining their health status.
- Legislation has helped in reducing the problems of who has the rights to medical developments and other products that would benefit clients.

Critical Thinking Questions

1. What role does culture play in the health and medical professions and how does it evolve?
2. Why are ethical codes developed in medical and human care professions?
3. Explain the connection between medical research and medical care.
4. What is the importance of the Belmont Report?
5. Explain why disclosure to clients is important.
6. How might the Bayh-Dole Act help in the delivery of better health care?

Applying Concepts

1. Part of maintaining ethical standards is making the right decisions when there seems to be a degree of uncertainty. Consider the position that athletic trainers are often put in with regards to injured athletes at the interscholastic or intercollegiate levels. Often an athletic trainer is asked to

(continued)

compromise their ethical stance of care of the athlete due to the influence of the athlete, coach, or in some cases the parents. For example, when an athlete at either of these two levels (regardless of the sport) receives a dislocated shoulder the discussion quickly moves to the severity of the dislocation and how soon can the athlete return to competition. The issue can be further complicated by when the injury occurred and the pressure to return the athlete to competition especially when the injury happens anywhere between the midpoint of the season to the end of the season. This is where pressure to rush the athlete back to action often comes from the coaching staff. Likewise, pressure also comes from the athlete as well if they sense that their immediate future to continue competing in the sport is threatened. For the high school athlete this means school losing interest in offering a scholarship to the athlete. At the intercollegiate level, the athlete could be facing a financial decision, whereby their draft status could be compromised by their sitting out during critical competitions in the second half of the season. Often the athletic trainer is put in a situation where they are asked to compromise their values system of care for an athlete on several levels. What are the inherent problems in this situation with athletes returning too soon to competition?

2. The idea of giving options that are viable to patients is an ethical decision that will need to be made by clinicians. Take for instance the choice of recommending a treatment procedure for a patient with allergies. Traditionally, the choice would be to recommend antihistamines for a patient. However, there are other therapies available and many patients are choosing to see acupuncturist for permanent allergy relief. Explain why both options should be made to patients and the problems and successes each have for this problem.

3. Real world problems often exist for researchers attempting to further their line of research. One of them is often funding of the research itself. For some practitioners they are faced with problems that comprise their ability to continue their research and ultimately their jobs. Take for example a research team that is devoted to the preservation and the extension of life and is doing research on the stresses on the body to extreme environmental conditions. The group has submitted several grant proposals to a variety of agencies including the Federal Government to fund their research. The only grant awarding agency at this time that will approve their research and give them funding is the United States Army. While the nature of the research is designed to enhance life, the factor of military interest always carries with it the potential of destruction of human life. Discuss the ethical decisions that need to be made here including the subject selection process if the grant is accepted.

REFERENCES

Baudrillard J. *Seduction*. New York: St. Martins Press; 1990.

Bourdieu P. *Outline of a Theory of Practice*. Cambridge, UK: Cambridge University Press; 1995.

Kuhn T. *The Structure of Scientific Revolutions*. 2nd ed. Chicago, IL: University of Chicago Press; 1970.

McGuire Dunn C, Chadwick G. *Protecting Study Volunteers in Research: A Manual for Investigative Sites*. CenterWatch, Inc., University of Rochester Medical Center; 1999:2–4.

McPherson JM. *Battle Cry of Freedom: The Civil War era*. New York: Ballantine Books; 1988.

Council on Governmental Relations. (2008). The Bayh-Dole Act: a guide to the law and implementing regulations. University of California technology transfer. Available at: http://www.ucop.edu./ott/faculty/bayh.html. Accessed October 24, 2008.

National Institutes of Health. "period" (2008). Developing sponsored research agreements: considerations for recipients of NIH research grants and contracts. NIH Guide. Available at: http://www.grants.nih.gov/grants/guide/notice-files/not94-213.html. Accessed October 24, 2008.

World Medical Association. (2008). World Medical Association declaration of Helsinki: ethical principles for medical research involving human subjects. Available at: http://www.wma.net/e/policy/b3.htm. Accessed October 24, 2008.

NCPHS. (1979). The Belmont Report: ethical principles and guidelines for the protection of human subjects of biomedical and behavioral research. Department of Health, Education, Welfare. Available at: http://www.bop.gov/news/BelmontReport.jsp. Accessed October 24, 2008.

SUGGESTED READING

1. National Bioethics Advisory Commission. Ethical and Policy Issues in Research Involving Human Participants. Vol 1: Report and recommendations of the National Bioethics Advisory Commission. Bethesda, MD: National Bioethics Advisory Commission; 2001.

2. Jones J. *Bad Blood: The Tuskegee Syphilis Experiment: A Tragedy of Race and Medicine*. New York: The Free Press; 1981.

3. National Science Foundation.*Proposal and Award Policies and Procedures Guide (PAPPG)*. NSF 10-1 January 2010; 2010.

4. National Institutes of Health. NIH Online Course: Human Participant Protections Education for Research Teams. Avialable at: http://cme.cancer.gov/c01/nih_intro_02.htm.

5. (NA). Nuremberg Doctors' Trial. *BMJ*. 1996;313(7070):1445–1475.

6. The Nuremberg Code. Available at: http://ohsr.od.hih.gov/nuremberg.php3.

7. The *Journal of Research Administration*. Commemorative Anniversary Edition. Volume XXXVII, 2007.

8. Online Ethics Center. Available at: http://www.onlineethics.org.

9. "Nazi Medical Experimentation". *US Holocaust Memorial Museum*. Available at: http://www.ushmm.org/wlc/article.php?lang=en&ModuleId=10005168. Accessed

January 5, 2010."Medical Experiment". *Jewish Virtual Library*. Available at: http://www.jewishvirtuallibrary.org/jsource/Holocaust/medtoc.html. Accessed January 5, 2010."The Doctors Trial: The Medical Case of the Subsequent Nuremberg Proceedings". *United States Holocaust Memorial Museum*. Available at: http://www.ushmm.org/research/doctors/indiptx.htm. Accessed January 5, 2010.

FURTHER READING

Bulger JW. An approach towards applying principlism. *Ethics Med*. 2009;25(2):121–125.
Fortin S, Alvarez F, Bibeau G, et al. Contemporary medicine: applied human science or technological enterprise? *Ethics & Med*. 2008;24(1):41–50.
Fuchs S. Relativism and reflexivity in the sociology of scientific knowledge. In: Ritzer G, ed. *Metatheorizing (Key Issues in Sociological Theory)*. Newbury Park, CA: Sage; 1992.
Goldblatt D. Ask the ethicist: must physicians respect an incompetent patient's refusal of treatment? *Med Ethics*. 2006;13(2):3.
Hoffmann D. The legal column: choosing paternalism. *Med Ethics*. 2006;13(2):4, 12.

PART II

SEEKING ANSWERS: HOW THE QUESTION DRIVES THE METHODS

FINDING THE EVIDENCE: INFORMATIONAL SOURCES, SEARCH STRATEGIES, AND CRITICAL APPRAISAL

Read not to contradict and confute, nor to believe and take
for granted… but to weigh and consider.

—*Francis Bacon (1561–1626, as quoted in* The Quotations
Page, *www.quotationspage.com)*

CHAPTER OBJECTIVES

After reading this chapter, you will:

- Be able to describe the role of the reference librarian.
- Understand the concept of the Invisible Web.
- Be able to use Boolean logic as part of your search strategy.
- Appreciate the notion search strategies for purposeful Web-based navigation for deliberate inquiry.
- Learn how to critically review and appraise scientific literature as evidence.
- Understand the benefits of peer-review in journal article publication.
- Recognize that various factors influence and determine the quality of informational sources.
- Appreciate the benefits and limitations of the journal impact factor.

KEY TERMS

boolean search	Invisible Web	pubMed
database	peer-review	search engine
evidence	proof	URL
hierarchy	prop	

INTRODUCTION

Before attempting to effectively interpret, critically appraise, apply, or conduct research, it is prudent to be familiar with how and where to find the plausible **"evidence"** to be had in various informational sources. Evidence consists of informational particulars of the theoretical, hypothetical, anecdotal, or empirical nature that can be corroborated, substantiated, or confirmed. In a research paradigm, data are gathered as evidence to either support or refute scientific viewpoints. In this manner, evidence can be used to corroborate or contradict previous research findings. Consequently, evidence is sometimes erroneously inferred as *proof* rather than *prop* for theoretical perspectives.

Evidence is evaluated based on a **hierarchy** of its derivational and presentational formats. Chapter 7 discusses the hierarchy of evidence in terms of its derivation (i.e., research design and research methodology). This chapter discusses the hierarchy of evidence in terms of its presentation/publication (i.e., prestige or importance of a refereed scientific journal in its field).

INFORMATIONAL SOURCES AND THE REFERENCE LIBRARIAN

The type of evidence you seek and the various types of informational source(s) you choose will depend on your question (see Chapter 1). As explained in Chapter 1, the research question drives the research methods. Once the question is clear, the search for evidence in the existing literature begins. Many undergraduate students begin their search of scientific literature by asking the help of a reference librarian. While a reference librarian will be able to assist you by pointing you toward your most likely resources, he or she will not necessarily be able to answer your question(s). Perhaps even more to the dismay of the frustrated student, the aspiration of the reference librarian is not to provide tangible results by conducting a comprehensive search on your behalf.

The goals of the reference librarian are to assist you in finding suitable informational sources and to provide guidance and instruction for using effectual search strategies. Reference librarians are generalists in a broad list of pedagogic categories and academic disciplines. They can provide instruction and guidance in navigating print periodicals, electronic and digital reference systems, commercial **search engines**, new standards for reference metrics, as well as more traditional topics such as organizing print and electronic resources, proper citation style formats and preventing plagiarism. The role of the reference librarian is important and while they can offer a vast amount of guidance and direction in conducting your search for evidence, they do not represent the culmination of your search.

✔ CONCEPT CHECK

The goals of the reference librarian are to assist you in finding suitable informational sources and to provide guidance and instruction for using effectual search strategies.

ELECTRONIC SOURCES AND DATABASES

It is a common practice among students and practitioners, alike, to search for credible information by utilizing freely accessible Web search engines (i.e., Google, Dogpile, etc.) or Wikipedia (i.e., the free content, collaboratively written Web-based encyclopedia). Web search engines can produce a variety of results in a relatively short time frame; however, Web search engines usually do not yield many journal articles. While the user-friendly appeal of such sites may seem obvious, Web search results should be considered with careful reservation.

Web searches can produce numerous informational Web sites and nonrefereed online documents. Often the information provided in general Web sites and nonrefereed documents is questionable in terms of the accuracy and reliability of information content. Web sites can provide a plethora of valuable information together with misinformation, out-of-date conclusions, and/or prejudiced opinion. By comparison, peer-reviewed journal articles found in **databases** can usually be trusted to have a prudent level of credibility and validity. Unfortunately, many people do not realize that journals databases are generally inaccessible to search engine indexes. Those areas of the Internet that are inaccessible to search engines are collectively known as the **Invisible Web**. Databases, for instance, are found on the Invisible Web and can be located by guessing or determining the Uniform Resource Locators (**URLs**) for specific organizations likely to hold answers to your question(s).

Databases are electronic libraries of indexed journals, books, and nonjournal bibliographic literature and documents that are overseen, managed, and updated on a regular basis. For example, **PubMed** is a journals database provided as a service of the U.S. National Library of Medicine and the National Institutes of Health. PubMed is a database of journal abstracts and citations and includes links to full text articles and other related resources. Refereed journals publish articles that have undergone **peer-review** prior to acceptance for publication. The peer-review process is one by which a panel of experts judge the content and correctness of one's work before accepting a research document for journal publication. Peer-review is a time-consuming and arduous practice thought to be necessary and meritorious to test and safeguard the quality of scholarly work.

✔ **CONCEPT CHECK**

Those areas of the Internet that are inaccessible to search engines are collectively known as the Invisible Web.

SEARCH STRATEGIES

Regardless of your preferred search strategy, it is important to remember that all searches are time-consuming to some extent. The effectiveness of your search strategies and the narrowness of your topic(s) will largely influence the amount of time it takes to generate good, usable results. Notwithstanding the chance benefits of luck and guessing, search results are only as good as the search strategies employed. It is prudent to understand the limits of hit and miss tangential style searches, and the value of planned investigation. Planned investigation begins with the understanding that searching and reviewing the literature is a purposeful and, sometimes, tiresome process. Guidelines and suggestions for search and review strategies are provided in Chapter 1.

There are online tutorials for search strategies, as well as Internet searching classes and books to aid in purposeful Web-based navigation for deliberate inquiry. While these instructional materials and classes can offer valuable recommendations and instructions, it may helpful to consider a few basic guidelines before beginning your search. Simple, self-explanatory steps include:

- Be patient and prudent.
- Keep an open mind.
- Use common sense.
- Learn as you go.
- Vary your approach, as necessary.
- Keep good records.

You may also wish to consider using Boolean logic as part of your search strategy. **Boolean searching** is based on the notion of logical relationships among search terms. Specifically, from a computer programming perspective, the operator terms of "OR," "AND," and "NOT" effect strict logically collated outcome or search results. Stated differently, each of the operator terms (i.e., OR, AND, NOT) used to combine search terms instructs a different operation or a set of search directions for the computer to follow.

Let us consider this concept in the following example using the search terms of "ankle" and "knee." The terms could be combined as such: ankle **OR** knee, ankle **AND** knee, ankle **NOT** knee. Search results based on these combinations would vary logically in this manner:

- ankle **OR** knee: would generate results in which *at least one* of the search terms was found
- ankle **AND** knee: would generate results in which *both* of the search terms were found
- ankle **NOT** knee: would generate results in which *only* the term "ankle" was found, but not if the term "knee" was found, even if the term "ankle" was found with it.

✔ CONCEPT CHECK

The effectiveness of your search strategies and the narrowness of your topic(s) will largely influence the amount of time it takes to generate good, usable results.

CRITICAL REVIEW AND APPRAISAL

When your search begins to generate results, you will need to sort out and organize the "evidence" as it accumulates. This process involves determining relevance and readability of the literature, as well as quality and importance of the informational source(s). A systematic and orderly plan to peruse and critique germane literature is a necessary component of effective, efficient search and review strategies. Restated, you absolutely must have a plan as to how you will review and appraise the scholarly evidence that results from your search. Similarly, you must have a plan as to how you will read the various types of research papers. Scanning, or reading quickly, is quite different from reading critically; however, both are valuable research skills for making inquiry and following a line of investigation. General appraisal should precede critical appraisal. In this context, appraisal refers to judgments on the relevance and readability of the evidence. Articles are evaluated for correctness and appropriateness of content. Erroneous and poorly chosen articles are eliminated in the appraisal process.

During preliminary evaluation, the suitability of a paper is determined by a quick read of the abstract. The abstract is an abbreviated summation of the main points of importance from the paper. The abstract provides a synopsis of the article by stating the purpose, methods, results, and a list of key terms. Depending on the journal format and specific author submission guidelines, more or less information may be included in the abstract. In addition to reading the abstract, the paper is scanned for appropriateness of content, comparable context, date of publication, highly regarded authors, reputation of journal, and references. Articles of uncertain yet potential relevance are kept until they can be eliminated without question.

Subsequent scrutiny and critical appraisal occur through a more serious and careful review. Critical review involves structured reading to answer questions, identify key points, and recognize significance. Reading critically and creatively is a skill that requires one to examine the content and context of the paper so as to extract important information about scientific contributions from writings using vocabulary and journal formats specific to a field or profession. Rather than merely annihilating the work, your goal is to identify areas of strength as well as areas for improvement. This process takes time. Seasoned professionals often read a paper more than a few times in order to discern the scientific contributions and nuances of an article. With this in mind, most people should plan to devote sufficient time to each paper they read for critical review.

Following critical review and appraisal, it may be helpful to skim the major parts of the paper before attempting to analyze or critique the paper. First, read the entire paper to get a sense of the "big picture" and identify any unfamiliar terminology or phrases. Next, read one section at a time for comprehension. Read to figure out answers to the following questions to help you locate information in the paper:

1. *Topic:* In your own words, clearly state the main topic and focus of the study. What was the article about? What was the issue or research problem in the article?

2. *Purpose:* In your own words, clearly state the point of the article. Briefly put in plain words why the study or experiment was done. Hint: The rationale for conducting a research study is typically to determine or investigate or explore the connection between or among variables of interest.

3. *Methods and Procedures:* In your own words, briefly describe what was being measured in the study and how it was tested. What was the general idea behind the nitty-gritty "nuts and bolts" of the study? What thing or list of things were being questioned or measured (*variables of interest*)? How were these variables measured or evaluated? Hint: identify the independent and dependent variables of interest; state how the variables were measures; summarize what was done and how it was done step by step to collect and/or test the variables of interest; provide appropriate, objective detail.

4. *Results:* What were the statistical findings from the study or experiment? If some thing of interest was measured, what was the outcome? How did

one variable influence or change another? Hint: identify the statistical relationship between the independent variable(s) and dependent variable(s) of interest in the population sampled or observed; report significant results, only; include numbers and important statistical findings that you understand; report numbers using precise statistical results (i.e., percentages, means, standard deviations, Chi-square, P values, etc.)

5. *Conclusions:* In your own words, explain the "take-home message" of this article. What did the authors deduce from the results of their study? Hint: conclusions are based on the results of the study.

6. *Theoretical Significance:* Clearly explain why you choose this particular article? Explain what you learned from the article and how it connects to the theories and research perspectives compared to other works? Hint: establish the relevance of the article and/or study.

7. *Critical Appraisal:* Objectively review and comment on the methodology of study.

We offer the following to our students as a reasonable gauge for determining when you have successfully finished reading a research paper: When you can make out the purpose, the independent and dependent variables of interest, the methods, and the results of the study, then you have finished reading the paper.

Lastly, you should summarize the information from each section into a review of the paper. Using the sections and questions listed above as your guide; make notes so that you can summarize the information in your own words for inclusion in an annotated bibliography. An annotated bibliography is similar to a reference list but, in addition to the bibliographic citations, includes a summary and/or evaluation of each of the sources you have searched and reviewed.

Part of critical review involves having appreciation for the quality of the informational source as well as the importance or influence of the journal. Credibility in scholarly informational sources can be influenced by judgments of hierarchy and impact. In an evidence-based context, the quality of an informational source as evidence is associated with the ranking or hierarchy of the evidence. A similar, yet different concept is the notion of impact factor. Impact factor is considered as a determinant of journal status associated with journal citation reports. A basic explanation of each of these factors is provided to assist you in your critical review and appraisal process.

Quality of Informational Sources

While it is beyond the scope of this chapter to consider the confluence of factors that influence and determine the "quality" of informational sources, it is nonetheless timely to raise this consideration. We feel we would be remiss if we were not to mention this issue and to remind the reader of the importance of establishing the existence of any rules for informational sources and/or expectations for quality of "evidence" in those informational sources. For example, perhaps the use of Web sites as informational sources is frowned upon or even disallowed. Or, perhaps, only peer-reviewed journal articles published within the last 5 years are approved for inclusion in your search results.

University libraries sometimes provide Web sites and informational brochures with guidelines for evaluating and critically analyzing the quality of informational sources, including Web sites. Likewise, employers, academic departments, graduate schools, or instructors may provide detailed directions and guidelines that clarify requirements for use of various informational sources. It is beneficial to know expectations regarding the quality of informational sources prior to initiating search strategies; be that as it may, it is imperative to confirm quality requirements before finalizing critical review and appraisal. As a rule, scholarly journals are usually preferred over nonscholarly periodicals and/or popular magazines when conducting a search for credible evidence.

The quality of informational sources and the notion of hierarchies of evidence as they relate to the strength of evidence in making decisions about patient care will be presented in detail in Chapter 7. For now, it suffices to note that differences in research methods (e.g., sampling) and data analysis will influence the quality or strength of evidence. Chapter 7 explores the concept of "evidence," what constitutes evidence, and how the strength of evidence can be weighed, interpreted, and applied as it applies to the advancement of healthcare practice and patient care.

✔ CONCEPT CHECK

University libraries sometimes provide Web sites and informational brochures with guidelines for evaluating and critically analyzing the quality of informational sources, including Web sites.

Impact Factor as a Determinant of Importance/ Influence of Journal

Journal impact factor (JIF) is widely considered a determinant of journal status associated with *Journal Citation Reports*. Expressly, impact factor is a mathematical rating system based on the numbers of journal citations and article publications within a 2-year time frame. This is a controversial, yet influential measure of journal evaluation, not to be confused with the hierarchy of evidence that applies to quality of evidence as determined by the pecking-order level of the informational source.

Each year, scientific journals are ranked according to impact factor in an attempt to establish their relative order of importance or influence within a professional field or scientific discipline (i.e., physical therapy). The use of JIF has allowed for journal comparison in professional fields. Consequently, JIF has become associated with prestige of publication status. Of recent years, debate has ensued over whether JIF is merely a reflection of reputation as determined by citation frequency. The crux of the issue is the distinction between quality (based on rigor of peer-review) and perceived status (based on JIF). Simply stated, the quality of the peer-review process is arguably not an extension of JIF (Wu et al., 2008; Kurmis, 2003; Benitez-Bribiesca, 2002). So, what is JIF and what does it tell us? Journals with high impact factors are regularly assumed to be more prestigious, but are those assumptions accurate?

The impact factor of a journal for any specific year is mathematically calculated by dividing the number of times a journal was cited in the previous 2 years by the number of articles it published in the same 2 years (Garfield, 2006). For example, a journal with a current impact factor of 1 would have a 1:1 citation-to-publication ratio, or an average of 1 citation for each article published in the previous 2 years. Arguably, this metric comparison does not tell us anything about the reputation of the peer-review process for scientific literature and a great deal of challenge and dispute has erupted around questions of validity and misuse.

JIF rankings are limited to the extent that frequency in citation and publication do not necessarily equate to scientific expertise, quality of scholarship, or an active research agenda. It has been argued that the originally intended value and purpose of JIF (Garfield, 2006) have been bastardized to encompass author impact. Professionals in scientific and academic research communities are often required to achieve a tally of scholarship requirements. In other words, there is a requirement to produce a certain number of publications within a certain time frame. This expectation for an active and productive research agenda is regularly referred to as the "publish or perish" peril of the academic tenure process. Additionally, it has become increasingly more common for institutions to require that a certain number of the publications happen in journals with rankings at or above a certain JIF.

Critics argue that depending on the mass of the scientific discipline and the extensiveness of the circulation of the journal, the JIF ranking could be skewed (Seglen, 1997; Hoeffel, 1998; Opthof, 1999; Yu et al., 2005; Garfield, 2006; Monastersky, 2005). For example, it is conceivable that a quarterly published journal with a wide circulation in a major, well-established professional organization would have more opportunity for citation than a semiannually published journal with a fairly small circulation in an emergent, yet obscure and highly specialized scientific discipline. More frequent publication equates to a larger number of articles published each year. Wider circulation reaches a bigger readership, and name recognition happens with bigger readership. Thus, it is plausible that a high impact factor would be more likely for the quarterly published journal with extensive readership and assumption(s) of high status in a major, well-established professional organization than for the semiannually published journal with a fairly small circulation in an emergent, yet obscure and highly specialized scientific discipline.

Human judgment is arguably the Achilles' heel of JIF, and this quandary fuels the publication debate over journal popularity versus journal influence and importance. In other words, how many (e.g., quantity, impact) versus whom your work reaches and the process by which it gets to that point (e.g., quality, influence).

✔ CONCEPT CHECK

Impact factor is a mathematical rating system based on the numbers of journal citations and article publications within a 2-year time frame. This is a controversial, yet influential measure of journal evaluation, not to be confused with the hierarchy of evidence that applies to quality of evidence as determined by the pecking-order level of the informational source.

CHAPTER SUMMARY

Resourcefully and capably locating credible informational sources can prove to be a tedious endeavor. Organized search strategies along with a practiced system for critical review and appraisal can greatly improve the overall outcome when attempting to find, read, and interpret scientific literature. Strategies such as Boolean searching and carefully comparing the reference lists of peer-reviewed research articles can help as you learn to piece together the literature as evidence. Learning to decipher how the evidence fits together requires patience, prudence, intellectual curiosity, and a willingness to look beyond the obvious. There are no shortcuts to finding the evidence; and, the results of your search will only be as good as the strategies you employ as you learn to better locate, critically review, and appraise the literature.

KEY POINTS

- In a research paradigm, data are gathered as evidence to either support or refute scientific viewpoints.
- Evidence is evaluated based on a hierarchy of its derivational and presentational formats.
- The role of the reference librarian is important and while they can offer a vast amount of guidance and direction in conducting your search for evidence, they do not represent the culmination of your search.

- Often the information provided in general Web sites and nonrefereed documents is questionable in terms of the accuracy and reliability of information content.
- The peer-review process is one by which a panel of experts judge the content and correctness of one's work before accepting a research document for journal publication.
- There are online tutorials for search strategies, as well as Internet searching classes and books to aid in purposeful Web-based navigation for deliberate inquiry.
- The abstract is an abbreviated summation of the main points of importance from the paper, and provides a synopsis of the article by stating the purpose, methods, results, and a list of key terms.
- JIF is widely considered a determinant of journal status associated with *Journal Citation Reports.*

Critical Thinking Questions

1. Why might it be beneficial to consult a reference librarian before beginning your search for evidence?
2. What is an annotated bibliography?
3. How is JIF calculated?
4. What is the debate surrounding JIF?

Applying Concepts

1. Discuss the steps you might follow to gather evidence if you were interested in learning more about whether or not muscle atrophy due to nerve damage can be prevented.
2. Review the Web pages for your university library or for your alma mater library. Locate and compare library Web pages guidelines for evaluating and critically analyzing the quality of informational sources, including Web sites.
3. Select a peer-reviewed journal article of interest to you. Exchange articles with a classmate, and read them one at a time for the purpose of critical review. Prepare an annotated bibliography. Compare your bibliographic citations and summaries for accuracy and comprehensiveness.

REFERENCES

Benitez-Bribiesca L. The ups and downs of the impact factor: the case of Archives of Medical Research. *Arch Med Res*. 2002;33(2):91–94.

Garfield E. The history and meaning of the journal impact factor. *JAMA*. 2006;295(1):90–93.

Hoeffel C. Journal impact factors. *Allergy*. 1998;53:1225.

Kurmis AP. Understanding the limitations of the journal impact factor. *J Bone Joint Surg Am*. 2003;85:2449–2954.

Monastersky R. The number that's devouring science. *Chron High Educ*. 2005. October 14. Available at: http://chronicle.com/free/v52/i08/08a01201.htm.

Opthof T, Submission, acceptance rate, rapid review system and impact factor. *Cardiovasc Res*. 1999;41:1–4.

Seglen PO. Why the impact factor of journals should not be sued for evaluating research. *Br Med J*. 1997;314(7079):498–502, Available at:
http://www.bmj.com/cgi/content/full/314/7079/497.

Wu X-F, Fu Q, Rousseau R. On indexing in the Web of Science and predicting journal impact factor. *J Zhejiang Univ Sci B*. 2008;9(7):582–590. [Electronic version].

Yu G, Wang X-Y, Yu D-R. The influence of publication delays on impact factors. *Scientometrics*. 2005;64:235–246.

CHAPTER 7

THE HIERARCHY OF EVIDENCE

"First learn the meaning of what you say, and then speak."

—*Epictetus (AD 55–135), as quoted in The Classic Quotes*
Collection on The Quotations Page
(www.quotationspage.com)

CHAPTER OBJECTIVES

After reading this chapter, you will:

- Understand when clinical experience should drive patient care decisions.
- Be able to describe the hierarchies of evidence as they relate to the strength of evidence in making decisions about patient care.
- Be able to explain how differences in research methods and data analysis across the spectrum of patient care can result in some differences as to how the hierarchy of evidence is described.
- Learn why larger samples are more likely to estimate true population values and result in narrower confidence intervals than small samples.
- Understand the principal difference between an RCT and a prospective cohort study.
- Understand why the RCT is a superior research design.
- Describe and explain the acronyms SpPIN and SnNOUT as they relate to diagnostic studies.
- Learn that there is more than one model of a research method hierarchy.

KEY TERMS

diagnosis	patient values	treatment plan
hierarchy	prevention	treatment response

information technology   prognosis   treatment outcomes
paradigm   strength of evidence

INTRODUCTION

The **paradigm** of evidence-based medicine or evidence-based clinical practice has been introduced in earlier chapters. The purpose of this chapter is to explore the concept of "evidence" as it applies to the advancement of healthcare practice and patient care. Before delving into what constitutes evidence and how the **strength of evidence** can be weighed, interpreted, and applied, let's consider the alternative to evidence in defining and advancing clinical practice.

Isaacs and Fitzgerald (1999) tackled the subject of alternatives to evidence-based medicine in their short and light-hearted paper entitled "Seven alternatives to evidence based medicine." Although entertaining, this paper confirms the necessity of evidence in the pursuit of improved patient care.

The first alternative, *Eminence based medicine,* suggests that experience, seniority, and recognition are sufficient to train and advance the practices of junior colleagues. While senior clinicians and faculty often are well positioned for this task *because* of their efforts to continue to critically review the best current literature many of us have encountered those who continue to make "the same mistakes with increasing confidence over an impressive number of years." Thus, while clinical experience is an important consideration, only when combined with appraisal of the best available literature should it drive patient care decisions and the advancement of health care. Isaacs and Fitzgerald continued by identifying *Vehemence based medicine, Eloquence based medicine,* and *Providence based medicine* as alternatives to evidence-based medicine. Certainly, proclaiming your opinion more loudly or smoothly may work in politics or the sale of used vehicles but has not been shown to benefit the patient or advance the practice.

These authors conclude by identifying *Diffidence based medicine, Nervousness based medicine,* and *Confidence based medicine.* In the first case nothing is done due to a lack of plausible solutions to the problem and, in second, too much is done since one does not want to miss a **diagnosis** or fail to use every opportunity or tool to foster recovery. It is rare indeed that a condition exists for which the medical literature fails to provide evidence of some merit to offer guidance. Equally true is that the literature provides guidance on diagnostic procedures and interventions that provide no benefit to the patient. More is not necessarily better. Lastly, we return to confidence. Certainly, confidence gained from experience and continued study of the literature helps the clinician cope with the stresses of providing optimal care and eases the anxiety of the patients we treat. However, as alluded to under *eminence-based medicine* we need to question on what our confidence should be based.

Thus, we are really left without an alternative to evidence-based medicine. However, one might ask that, given the long history hasn't evidence always been at the foundation of medicine? There is not an answer to this rhetorical question; however, let's consider what has changed since the term evidence-based medicine, was introduced a few decades ago that has brought so much attention. While there have been and continue to be incredible advances in science and medicine, the growing focus on evidence-based medicine has been fueled by the advances in **information technology**. Most of those reading this text likely cannot remember the days before the Internet. For some of us, however, our research and professional development was built on trips to the library to search through pages in the volumes of *Index Medicus* and similar references, requests for interlibrary loan and analysis by hand. Today we can search, acquire, read, synthesize, and analyze ever-increasing amounts of information within the comfort of our home or office. Technology has provided the access and more importantly the time to review and assess more literature than has ever been possible. Moreover, unlike the dog chasing the car, we know, or can learn what to do with the volume of information when we catch it. In fact, a primary reason for this book is to assist students and clinicians learn how to appraise and apply the volume of information now at their fingertips.

✔ CONCEPT CHECK

While clinical experience is an important consideration, only when combined with appraisal of the best available literature should it drive patient care decisions and the advancement of health care. Thus, medical decisions become evidence based.

EVIDENCE ACROSS PATIENT CARE

The care of patients spans a spectrum of interactions including screening examinations, diagnostic procedures, providing a **prognosis**, developing a **treatment plan**, and the implementation of **prevention** efforts. Research efforts in each of these areas can inform and improve clinical practice. In the later chapters of this book the differences in research methods, for example, to determine the usefulness of a diagnostic procedures versus the anticipated response to a treatment will be described in detail. However, the differences in research methods and data analysis across the spectrum of patient care also result in some differences as to how the **hierarchy** of evidence is described. For the purposes of this chapter the hierarchy of evidence related to **treatment responses** and prevention is presented first and developed to the greatest extent. The hierarchy of evidence related to diagnostic procedures and prognosis will be presented in a manner that compares and contrasts the "levels" of evidence with those of **treatment outcomes**. The evaluation of screening effectiveness often involves cost-benefit assessment and lies beyond the scope of this chapter. An excellent overview of these issues was provided by Katz (2001).

 CONCEPT CHECK

It is important to keep in mind that differences in research methods and data analysis across the spectrum of patient care can result in differences as to how the hierarchy of evidence is described.

IS ALL EVIDENCE EQUAL? LEVELS OF EVIDENCE

Evidence-based medicine is a relatively new paradigm across healthcare. While the term seems self-explanatory one of the purposes of this book is to help the reader through the nuances of the research and statistical methods employed in clinical research. The reality is that not all evidence is created equally. Differences in the strength of evidence come from two sources, sampling and research methods. The issue of sampling is quite straightforward; larger samples are more likely to estimate true population values and result in narrower confidence intervals than small samples. Thus, data from a large clinical trial with solid research methods will provide more compelling evidence than a small study of similar methodological quality.

The second influence on the strength of evidence, research method, requires more explanation. The following subsection explains two models of a research method hierarchy.

✔ **CONCEPT CHECK**

Data from a large clinical trial with solid research methods will provide more compelling evidence than a small study of similar methodological quality.

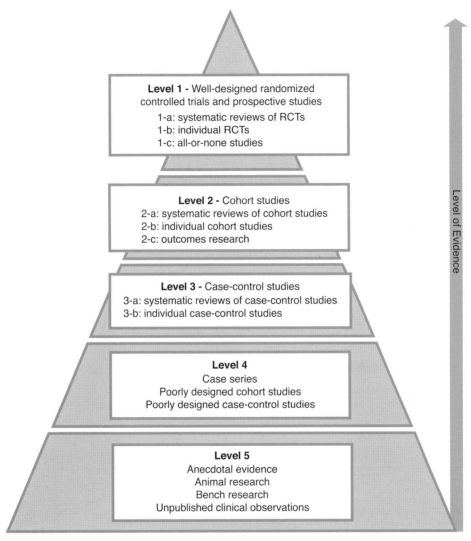

FIGURE 7-1   The Oxford Center for Evidence-Based Medicine hierarchy. (Adapted with permission from http://www.cebm.net/index.aspx?o=1025. Oxford Center for Evidence-Based Medicine—Levels of Evidence [March 2009]. Accessed May 10, 2010.)

Hierarchy of Treatment Outcomes

Two models related to the hierarchy of treatment outcomes studies are presented here for comparison (Figure 7-1 and Box 7-1). Although the elements are quite similar, subtle differences warrant discussion.

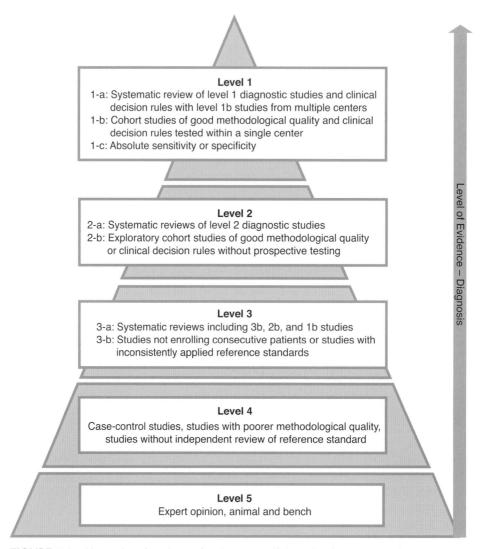

FIGURE 7-2   Hierarchy of evidence for diagnosis. (Adapted with permission from http://www.cebm.net/index.aspx?o=1025. Oxford Center for Evidence-Based Medicine—Levels of Evidence [March 2009]. Accessed May 10, 2010.)

Within Patient Randomized Treatment Order Trials

Beginning from the top of Box 7-1, within patient, randomized treatment order trials, also referred to by Guyett et al. (2001) as an *N* of 1 randomized trial, can provide the strongest evidence or treatment effect. Within patient, randomized treatment order

| BOX 7.1 | A hierarchy of strength of evidence for treatment decisions. |

Within patient, randomized treatment order trial
Systematic review of clinical trials with random assignment to treatment
Clinical trial with random assignment to treatment
Systematic review of nonrandom assignment of treatment trials
Single trial with nonrandom assignment of treatment
Laboratory studies related to physiological and biomechanical mechanisms
   underlying disease, injury, or treatment
Opinion developed through informal clinical observations

trials are studies in which patients receive all interventions under consideration in random order over the duration of the investigation. Since patients essentially serve as their own control, within patient, randomized treatment order trials studies minimize the influence of differences between patients in terms of responsiveness to intervention. While potentially providing strong evidence, these studies require that the condition being treated be relatively stable and that the effect of an intervention does not influence the response to the other interventions being investigated.

Yelland et al. (2007) provides an example of such a study. These investigators studied the effects of celecoxib, SR paracetamol, and placebo on pain, stiffness and functional limitation scores, medication preference and adverse effects in patients suffering from osteoarthritis of the knee. Each patient completed three cycles of paired treatment periods (2 weeks for each treatment over the course of 12 weeks) in a randomized order. The value in within patient, randomized treatment order trials studies is readily apparent when one considers that patients will differ considerably in their reports of pain, stiffness and functional limitation despite having similar radiographic changes. Moreover, while symptoms may worsen over time, large changes in a 3-month period are unlikely. Furthermore, the effects of the medications studied are not likely to result in long-term changes. Thus the within patient, randomized treatment order trials design provides strong evidence and minimizes the number of patients needed as there are no comparison groups.

Within patient, randomized treatment order trials studies are not common, however, simply because few conditions treated by physical therapists, occupational therapists, and athletic trainers are stable across long periods of time and because the natural history and interventions directed at change are not reversible. Consider, for example, the management of an acute lateral ankle sprain. First, natural history projects improvement in pain, loss of motion, and function over time without intervention. Secondly, once impaired motion is improved it remains improved. Thus, investigations into the treatment of conditions such as the lateral ankle sprain require other research designs such as a randomized-controlled clinical trial to be discussed shortly.

Systematic Reviews of Randomized Trials

Since within patient, randomized treatment order trials cannot be conducted in many circumstances and are rare in many healthcare specialty areas we move on to the next highest levels of evidence. Atop the second hierarchy (see Figure 7-1) we find systematic reviews with or without meta-analysis as part of what has been labeled "level 1" evidence by Oxford Center for Evidence-Based Medicine, a topic to be elaborated on shortly. Systematic review is quite important and we have devoted Chapter 18 to the explanation of the systematic reviews and quality assessment of systematic reviews. Briefly however, systematic reviews are research efforts where data are acquired from existing literature through a planned and thorough search process. Data acquired through systematic review may undergo statistical analysis through a process called meta-analysis. Because data from multiple studies are combined statistical power is increased providing for narrower confidence limits and greater confidence in the conclusions drawn from the analysis. It is not always possible to combine data from multiple studies to perform meta-analysis, a discussion reserved for Chapter 18. However, qualitative assessment of the data from multiple studies often provides strong evidence to guide clinical decisions.

The research process in systematic review is presented in the methods section of the paper as is typical of reports generated from all other research efforts. As with other types of research, the research methods employed can bias the data and thus the conclusions drawn following analysis. In Chapters 13–18 the appraisals of research methods of studies into diagnostic testing, prevention, treatment outcomes, and systematic review, respectively, are provided. At this point in our discussion it is important to simply appreciate that all clinical research is not of similar methodological quality. Thus, although a research report may be characterized as a systematic review or some other type of paper on the hierarchy, such classification assumes a reasonable degree of methodological quality. As a clinical research consumer it is imperative that one develop the skills to critically appraise the methodological quality of the research they read.

Randomized-Controlled Clinical Trials

The next level on the evidence hierarchy consists of randomized-controlled clinical trials (RCTs). An RCT assembles a sample of patients and then assigns individuals to a treatment group through an unbiased or random allocation. Well-conducted RCTs that result in narrow confidence also rate as level 1 evidence. These studies prospectively assign patients to treatment groups and measure specific outcomes in order to assess the benefit of a particular intervention. Mechanisms used to evaluate the methodological quality of randomized-controlled clinical trials are described in later chapters. However, it is important to note two aspects of design that differentiate randomized-controlled clinical trials from designs that fall lower on the hierarchies. First, as noted previously randomized-controlled clinical trials are prospective that is in contrast to case series or case studies as examples where patients are identified after a course of care for analysis. Prospective designs allow for greater control over factors that confound the identification of cause–effect relationships. Take, for example, an effort to determine if a protocol of three times per week treatment with low-power laser reduces the need for surgery in the treatment of carpal tunnel syndrome. If one were to address the question prospectively, uniform instructions could be provided to all of the patients receiving real and sham laser treatment regarding medication use, right splint use, and exercise. Thus, if the intervention was found to be successful, the differences between treatment and sham could not be attributed to differences in medications, brace use, or exercise. However, if one addressed the question retrospectively by reviewing the charts of patients treated for carpal tunnel syndrome to determine whether those receiving laser were less likely to undergo surgery, several potentially confounding factors may exist, clouding the ability to attribute differences solely to laser intervention.

In a similar vein, RCTs assign patients to groups without bias; all patients have the same likelihood of assignment to a particular group. When patients are studied in groups (often referred to as cohorts) the influence of factors such as environment is not distributed equally across all groups. For example, the results of laser treatment might be studied by comparing outcomes of care at a specialized hand clinic that uses laser in a treatment protocol to the outcomes of patients treated in a busy physical therapy clinic in a large hospital where laser is not used. Patients treated in the hand clinic may be biased when assessing their response to treatment by the individualized attention and clinic environment thus leading to misleading conclusions regarding the efficacy of laser. Thus, while cohort, case series, and case studies can provide important information, randomized-controlled clinical trials represent the strongest single study research design when assessing responses to treatments.

All-or-None Studies

The Oxford Center for Evidence-Based Medicine hierarchy identifies "all or none" studies (level of evidence 1c), which is missing from the listing in Box 7-1. Such studies are often linked to mortality where prior to an intervention all patients died while now some survive or where prior to intervention some patients died and now all survive. Certainly, death or survival is not the only measure that lends to the completion of all-or-none reports but absolute outcomes are uncommon.

Box 7-1 categorizes all studies that are not RCTs collectively while The Oxford Center for Evidence-Based Medicine classifies such studies based on whether the study was prospective or retrospective and cohort based or case based. Systematic reviews of nonrandom assignment of treatment studies on the hierarchy generally provide stronger evidence than individual reports, if for no other reason than the fact that more patients are studied. As with systematic reviews of RCTs, a thorough systematic review of nonrandom assignment of treatment studies regardless of the specific methods of the study is more likely to provide data to influence clinical decisions than a single report.

Cohort Studies

Cohort studies, which may be prospective or retrospective in design, involve the study of groups based on exposure or intervention and assessed for differences in outcomes. The principal difference between an RCT and a prospective cohort is that in the RCT individuals or, in some case, groups are randomly assigned to interventions, while cohort studies lack random assignment. In some cases the random assignment of a group to intervention is possible. Retrospective cohort studies identify groups based on exposure or intervention at some point in the past and then follow the groups forward. Thus, random assignment is not possible.

At this juncture one may ask, "If the RCT is a superior research design then why consider prospective cohort studies?" To answer this question to a reasonable degree let's consider circumstances where random assignment of individuals to exposure or intervention would be difficult or impossible. Consider, for example, the investigation of a pre-practice exercise regimen purported to reduce lower extremity injuries in a team sport (Myklebust et al., 2007). Since teams generally warm-up together assigning teams to receive or not receive the intervention poses significant challenges. Moreover, the culture of sport may preclude participation of organizations and teams if random assignment to control is perceived negatively. Thus, cohorts might be identified for study rather than seeking to randomly assign individual or groups to treatment.

If in this example a decrease in injuries was observed at the conclusion of the study, one could conclude that the intervention was effective. The challenge for the investigator and research consumer is confidence that the conclusion drawn reflects the true effect. In this scenario differences in coaching, practice and game facilities, equipment, climate, or a number of other factors including simply being studied (Hawthorne effect) could be responsible for the observed effect. Certainly, one would have greater confidence in the conclusions if efforts were taken before the study to maximize the similarities across the cohorts on all other factors except for the intervention of interest. When done well prospective cohort designs can maximize efficiency, reduce research costs, and yield important information. The appraisal of such studies, however, can be more difficult for the research consumer since variables with effects that are likely to be normally distributed in an RCT can influence the behavior and response to intervention of a group.

The results of retrospective cohort studies can also be affected by numerous factors outside the investigators control. Such studies, however, may offer efficiencies in time and costs that lead to more rapid advances in science. Moreover, in some circumstances it is not permissible to randomly assign research participants to specific patterns of behavior. Deberard et al. (2008), for example, investigated long-term multidimensional outcomes of lumbar discectomy within a cohort of Workers' Compensation patients from Utah to identify presurgical biopsychosocial factors related to poor outcomes. Subjects were interviewed a minimum of 2 years post surgery. Through this work several factors that contribute to poorer postsurgical outcomes were identified without enrolling a large number of patients into a prospective investigation requiring more than 2 years to completion while removing the influence of knowing that one is "being studied."

✔ CONCEPT CHECK

The principal difference between an RCT and a prospective cohort is that in the RCT individuals are randomly assigned to interventions while in a cohort study groups are investigated. Random assignment in retrospective cohort studies is not possible because researchers identify groups based on exposure or intervention at some point in the past and then follow the groups forward.

Outcomes Studies

Population-based "outcomes research" (level 2c in Figure 7-1) is similar to cohort studies but has been defined as research that:

> seeks to understand the end results of particular health care practices and interventions. End results include effects that people experience and care about, such as change in the ability to function. In particular, for individuals with chronic conditions—where cure is not always possible—end results include quality of life as well as mortality. By linking the care people get to the outcomes they experience, outcomes research has become the key to developing better ways to monitor and improve the quality of care. (Agency for Healthcare Research and Quality, U.S. Department of Health and Human Services, http://www.ahrq.gov/clinic/outfact.htm, accessed October 21, 2009)

Case-Control Studies

Case-control studies are similar to retrospective cohort studies or imbedded within a prospective cohort study. In case-control studies, however, comparisons are made between groups of subjects based on an outcome rather than an exposure or intervention. Take, for example, the finding that drinking moderate amounts of alcohol, particularly red wine, reduces the incidence of heart attack (Yusuf et al., 2004; Carevic et al., 2007). This finding resulted from retrospectively studying groups of people who did or did not suffer a cardiac event and attempting to identify factors that increased or decreased risk. Several factors including smoking, obesity, diet, and exercise habits along with alcohol consumption alter risk. The data, however, suggest that alcohol consumption has a cardioprotective effect. Our purpose here is not to debate the benefits and potential harms of alcohol consumption but to consider the means by which this finding was originated. Consider addressing the question of whether red wine reduces the incidence of heart attack in an RCT. First, subjects would have to agree to drink or not drink as part of the study. Certainly, many individuals make this personal choice and would be adverse to changing their behavior for a long time in order to participate in the research. Next consider what a long time means—the following of subjects until they experienced a cardiac event or died of other causes; truly an impossible study. Thus, while shorter-term RCTs related to the mechanisms behind the observed benefits have been conducted (Jensen et al., 2006; Tsang et al., 2005) much has been learned about cardiovascular risk factors from case-control studies. Cohort and case-control studies have an important place in research. The research consumer, however, must again be aware of factors out of the investigators control that might bias the results.

Case Series and Case Studies

Case series and case studies provide detailed descriptions of a series or single case. By design, these reports provide no statistical comparison but rather describe the course of care and the outcome of one or more cases. Because only a single of few cases are reported, it is not possible to make inferences with regard to cause and effect or generalize the outcome of the cases with confidence. Case reports and case series do, however, inform practice under unique circumstances or when the focus of the report is on rare conditions. For example, Fiala et al. (2002) reported on the management of an intercollegiate soccer player with hemophilia. Hemophilia at one time would have disqualified the subject of the case from participation. However, changes in medicine and regulations resulted in circumstances that allowed for this athlete to participate. Thus, the subject of the case was truly unique. In effect, the report established a standard of care for the athletic training and sports medicine management of athletes in collision sports where none existed. Similarly, Seiger and Draper (2006) reported on the use of pulsed diathermy and manual therapy in the restoration of ankle motion patients suffering from posttraumatic capsular restriction following open reduction with internal fixation. This report demonstrated the safety of pulsed diathermy in the presence of metal implants and suggests that the combination of pulsed diathermy and manual therapy can effect changes in motion that are known to be difficult to achieve. Due to the experimental nature of the pulsed diathermy application it was more appropriate to begin treating a small number of patients. Moreover, due to the relative rarity of appropriate patients the completion of a prospective cohort or RCT would have taken years to complete. Thus, this case series provide clinicians with important evidence of safety and an alternative approach to treating patients with loss of motion at the ankle.

Bottom of the Evidence Hierarchies

At the bottom of the evidence hierarchies we find two distinctly different types of research. Box 7-1 labels these works as laboratory studies related to physiological and biomechanical mechanisms underlying disease, injury, or treatment while the Oxford Center for Evidence-Based Medicine identifies these studies as bench research and animal research. The term "bench science" is a broad term. It is important to recognize the contributions to understanding human performance and the human response to exercise that have resulted from research in "healthy" subjects. It is also necessary to recognize that the responses of patients may differ from healthy subjects in their responses to exercise and physical activity.

Clearly, major health care advances have also resulted from basic and animal science and much of this work is highly technical. The point to make here is that conclusions drawn from bench (a.k.a. basic) science and animal research cannot be generalized directly to human patients. For example, promising research in medication development may not yield expected benefits when tested through human trials. This work is vital to advancing health care and forms the foundation of human clinical trials; however, it is not evidence on which most clinical decisions can be based.

In Figure 7-1, the last categories of Level 5 of Evidence are "opinion developed through informal clinical observations" and, under anecdotal evidence, "unpublished clinical observations." Recall that the hierarchies of evidence relate to the strength of evidence in making decisions about patient care, not the sophistication of the research methods and data. Clinician experience plays an important role in decision making. However, when research evidence is available it is expected that the information be integrated. Experience and observation alone cannot yield consistent, high quality healthcare. Discussion of these latter categories leads us back to where this chapter begins, discussion of alternatives to evidence-based practice. We all learn from our teachers, mentors, and the experienced clinicians around us. On occasion we encounter an observational pearl of wisdom but for the most part excellent teachers have appraised and synthesized the best available research for their own applications. Professional growth requires that we question what we have been taught and continue to seek new understanding. Listen to, but carefully evaluate anecdotal evidence. Recall the words of Epictetus (AD 50–138) (see the beginning of the chapter). Things may not be as they appear. Such is likely true of anecdotal evidence.

Hierarchy of Evidence for Diagnosis

The Oxford Center for Evidence-Based Medicine identified five levels of evidence of diagnostic studies paralleling those of treatment and prevention studies (Figure 7-2).

Level 1a evidence consists of systematic reviews of high-quality individual trials with homogeneous findings and clinical decision rules (CDR) derived from high-quality cohort studies or prospectively validated CDRs from multiple centers. Level 1b studies consist of those cohort studies and CDRs validated in a single setting. A detailed discussion related to the assessment of methodological quality of studies of diagnostic tests is presented in later chapters. These chapters will also describe the process through which specificity and sensitivity are calculated. When the sensitivity or specificity of a test approaches 1.0 the test will be nearly perfect at ruling out or detecting a disease or condition respectively. The acronym SpPIN refers to tests with near perfect specificity (high specificity rules in) while SnNOUT refers to tests with near perfect sensitivity (high sensitivity rules out). Studies revealing "absolute" SpPIN or SnNOUT constitute level 1c evidence.

Level 2a evidence consists of systematic reviews of 2b evidence that consists of exploratory (small sample) reports with good reference standards and CDRs not validated prospectively at one or more centers.

Level 3 evidence consists of systematic reviews (3a studies) of 3b reports that involve the enrollment of nonconsecutive patients or fail to consistently apply reference standards.

Similar to the hierarchy of treatment and prevention level 4 evidence comes from case-control studies or diagnostic studies without independent review of the reference standard, a topic reserved for later chapters.

Likewise level 5 evidence stems from expert opinion and bench and animal science.

✔ CONCEPT CHECK

The acronym SpPIN refers to tests with near perfect specificity (high specificity rules in) while SnNOUT refers to tests with near perfect sensitivity (high sensitivity rules out). Studies revealing "absolute" SpPIN or SnNOUT constitute level 1c evidence.

Hierarchy of Evidence for Prognosis

The hierarchy of evidence related to prognostic studies (see Figure 7-3) is similar to that of diagnostic studies.

There are strong similarities in level 1 evidence with all or none of the case series replacing absolute SpPIN or SnNOUT in level 1c. Level 2 differences consist of "outcomes research" at level 2c that does not exist for diagnostic studies. Outcomes research was discussed in relation to intervention studies previously. No level 3 evidence exists for studies of prognosis and level 4 also consists of case-series studies. Level 5 evidence is generally consistent across all categories of research.

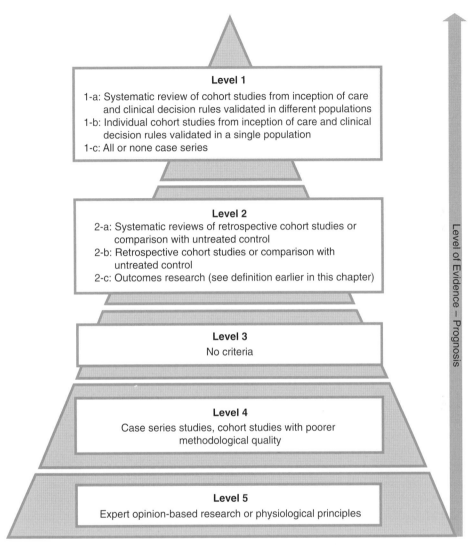

FIGURE 7-3   Hierarchy of evidence for prognosis. (Adapted with permission from http://www.cebm.net/index.aspx?o=1025. Oxford Center for Evidence-Based Medicine—Levels of Evidence [March 2009]. Accessed May 10, 2010.)

RELEVANCE OF EVIDENCE TO PROBLEM

This chapter has reviewed the types and hierarchies of evidence that clinicians can access to help them best treat their patients. Before closing out the chapter some perspective is in order to prepare for a more detailed discussion of research related to diagnostic procedures, prognosis, and responses to intervention. At several points in the hierarchies discussed, issues of the validity of data, the applications of data analysis, and methodological quality were mentioned. These are important considerations for the clinician since a poorly conducted study while being classified, for example, as an RCT might constitute weaker evidence than a well-conducted prospective cohort study. These issues are really intertwined as poor methods increase the likelihood of biased data threatening internal as well as external validity. These issues are discussed in far greater detail in ensuing chapters since the methods employed and thus the assessment criteria studies of diagnostic procedures differ markedly from studies of treatment effects.

As a preview to future discussions related to the interpretation of clinical research one should be prepared to ask the following about the papers we read:

- Are the results accurate, correct, and unbiased?
- Do the results apply to the patient I am treating?
- Will the results help me?

Consider these questions as you read the remaining chapters in Part II of this book, develop skills in the retrieval and appraisal of the clinical literature, and apply your reading to the care of individual patients. Certainly, caution is warranted if the validity of the data reported is of concern. Moreover, one must consider the whole of the patient they are treating when applying the results of students. Individuals may differ in age, gender, race and culture, the presence of co-morbidity, and a host of other factors from the subjects in a research report. Rarely are there clear recommendations to be made as to whether the results of a clinical trial apply to the individual patient. Recall that the practice of evidence-based medicine requires the integration of the best available evidence with clinical experience and **patient values**. Consideration of the first two questions then leads to the most important: Will (and perhaps how) the results help me? When the evidence is very strong and the patient presentation is clearly consistent with those studied in clinical trials the evidence will most certainly be of help in developing and explaining a plan of care. The real dilemma comes when the evidence is less strong or conflicting and when the patient differs from those described in the research. The patient is seeking care and decisions must be made. We may elect to cast aside evidence that poses more questions than answers, yet we must continue to pursue the research that will ultimately best inform our decisions.

CHAPTER SUMMARY

This chapter has provided an overview of how the sources of evidence used to make clinical decisions are generated and how the importance of the evidence based on the methods used to gather data is viewed. Two commonly cited hierarchies (with that of the Oxford Center for Evidence-Based Medicine being divided by category in Figures 7-2 to 7-3) are presented, primarily to highlight the similarities in presentation, but also to address subtle differences. The practice of evidence-based health care requires the consideration of the best available evidence along with clinical experience and patient values in recommending a course of care. Within patient, randomized treatment order trials and "level 1" evidence should be weighted more heavily in clinical decisions than sources lower on the hierarchy. The clinician, however, must appreciate that this level of evidence is not always available and carefully consider how strongly the available research will influence their decisions. Not all evidence is created equal, nor can be applied equally for all patients. All evidence, however, is worthy of consideration for the patients seeking our care.

KEY POINTS

- Confidence gained from experience and continued study of the literature helps the clinician cope with the stresses of providing optimal care and eases the anxiety of the patients we treat.
- Within patient, randomized treatment order trials and "level 1" evidence should be weighted more heavily in clinical decisions than sources lower on the hierarchy.
- Within patient, randomized treatment order trials are studies in which patients receive all interventions under consideration in random order over the duration of the investigation.
- Hierarchies of evidence relate to the strength of evidence in making decisions about patient care, not the sophistication of the research methods and data.
- Differences in the strength of evidence come from two sources, sampling and research methods.
- Case series and case studies provide detailed descriptions of a series or single case.
- Poor methods increase the likelihood of biased data threatening internal as well as external validity.
- Clinicians must carefully consider how strongly the available research will influence their decisions.
- All evidence is worthy of consideration for the patients seeking our care.

Critical Thinking Questions

1. When should clinical experience drive patient care decisions?
2. The practice of evidence-based health care requires careful consideration of what three aspects when recommending a course of care?
3. How has the focus on evidence-based medicine been fueled by the advances in information technology?
4. What are the limitations to conducting a within patient, randomized treatment order trial?
5. When will the sensitivity or specificity of a test be nearly perfect at ruling out or detecting a disease or condition respectively?

Applying Concepts

1. Form groups and discuss how the differences in research methods and data analysis across the spectrum of patient care also result in some differences as to how the hierarchy of evidence is described. Provide clinical examples along with examples from the literature to support your viewpoint.
2. Form groups and discuss the question of, "If the RCT is a superior research design then why consider cohort studies?" Remember to consider circumstances where random assignment of individuals to exposure or intervention would be difficult or impossible, and provide clinical examples along with examples from the literature to support your viewpoint.

REFERENCES

Carevic V, Rumboldt M, Rumboldt Z. Coronary heart disease risk factors in Croatia and worldwide: results of the Interheart study (English abstract). *Acta Med Croatica.* 2007;61(3):299–306.

DeBerard MS, Lacaille RA, Spielmans G, et al. Outcomes and presurgery correlates of lumbar discectomy in Utah Workers' Compensation patients. *Spine J.* 2009;9:193-203.

Fiala KA, Hoffmann SJ, Ritenour DM. Traumatic hemarthrosis of the knee secondary to hemophilia A in a collegiate soccer player: a case report. *J Athl Train.* 2002;37(3):315–319.

Guyatt GH, Haynes B, Jaeschke RZ, et al; for the Evidence Based Medicine Working Group. EBM: Principles of Applying User's Guide to Patient Care. Center for Health Evidence, 2001. (Available at: http://www.cche.net/text/usersguides/applying.asp. Accessed May 10, 2010.)

Isaacs D, Fitzgerald D. Seven alternatives to evidence based medicine. *BMJ*. 1999;319:1618.

Jensen T, Retterstøl LJ, Sandset PM, et al. A daily glass of red wine induces a prolonged reduction in plasma viscosity: a randomized controlled trial. *Blood Coagul Fibrinolysis*. 2006;17(6):471–476.

Katz DL. *Clinical Epidemiology & Evidence-based Medicine*. Thousand Oaks, CA: Sage Publications; 2001.

Myklebust G, Engebretsen L, Braekken IH, et al. Prevention of noncontact anterior cruciate ligament injuries in elite and adolescent female team handball athletes. *Instr Course Lect*. 2007;56:407–418.

Seiger C, Draper DO. Use of pulsed shortwave diathermy and joint mobilization to increase ankle range of motion in the presence of surgical implanted metal: a case series. *J Orthop Sports Phys Ther*. 2006;36(9):669–677.

Tsang C, Higgins S, Duthie GG, et al. The influence of moderate red wine consumption on antioxidant status and indices of oxidative stress associated with CHD in healthy volunteers. *Br J Nutr*. 2005;93(2):233–240.

Yelland MJ, Nikles CJ, McNairn N, et al. Celecoxib compared with sustained-release paracetamol for osteoarthritis: a series of N-of-1 trials. *Rheumatology*. 2007;46:135–140.

Yusuf S, Hawken S, Ounpuu S, et al. Effect of potentially modifiable risk factors associated with myocardial infarction in 52 countries (the INTERHEART study): case-control study. *Lancet*. 2004;364(9438):937–952.

CHAPTER 8

QUALITATIVE INQUIRY

There are in fact two things, science and opinion; the former begets knowledge, the latter ignorance.

—*Hippocrates, Law Greek physician (460 BC–377 BC) from Classic Quotes as quoted in The Quotations Page (www.quotationspage.com)*

CHAPTER OBJECTIVES

After reading this chapter, you will:

- Be able to describe the nature of qualitative inquiry.
- Be able to contrast the difference between inductive and deductive vantage points of where to begin research projects.
- Understand the various perspectives and theoretical traditions that use qualitative research methods.
- Understand that the interpretation of the world should happen in natural settings when practicable and practical.
- Understand the various types of qualitative data collection.
- Develop respect for the rigors of qualitative inquiry.
- Appreciate the time-intensive makeup of qualitative inquiry.
- Explain the role of observation in qualitative inquiry.
- Understand the role of theory development in qualitative inquiry.
- Understand the various rigors of qualitative research.
- Understand that qualitative research requires multiple views, research methods, and realities to bring a better understanding to the social world.

KEY TERMS

credibility	ethnography	interpretivism
dependability	grounded theory	observation
deductive	hypotheses	paradigm
epistemology	inductive	phenomenology

INTRODUCTION

This chapter introduces you to the notion of a qualitative research **paradigm**. Qualitative inquiry allows for the exploration of naturally occurring social phenomena in actual contexts (Wilson, 2007). Within scientific endeavors, the qualitative research paradigm has long served the needs of social scientists who were interested in the rigors of systematic and disciplined data collection and analysis but who did not want to sacrifice the complexity of the data under investigation for the purposes of scientism (Mills, 1998; Ross, 1992). We will introduce you to a number of perspectives and theoretical traditions, and methods for conducting qualitative research and qualitative data collection. Considerations of reliability and validity will also be discussed.

WHAT IS QUALITATIVE INQUIRY?

Qualitative research is a descriptive/explanatory paradigm of investigation. A number of research techniques and strategies were constructed within that paradigm so that rich description and explanation of social phenomena could be the objective of the investigations (e.g., Berger & Luckmann, 1967; Blumer, 1969; Creswell, 1998; Fosnot, 2005; Garfinkel, 1967; Goffman, 1969; Geertz, 1983; Holtgraves, 2002).

The methods of inquiry found within this paradigm allow for a detailed and rich description of the data, as well as an in-depth explanation of trends and patterns uncovered during the investigation (Wilson, 2007). Agar (1986a,b) states that with the qualitative research paradigm, qualitative methodologies such as **ethnography** are neither subjective nor objective, rather they are interpretive by nature (Wilson, 2007). That is, they are oriented toward the explication of social phenomena rather than just the determination that these phenomena exist and that they tend to correlate with numerous variables. Similarly, Creswell (2003) suggests that qualitative methods not only enable the interpretive investigation of social phenomena in natural settings, he also emphasizes that since these methods deal with emergent data, there is a better chance that a sufficient explication of the phenomena can occur because these methods allow the data to guide the research and the research questions.

Qualitative research involves the **observation** and analysis of information in natural settings to explore phenomena, understand issues, and answer questions.

The purpose of qualitative inquiry can be to explain, predict, describe, or explore the "why" or the nature of the connections among unstructured information. The focus of qualitative inquiry is the **inductive** process rather than the **deductive** outcome. Nominal data from qualitative inquiry provides unencumbered information; thus, the researcher must search for narrative, explanatory patterns among and between variables of interest, as well as the interpretation and descriptions of those patterns. Rather than starting with **hypotheses**, theories, or precise notions to test, qualitative inquiry begins with preliminary observations and culminates with explanatory hypotheses and **grounded theory**.

The process of qualitative work is one where the hypothesis(es) form or develop as the research progresses during the study (Lincoln & Guba, 1985). In other words, the overriding or guiding theory may be augmented or changed entirely as the study runs its course and data are collected (Wilson, 2007). One of the unique features of qualitative research designs is that it is data-driven versus hypothesis-driven. Subject(s) are often studied in their natural environment and the data responses come unfiltered from the subject(s) (Patton, 1990). This means the data are collected in natural settings where it is to be found: workplace, street, gym, or home. The most familiar characteristic of qualitative inquiry is that it provides detailed data and rich interpretation of that data, often without the need for statistical procedures (Wilson, 2007).

The task of the researcher in qualitative inquiry is to observe to the point of saturation. The idea is not about large numbers; it is about observing a phenomenon until all observations have been repeated and main themes fit into emerging categories. The well-conducted progression of qualitative inquiry is extremely time-intensive due to the fact that the researcher is constantly observing, documenting, and analyzing.

OBJECTIVES OF QUALITATIVE RESEARCH

The objectives of qualitative research can be divided into five general groups: taking a learning role, understanding procedural affairs, presenting a detailed view, focusing on the individual, and understanding the mundane (Damico et al., 1999a,b). Understanding these objectives of qualitative research allows for the researcher to effectively employ qualitative methods to explore natural social phenomena without losing sight of the context in which they occur. Damico et al. (1999a,b) describe seven strengths of qualitative research, which make it ideal for understanding human interaction:

1. Qualitative research is designed to study phenomena in natural settings. By investigating how an individual acts in a natural context, functions and variables can be uncovered that would not be accessible under contrived circumstances.

2. Qualitative research sustains a preference for the open and relatively unstructured research designs. This allows for a certain amount of flexibility on the researcher's part when identifying patterns and functions.
3. Qualitative research is designed to use the researcher as the key instrument of data collection. That is, the researcher is able to take a relatively open stance in the collection and analysis of data.
4. Qualitative research is designed to collect descriptive data. That means being able to provide a more detailed description (rather than just numbers) of how discourse markers are used and what they are.
5. Qualitative research is designed to orient to a more focused description than a broader one. Instead of generalizations, qualitative research seeks to understand behaviors within a specific context. While the findings may only apply to the particular situation, the patterns that emerge may apply to understand behaviors of individuals.
6. Qualitative research is designed to focus on the process of accomplishing social action rather than the product of social action as the outcome of analysis. That is, the research focuses on how things happen and not just that they happen.
7. Qualitative research is designed to focus on the participants' perspectives to achieve a deeper understanding of the data. The interpretation of the data allows the researcher to not just focus on what has been observed, but to understand how the observed behaviors contribute to the participant's' abilities.

Finally, Rempusheski (1999) described qualitative research and its potential in the investigation of Alzheimer disease since qualitative research has the advantage of being able to explore and describe a topic, especially when discovering and identifying new areas of interest within a known topic. Utilizing qualitative methods is an ideal way of understanding and uncovering the unknown about a particular topic or population of individuals.

✔ CONCEPT CHECK

The well-conducted progression of qualitative inquiry is extremely time-intensive because the qualitative researcher is constantly observing, documenting, and analyzing.

TYPES OF QUALITATIVE RESEARCH

Qualitative inquiry is also referred to as **interpretivism** (Lincoln & Guba, 1985). Many students and clinicians of human movement sciences are unfamiliar with interpretivism. Although widely used and accepted in the social sciences, qualitaive inquiry remains largely disregarded in the fields of medicine and human movement sciences in favor of the more widely recognized **epistemological** category of quantitative inquiry. Quantitative inquiry, which is largely based on causal associations and statistical models, is discussed in Chapter 9.

As described by some of the overall themes that follow in this paragraph, Wilson (2007) explained that the underlying premise of intrepretivism is that to understand the meaning of an experience for particular participants, one must understand the phenomena being studied in the context of the setting for the participants of interest. During qualitative inquiry, the researcher attempts to find meanings attached to and/or associated with the institution, phenomena, or group culture under investigation. Thus, the process of qualitative inquiry is a process by which inferences and generalizations are extrapolated to explain underlying patterns and intricacies of observable situations or occurrences. Stated differently, qualitative research is an interpretive progression of investigation and examination. The qualitative researcher reports extensive detail to interpret or understand phenomenon directly observed or experienced. Results of qualitative inquiry are expressed with word descriptions rather than numerical statistics to capture and communicate the essence of that which is being studied.

Qualitative fieldwork often does not follow the same procedures of investigation that would be used by a chemist or an exercise physiologist; however, observations and analyses are purposeful and take place within philosophic paradigms that provide theoretical frameworks to guide the inquiry process for each type of qualitative research. The main types of qualitative inquiry include grounded theory, case study, interviews, observation, participant observation, and artifact analysis. Qualitative research provides an extensive narrative interpretation of results unique in context and dependent on the manner in which the data were collected.

It is important to re-emphasize the point that qualitative inquiry leads to new theory, whereas quantitative data provides support to answer questions and supports or refutes a pre-existing theory. As stated earlier, the goal of the qualitative researcher is to observe phenomenon, occurrences, or experiences to the point of saturation and repetition. The starting point for qualitative inquiry is inductive in nature. By comparison, quantitative inquiry is deductive and causal in nature. Various types of qualitative perspectives and data collection methods are presented in the next sections.

✔ CONCEPT CHECK

Results of qualitative inquiry are expressed using word descriptions rather than numerical statistics to capture and communicate the essence of that which is being studied.

METHODS OF QUALITATIVE INQUIRY

Grounded Theory

Grounded theory research is a method of qualitative inquiry that results in the generation of a theory. The theory can be thought of as a by-product of the data because it develops and perhaps even changes during the qualitative inquiry process. Major and minor themes emerge from the data as the researcher uses informed judgments to analyze it and offer expounding theory to explain or describe the observations. The resultant theory evolves and is derived from the data; thus the theory is considered anchored or "grounded" in the research. Hence the term "grounded theory research." One widely held example is that of Aristotle's (fourth century BC) careful and detailed observations of the elements and heavenly bodies in motion that led to what we now refer to as gravitational theory.

Case Study

Case study research involves a thorough study of a single institution, situation (cultural group), or one individual (Yin, 1994). A case study provides detailed information about unique characteristics. The researcher collects data about the individual or situation by conducting firsthand observations, interviews, or other forms of data collection (qualitative or quantitative). Clinical case reports are examples of case study research in medical and human movement science disciplines. The purpose of a case study is to observe, collect, document, and analyze detailed information and knowledge about one individual. If this process is conducted over time (i.e., several months or years), then it is termed "longitudinal research."

Interviews

The use of interviews in qualitative research is central to the data collection process. Interviews are often recognized as the most common instrument for qualitative data collection. They allow the persons under study to contribute their knowledge and experience to the research project. Interviewing takes on many aspects where the researcher may do repeated interviews with the same person or people for the purpose of validating the data given during the interviewing process and as attempt to gain greater breadth and depth of the data given by key research informants. The format of the interview content may also vary. The researchers, in many cases, often start with a list of prepared closed and open-ended questions to ask informants but they will not limit themselves to the script if the informant goes into greater detail on subject related to the research project.

Observation

Qualitative researchers often observe the "cultural" landscape to view how the action of everyday life unfolds in the organization or group under investigation. This goes back to the idea within qualitative methods of studying groups in their natural setting and not manipulating the research environment.

Participant Observation

In some cases the researcher may have to become directly involved in the study itself by taking part in or at least being present for ordinary or important practices and rituals performed by the group under investigation. It is often acceptable for researchers to immerse themselves in group practices to better understand what the group does that makes the group unique, interesting, or insightful as compared with existing data or other groups. The obvious concern with immersion is that the researcher might risk becoming overly involved with the subjects(s) (i.e., group under investigation) and lose objectivity; however, this technique often gives a rare vantage point that is useful for understanding the group and its world.

Artifact Analysis

This is the evaluation of written or electronic primary and secondary sources for the topic being researched. Often the form of investigation is archival retrieval of data sources that aid in giving interpretation and meaning to the subject being studied because the gathering and evaluation of written documents may be relevant in providing background/historical information on a particular person or group, change of policy when examining previous interventions for a group, or strengthening and validating other types of collected qualitative data within the study.

TYPES OF QUALITATIVE DATA COLLECTION

A few of the more common types of qualitative data collection in medical and human movement sciences include questionnaires, interviews, and surveys. All the three of these types of data collection entail the use of well thought-out questions to obtain subjective and objective information from the perspective of the participant being questioned. However, it must be made explicitly clear that all three of these types of data collection tools have to be constructed with open-ended responses.

Qualitative questionnaires, interviews, and surveys differ from quantitative uses of these same data collection tools by allowing the subject to speak for themselves, give data to the researcher that might otherwise be missed by a more confining quantitative tool and it allows the subject to describe their own world views. In the quantitative paradigm subject responses to questionnaires, interviews, and surveys are designed around a Likert scale (numerical-ordinal scale [often seen as a 1 to 5 or 1 to 7 response scale to how the subject feels about or rates someone or something]) that confines the subject into responding how the researcher views the world. In turn, the researcher can take this numerical data, analyze it with statistical procedures such as correlations, multiple regressions, or chi-square. For example, a questionnaire might be useful in the collection of information such as opinions of best practices, satisfaction with exercise conditions, perceived mood states, and patient or client demographics. An interview is similar to a questionnaire in that it would utilize the same data collection technique as the questionnaire, but allows for the opportunity to rephrase questions and seek follow-up information with the participants. By comparison, a normative survey might be used to collect performance data or subject knowledge data from a large sample population thus giving results that could conceivably be judged against norms.

PERSPECTIVES AND THEORETICAL TRADITIONS

In this section a number of perspectives and theoretical/disciplinary roots will be reviewed and presented with practical examples for future consideration for use in evidence-based approach (EBA) research. The following qualitative perspectives will be reviewed: **phenomenology** (philosophy), ethnography (anthropology and sociology), symbolic interactionism (social-psychology), systems theory (interdisciplinary systems), and orientational qualitative (ideologies and political economy) (Patton, 1990).

Phenomenology

Phenomenological research focuses on the study of a question (Patton, 1990). Phenomenology refers to how people describe things and how they experience them via their senses and the role of the researcher(s) is to then study and describe these experienced situations. Phenomenology is used as an approach to enhance meaning and details about the subject of inquiry. In essence, phenomenology is at the heart of qualitative inquiry because the qualitative researcher seeks to find meaning in the data and develop explanations, trends, and patterns of behavior from the particular data set so as to understand the phenomena observed. This means the researcher often has to take part as a participant in the study, and in some way experience what others in the group are describing as their reality or life experience. Within this perspective the researcher develops an understanding for the group experiences by immersing themselves in the project or situation.

> EXAMPLE

Exploring the world of the professional athlete

For example, the late journalist/sports writer George Plimpton conducted phenomenological experiments where he explored what is it like to be a professional athlete and how is their world differs from those who are not included in the fraternity of the professional or world-class athlete. Plimpton pitched to, and attempted to hit pitches from, Major League Baseball players, sparred with a world champion boxer, and went through summer camp on a professional football team as a quarterback (Plimpton, 2003, 2006). He wanted to know based on his articles and books on the subject what it was that topflight athletes felt, went through, and how they prepared for one-on-one competition. Likewise, health professionals investigating the phenomena of drug use in small groups and the transference of disease have used this approach to better understand why these individuals would put themselves at such health risks by sharing hypodermic needles. These professionals would not only interview drug users who shared needles but were present when people shared needles and were able to obtain the rationales and meanings from users while they were shooting up to derive the meaning from sharing in this small group situation.

Ethnography

Ethnographic research focuses on the study of the group and their culture. Ethnography is closely associated with the fields of anthropology and sociology. Ethnographers utilize firsthand observation and participant field research methods as a means of investigation. Ethnographic research is often associated with studying cultural or cultural groups, but it is not limited to this inquiry and includes topics of investigation such as office settings/corporate culture, youth sport groups, cults, community-based groups, feminism/sexism in communities or institutions, policy application and delivery, and racism (Agar, 1986a,b). Ethnographers start with a premise about group culture. The tradition here is to immerse oneself in the culture for usually a year, conduct interviews, be a participant observer, and conduct other fieldwork connected to the group. Examples of fieldwork would include tasks such as reviewing other primary and secondary sources of written and archival data. The starting point for studying any cultural group is when people form a group they will generate their own values, traditions, policies/laws, and physical artifacts. For example, anthropologist Alan Klein studied the subculture of male body builders in Southern California in the mid-1980s. From his research, Klein (1993) presents a world where in public displays (competitions) these men are presented as the idealized male physique but the reality is that the athletes involved in this sport suffer from narcissism, questionable or confused sexual identities, as well as needs and rituals for human performance-enhancing aids to achieve the highest levels of athletic and commercial achievement within the sport (Klein, 1993).

Symbolic Interactionism

This perspective investigates symbols in relation to each other, and how people give meaning to their interactions with others. This perspective comes from the tradition of the social-psychologist. The push of this perspective is to derive meaning and interpretation from what others consider meaningful and is a shared experience. These shared meanings and experiences become reality, and develop the shared reality of the group. Erving Goffman's works on stigmas (Goffman, 1986) and dramography (Goffman, 1999) are key to understanding this perspective. One of Goffman's (1999) insights was that we live in a front stage (how we present ourselves and what we do)–back stage (who we are) world that we create. Front stage is the world in which we create and perform roles that the general public takes part in and views, while the back stage is the unseen or protected realm whereby people present their real selves to the group(s) in which they work and share their lives. In other words, the back-stage world "real self" is unknown to the public masses, while the front-stage world "Social Face" is shown and known in the general public. An example of this type of constructed social world study in the health professions can be found in Howard Becker's study (Becker et al., 1976), "Boys In White," which examines how medical students learn the role of how to become a medical doctor and the symbolic importance attached to wearing a white lab coat as a doctor or health professional when interacting with clients or other non–health professionals.

Systems Theory Approach

Systems theory approach examines how organizations operate and how policy is formed, and executed (Schultz, 1984). This perspective recognizes that organizations need to be studied as a whole unit. When considering the EBA, a systems perspective makes for a good qualitative match for implementing behavior intervention in an organizational setting and then checking for the effectiveness of that program over time (Patton, 1990). In order to evaluate the efficacy of an EBA system the following must be considered and investigated: communication hierarchies, client care, credentials of all staff, institutional policies, and fiscal responsibility within the institution to name a few areas that would need to be investigated. The interaction between the researcher(s) and the institution would also include observations along the lines of: in what manner do health professionals interact with one another; how professionals define their roles; how satisfied clients feel about their treatments at this particular facility. For researchers to observe and evaluate an EBA program they would need to include experts from a number of health fields to assist in the data collection and interpretation of the data. Other considerations within a systems approach would be to work on site for the data collection, describe how doctors, athletic trainers, physician assistants, physical therapists, registered nurses, and orderlies work together to meet the needs of the clients. Under this perspective the evaluative process is all-inclusive in order to reveal revenue streams, credentials, education levels, and roles and responsibilities on site. Questions that might be asked under a systems approach entering health provider facility that is attempting to follow an EBA system include: how is treatment and care administered by those within the system, types of care offered (consideration given to context-local, budgets, etc.); changes in the facility if the EBA system has been recently implemented; how responsive and adaptive is the staff to problems and situations that occur on site.

Orientational Qualitative

The orientational perspective examines how a particular ideology or phenomena manifests itself in a social situation or group (Patton, 1990). What differs from this perspective as compared to most other qualitative traditions is that researchers go into the project with an explicit theoretical perspective that determines what variables and concepts are most important and how the findings will be interpreted. A predetermined and defined framework determines this type of qualitative inquiry. For instance, in order to investigate if a medical caregiver is in line with the EBA framework, it needs to be investigated by the framework or mandates of what an ideal EBA system looks like and functions as a medical caregiver.

Historical

Historical research shares much in common with qualitative research designs. The development of social histories is often a feature of many of the qualitative perspectives used where the form of investigation is non-experimental and often analytical. The data resources used for investigation by historians include but are not limited to the following: archival records, interviews (past recordings of interviews and/or those recently conducted), oral histories, books, journals, newsprint, and film (Yow, 1994). Historical research deals with events that have already occurred. In historical research, the researcher provides a detailed narration in an attempt to relate meaning to past events. A study that uses data collected from deceased patients' hospital records to better understand how to treat a medical problem that has been dormant for a period is an example of historical research in medical science and human movement studies.

VALIDITY IN QUALITATIVE RESEARCH (CREDIBILITY)

The concept of validity in research can be explained as a judgment of the accuracy or correctness of the research findings. Validity speaks to the question, "How trustworthy and accurate are the data?" If findings are accurate, then they are considered to be valid. Validity in qualitative inquiry is not an issue of accuracy in methodology or numbers, but rather a question of whether the researcher sees what they think they see. Validity in qualitative research is referred to as **credibility**. Credibility in qualitative inquiry is based on a set of standards by which the honesty, accuracy, and **dependability** of the data can be judged. The intensive, firsthand presence of the researcher is the strongest support for the validity or credibility of the data collected through qualitative inquiry.

One technique that qualitative researchers can use to increase credibility of their data is triangulation. Triangulation is simply a multi-tiered approach to data collection whereby the researcher uses multiple methods (i.e., interviews and questionnaires), multiple data sources (i.e., interviews with two or more different participant groups), multiple theories (different layers of analysis), or multiple researchers (i.e., a diverse research team) to corroborate and analyze the data being collected. The basic idea of triangulation is that if similar findings are produced as a result of multiple methods, or multiple sources, or multiple researchers then such findings would be indisputably more credible than findings obtained from one method, one source, or one researcher. To the extent that there is agreement, the findings are strengthened and held to be more valid and repeatable, hence dependable.

✔ CONCEPT CHECK

The basic idea of triangulation is that if similar findings are produced as a result of multiple methods, or multiple sources, or multiple researchers then such findings would be indisputably more credible than findings obtained from one method, one source, or one researcher.

RELIABILITY OF QUALITATIVE RESEARCH (DEPENDABILITY)

The concept of reliability in research is associated with a judgment of the repeatability of research findings. If findings are repeatable, then they are considered to be reliable. In qualitative research, the notion of reliability is referred to as dependability. Dependability in qualitative inquiry is associated with consistency.

A few of the techniques that qualitative researchers can use to strengthen dependability of their data include asking the same question to a number of individuals and/or interviewing the same person (people) again (consistency), and taking more than enough diligent and detailed notes. Detailed notes must then be logged, chronicled, and transcribed. Detailed notes are essential in the systematic approach for observing a phenomenon until nothing new appears. The researcher observes and records the observations via notes until all observations have been repeated, and main themes fit into emerging categories that represent the social world that was researched or investigated.

HEALTH PROFESSIONAL AS BEING "ON" WHILE ON THE JOB

Any professionally trained individual who works with clients and other professionals during the work day is by their very role constantly on the job. What this means is that the health care professional has to react and interact with a number of other people and respond to either their professional or personal needs in a professional manner. Another way of considering this part of the profession is that while working in a health care facility you as an individual are in a mode of analyzing your social surroundings, thinking of how others can improve their health status, observing how other professionals interact with each other to solve problems or how professionals interact with clients. This is an ongoing process of conducting and collecting informal data by the individual to help themselves with their own ability to better deliver health care to their clients. In a way, qualitative data management skills become a mode of behavior while working with people in natural professional settings. You interview them in order to better understand what they are experiencing, compare data on clients from a variety of documents and tests, and you interact with other professionals concerning cases to look for emerging patterns in order to make sure the best health care is delivered to the client. These procedures are all central to qualitative researchers with the exception being that the qualitative researcher has more formal and systemized role in the type of data to be collected and analyzed, normally over a longer period of time.

THE HEALTH PROFESSION AND PROFESSIONALS AS A COMMUNITY WITH MULTIPLE ROLES

Consideration of thought regarding ethnographic work by anthropologist and sociologist with regard to health care professions is that they operate as a community and to a greater degree as a network. From the community standpoint a health care facility works as a community by professionals delivering care to clients at various levels of expertise and degrees of interaction with clients. However, this goes beyond just performing one's role as an orthopedic surgeon or a physical therapist, where doctor does the operation and the physical therapist (PT) works with the recovering clients. The bond between these two individuals goes beyond this in that there is a shared knowledge base concerning the treatment, previous experiences with different clients with the same problems, and the numbers of years the two have worked together in the same facility. The community constructed in a health care facility is not built around segregated roles of each profession but the integration of them. Additionally, each health care facility is interconnected by networks that each individual has with other people in their own field and those they know outside of their domain of health care. For example, the physician's assistant who has a network of contacts at a number of other health care facilities where three people in their network are long-time friends who are now medical doctors and certified athletic trainers working with sport medicine specialist. These network connections help build and strengthen the existing community within a particular facility.

QUALITATIVE AND QUANTITATIVE INTEGRATION

While these two research paradigms are different in their approach to data collection and analysis they are not incompatible. Both designs can benefit the practitioner in providing useful information in dealing with a client or patient. Implementing an experiment for drug development or exercise prescription gives insight as to ways to proceed using either technique with a client. The drug study can reveal results on the effectiveness and use of a new drug for a particular health problem, and an exercise prescription based on an exercise protocol can provide information on how to bring clients back to full mobility. However, qualitative measures can augment and help to answer questions in the delivery of either of these two tested prescriptions on patients. For instance, data collection on religious, ethnic, social class or other personal value, typology backgrounds, and personal views help in a better delivery and use of drugs as a prescription to clients. The same can be said for applying and modifying an exercise prescription to clients to achieve positive results in making them fully mobile once again. In a practical sense many experienced doctors analyze data and prescription options from this position considering data garnered from qualitative sources, quantitative sources, and personal experiences with the present case.

CHAPTER SUMMARY

This chapter provided an overview of qualitative inquiry. Common types of qualitative research as well as common types of qualitative data collection were presented. It is our intention that you will now have a clear understanding of what qualitative research is and what is involved to turn out credible and dependable results through a careful and detailed qualitative inquiry.

KEY POINTS

- Qualitative research is an interpretive progression of investigation and examination.
- The task of the researcher in qualitative inquiry is observation to the point of saturation.
- Qualitative inquiry is largely established through the collection of observable data.
- Qualitative data yields a research question or a new theory, whereas quantitative data answers a question and supports or refutes a pre-existing theory.
- Qualitative inquiry is also referred to as interpretivism.
- Validity in qualitative research is referred to as credibility.
- In qualitative research, the notion of reliability is referred to as dependability.

Critical Thinking Questions

1. What are the main types of qualitative research?
2. What are a few of the more common types of qualitative data collection in medical and human movement sciences?
3. What is triangulation in qualitative inquiry?

Applying Concepts

1. Select a qualitative research study of interest to you. In your own words, prepare a 1-page summary of the study including relevant details about the research question and the qualitative methods. Be sure to include critical analysis of strengths and areas for improvement in the study.

2. Consider an answerable research question of interest to you. Suggest a do-able qualitative research design to explore answers to this question. Be prepared to discuss plausible strengths, areas for improvement, and clinical applications of the design.

ACKNOWLEDGMENT

We wish to thank Timothy J. Bryant and Brent Thomas Wilson for their input and contributions to this chapter.

REFERENCES

Agar M. *Speaking of Ethnography*. Newbury Park, CA: Sage Publications; 1986a.

Agar MH. *Speaking of Ethnography. Vol. 2, Qualitative Research Methods Series*. Newbury Park, CA: Sage Publications; 1986b.

Becker HS, Geer B, Hughes EC, et al. *Boys in White: Student Culture in Medical School*. Edison, NJ: Transaction Publishers; 1976.

Berger PL, Luckmann T. *The Social Construction of Reality. A Treatise in the Sociology of Knowledge*. New York: Anchor Books; 1967.

Blumer H. *Symbolic Interaction*. Englewood Cliffs, NJ: Prentice-Hall; 1969.

Creswell JH. *Research Design: Qualitative, Quantitative, and Mixed Methods Approaches*. 2nd ed. Thousand Oaks, CA: Sage Publications, Inc.; 2003.

Creswell JW. *Qualitative Inquiry and Research Design. Choosing Among Five Traditions*. Thousand Oaks, CA: Sage Publications; 1998.

Damico JS, Oelschlager M, Simmons-Mackie NN. Qualitative methods in aphasia research: conversation analysis. *Aphasiology*. 1999a;13:667–680.

Damico JS, Simmons-Mackie NN, Oelschlager M, et al. Qualitative methods in aphasia research: basic issues. *Aphasiology*. 1999b;13:651–665.

Fosnot CT, ed. *Constructivism. Theory, Perspectives, and Practice*. 2nd ed. New York: Teachers College Press; 2005.

Garfinkel H. *Studies in Ethnomethodology*. New York: Prentice-Hall; 1967.

Geertz C. *Local Knowledge*. New York: Basic Books; 1983.

Goffman E. *Strategic Interaction*. Philadelphia, PA: University of Pennsylvania Press; 1969.

Goffman E. *Stigma: Notes on the Management of Spoiled Identity*. New York: Simon & Schuster; 1986.

Goffman E. *Presentation of Self in Everyday Life*. Gloucester, MA: Smith Peter Publisher; 1999.

Holtgraves TM. *Language as Social Action. Social Psychology and Language Use*. Mahwah, NJ: Lawrence Erlbaum Associates, Inc.; 2002.

Klein AM. *Little Big Men: Bodybuilding Subculture and Gender Construction*. Albany, NY: State University of New York Press; 1993.

Lincoln YS, Guba EG. *Naturalistic Inquiry*. Newbury Park, CA: Sage Publications; 1985.

Mills JA. *Control: A History of Behavioral Psychology*. New York: New York University Press; 1998.

Patton MQ. *Qualitative Evaluation and Research Methods*. Newbury Park, CA: Sage Publications; 1990.

Plimpton G. *Out of my League: The Classic Hilarious Account of an Amateur's Ordeal in Professional Baseball*. Guilford, CT: Lyons Press; 2003.

Plimpton G. *Paper Lion: Confessions of a Last String Quarterback*. Guilford, CT: Lyons Press; 2006.

Rempusheski VF. Qualitative research and Alzheimer's disease. *Alzheimer Dis Assoc Disord*. 1999;13(1):S45–S49.

Ross D. *Origins of American Social Science*. Cambridge, UK: Cambridge University Press; 1992.

Schultz SJ. *Family Systems Therapy: An Integration*. Northvale, NJ: Aronson; 1984.

Wilson BT. A functional exploration of discourse markers by an individual with dementia of the Alzheimer's type: A conversation analytic perspective. Unpublished doctoral dissertation, The University of Louisiana at Lafayette; 2007.

Yin RK. *Case Study Research: Design and Methods*. 2nd ed. Thousand Oaks, CA: Sage Publications; 1994.

Yow VR. *Recording Oral History: A Practical Guide for Social Scientists*. Thousand Oaks, CA: Sage Publications; 1994.

CHAPTER 9

QUANTITATIVE INQUIRY

*You can use all the quantitative data you can get, but you still
have to distrust it and use your own intelligence and judgment.*

*—Alvin Toffler from Cole's Quotables as quoted in The
Quotations Page (www.quotationspage.com)*

CHAPTER OBJECTIVES

After reading this chapter, you will:

- Understand the characteristics of quantitative inquiry.
- Appreciate the significance behind collecting data in a systematic manner.
- Comprehend how the concepts of central tendency are used in statistical analysis to test hypotheses.
- Be able to describe the basic steps of the scientific method.
- Be able to explain the difference between the types of measurement data.
- Understand the different research experimental designs.
- Understand the difference between Type I and II errors and the relevance to data analysis.

KEY TERMS

a priori power analysis	external validity	scientific method
confounding variables	independent variable	
dependent variable	research hypothesis	

INTRODUCTION

Quantitative inquiry forms the basis for the **scientific method**. Through the performance of controlled investigation, researchers may objectively assess clinical and natural phenomena and develop new knowledge. By collecting data in a systematic manner and using statistical analysis to test hypotheses, the understanding of human physiology and behavior may be advanced. Quantitative inquiry is central to advancing the health sciences. The aim of this chapter is to identify the characteristics of quantitative research. This chapter is presented based on classical test theory (pretest–posttest) rather than from the perspective of clinical epidemiology (case control, cohort, randomized-controlled clinical trial). The principles of clinical epidemiology are essential for applying research in clinical practice and are addressed in subsequent chapters specifically related to prevention, diagnosis, and treatment outcomes. The material presented here is, however, an essential foundation for laboratory and clinical research.

CHARACTERISTICS OF QUANTITATIVE INQUIRY

Scientific Method

The scientific method is the primary means by which new knowledge is acquired. To advance the understanding of nature, phenomena must be tested in objective, quantitative, and empirical ways. Central to the scientific method is the creation of research hypotheses that are based on existing knowledge and unconfirmed observations. Experiments are then designed and conducted to test these hypotheses in an unbiased manner. The scientific method requires that data be collected via observation or, in the health sciences, often via instrumented devices in a controlled manner. The basic steps of the scientific method are delineated in Table 9-1.

TABLE 9-1 Basic steps of the scientific method
1. *Observation* of a natural phenomenon.
2. Ask a *research question*.
3. Develop a *research hypothesis* that predicts the answer to the question.
4. Design and *conduct an experiment* to test your hypothesis.
5. *Answer the research question* on whether the experiment confirms or refutes the hypothesis.
6. Confirm your results by *replicating the experiment*.

Good scientists are keen observers of their surroundings. A scholarly health care practitioner will often observe phenomena or patterns during their clinical practice. These observations will often lead to a specific research question. The formulation of a good research question cannot be based simply on the clinical observation alone, but instead must be developed by framing the observation within the existing knowledge base of a specific discipline. This process should involve the clinician–scientist reviewing the existing literature to see what is already known on a given topic before the exact research question is finalized. Once the question is asked, a **research hypothesis** is formed that predicts the answer to the question. Like the formulation of the question itself, the hypothesis should be based on both the clinical observation and what is known in the existing literature.

✔ CONCEPT CHECK

The formulation of a good research question cannot be based simply on the clinical observation alone, but instead must be developed by framing the observation within the existing knowledge base of a specific discipline.

The design of an experiment to test the hypothesis must be done in an unbiased way to ensure objective results. Experiments most typically involve data collection before and after both an experimental intervention and a control condition. This allows for the assessment of the effect of experimental intervention on the outcome measure of interest in comparison to the effect of a control (often times consisting of no intervention or a placebo or sham intervention). The outcome measures are referred to as *dependent variables*, while the interventions are referred to as *independent variables*. The results of the experiment should provide a clear answer to the research question. This information should then be integrated into the existing body of knowledge.

A very important, but often underappreciated, step in the scientific method is the replication of an experiment to confirm the results found in the initial experiment. Ideally, the replication study is performed by a different group of researchers than who performed the initial study. This ensures that the findings can be generalized to a broader population. This is particularly important in the health sciences where diagnostic and therapeutic procedures are often administered by individual clinicians. For example, if a clinician develops a new physical exam test for a specific musculoskeletal condition and performs a well-controlled study that demonstrates that test's diagnostic accuracy, it is critical that the ability of other clinicians to use this test also be investigated. Without such confirmation, the results of the original study may not be confidently generalized into the routine practice of other clinicians.

Measures of Central Tendency

Hypothesis testing is typically performed to assess whether there is a difference in the scores of a dependent variable between either two or more groups (i.e., a group receiving an experimental treatment, a group receiving standard of care traditional treatment, and a control group receiving no treatment), or if there is a difference in the scores of a dependent variable over time within the same group of studies (i.e., pretest vs. posttest scores). This requires the comparison of representative scores across groups or testing sessions, and this is most often performed by comparing measures of *central tendency*. The most common measure of central tendency used in health care research is the *mean*, while the *median* and *mode* are utilized less often.

EXAMPLE

Mean, Median, and Mode

The following data set will be used to show examples of calculating the mean, median, and mode. These scores represent measures of knee flexion active range of motion in five patients who are 3 weeks post arthroscopic partial menisectomy:

Patient #1 = 118°   Patient #2 = 127°   Patient #3 = 123°
Patient #4 = 104°   Patient #5 = 116°   Patient #6 = 116°

The mean ($\bar{x}$) represents the arithmetic average of scores across all sampled subjects and is computed by summing the scores of all subjects and dividing by the total number of subjects. This is expressed mathematically as: $\bar{x} = \Sigma x_i / n$ where x_i represents the score of each individual subject and n is the total number of subjects.

To calculate the mean,

$$\bar{x} = \frac{\Sigma x_i}{n}$$

$$\bar{x} = \frac{(118 + 127 + 123 + 104 + 116 + 116)}{6}$$

$$\bar{x} = \frac{704}{6}$$

$$\bar{x} = 117.33$$

Sometimes one or even a few individual scores are much higher or lower than the other scores. In this case, the outlying scores can skew the data in such

(continued)

a way that the mean is not a good representative measure of the entire data set. The median (M_d) represents the individual score that separates the higher half of scores from the lower half of scores. It is the score that is in the middle of score of all observations. To determine the median, all scores are first ranked in ascending order from the lowest to the highest. The median score is determined with the formula: $M_d = (n+1)/2$. If there are an odd number of samples, the score that falls in the rank-ordered slot equal to M_d represents the median. If a data set has an even number of samples, the average of the scores from the rank-ordered slots immediately above and below M_d is computed that represents the median score.

To calculate the median, the scores are first rank ordered from the lowest to the highest:

104, 116, 116, 118, 123, 127

We then calculate the median rank:

$$M_d = \frac{n + 1}{2}$$

$$M_d = \frac{6 + 1}{2}$$

$$M_d = 3.5$$

Because there are six samples in the data set, the average of rank-ordered scores #3 (116) and #4 (118) is calculated, so the median value of this data set is 117. Half of the scores fall above and half fall below this value.

The mode (M_o) is the score that occurs most frequently out of all included observations. To calculate the mode, we observe that two subjects have a score of 116, while all other subjects have unique scores. Thus, the mode is 116.

We can thus see that in this data set, the mean (117°), median (117°), and mode (116°) are all very similar in their estimates of the central tendency of knee flexion range of motion scores. Now, let us look at a data set that produces markedly different estimates of central tendency. This data set represents the total billable health care costs of five patients who had an acute onset of low back pain:

Patient #1 = $748   Patient #2 = $12431   Patient #3 = $1803
Patient #4 = $1376   Patient #5 = $1803

To calculate the mean,

$$\bar{x} = \frac{\Sigma x_i}{n}$$

$$\bar{x} = \frac{(748 + 12431 + 1803 + 1376 + 1803)}{5}$$

(continued)

$$\bar{x} = \frac{18161}{5}$$

$$\bar{x} = 3632.20$$

We can see that a mean of \$3632.20 is not a good estimate of central tendency for this data set because four out of the five samples are less than half of the mean.

To calculate the median, the scores are first rank ordered from the lowest to the highest:

748, 1376, 1803, 1803, 12431

We then calculate the median rank:

$$M_d = \frac{n + 1}{2}$$

$$M_d = \frac{5 + 1}{2}$$

$$M_d = 3$$

The median is thus \$1803, the value ranked third out of the five samples. The mode in this case is also \$1803 because two patients had this value while no other patients had the same values. In this case, both the median and the mode are more representative of the central tendency of the data than the mean since the data is skewed because of the highest score being more than \$10,000 greater than the other four scores.

Estimates of Dispersion

Besides the estimates of the magnitude of subject scores, another important characteristic of a data set is the dispersion, or variability, of observed values. The *range* of scores represents the arithmetic difference between the highest and the lowest scores in a data set. A limitation of the range is that *outliers*, individual scores at the low and/or high extremes of the data set, can skew this estimate of dispersion.

A more robust estimate of dispersion is the *standard deviation*. The standard deviation (s) estimates how much the scores of individual subjects tend to deviate from the mean. The formula to calculate standard deviation is $s = \sqrt{(\Sigma(x_i - \bar{x})^2)/(n - 1)}$. The numerator of this equation is termed the *sum of squares*, and is used in a wide variety of statistical analyses.

EXAMPLE

Standard Deviation

Using the knee range of motion data from earlier in this chapter the standard deviation is calculated as follows:

Patient #1 = 118°   Patient #2 = 127°   Patient #3 = 123°
Patient #4 = 104°   Patient #5 = 116°   Patient #6 = 116°

$$\bar{x} = 117.33$$

$$s = \sqrt{\frac{\Sigma(x_i - \bar{x})^2}{n-1}}$$

$$s = \sqrt{\frac{(118-117.33)^2 + (127-117.33)^2 + (123-117.33)^2 + (104-117.33)^2 + (116-117.33)^2 + (116-117.33)^2}{6-1}}$$

$$s = \sqrt{\frac{0.45 + 93.5 + 32.1 + 177.7 + 1.8 + 1.8}{5}}$$

$$s = \sqrt{\frac{307.35}{5}}$$

$$s = \sqrt{61.47}$$

$$s = 7.84$$

The standard deviation of 7.84° is relatively small in relation to the mean of 117.33°. When a set of data has a *normal distribution*, 68% of data points for the entire data set will lie within ($\pm$) 1 standard deviation of the mean. Likewise, 95% of data points will lie within ($\pm$) 2 standard deviations of the mean and 99% of data points will lie within ($\pm$) 3 standard deviations of the mean. Figure 9-1 illustrates this concept using the knee range of motion data set.

Tests of inferential statistics (t-tests, analysis of variance) discussed in later chapters utilize the concepts of the variability in data sets to compare means. One important application to this context is that *variance* is defined as the standard deviation squared (s^2). Another important application is that a comparison of two means with these statistical tests is based on the probability of overlap in the normal distribution of the two data sets being compared.

Hypothesis Testing

Quantitative inquiry usually involves statistical analysis of the collected data. The statistical analysis is typically performed to test the hypothesis, or hypotheses, that the investigator has established. When establishing a *research hypothesis* (also called

(continued)

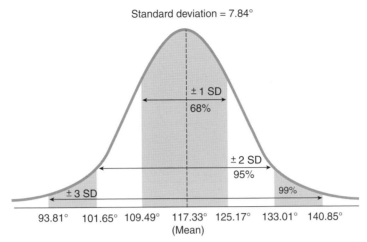

FIGURE 9-1 A normal distribution for a data set of knee flexion active range of motion with a mean of 117.33° and a standard deviation of 7.84°.

the *alternative hypothesis*), the investigator generally has an idea that the independent variable (the intervention being manipulated) is going to cause a change in the dependent variable (the characteristic being measured). For example, an investigator may form a research hypothesis that the application of a newly designed wrist brace will limit wrist flexion range of motion in patients with carpal tunnel syndrome. In contrast to the research hypothesis, the *null hypothesis* is that the independent variable will not cause a change in the dependent variable. Using the previous example, the null hypothesis would be that the newly designed wrist brace would *not* cause a change in wrist flexion range of motion in carpal tunnel syndrome patients.

Despite the fact that the use of the scientific method normally results in investigators generating a directional research hypothesis, inferential statistical analysis, the most common type of analysis, actually is a test of the null hypothesis. In other words, most statistical analyses are performed to determine if there is *not* a difference between two measures. Hypothesis testing will yield a yes or no answer as to whether or not there is a statistically significant difference between measures in the study sample. This result, however, may not be representative of the population at large. When this occurs, either a Type I or Type II error has occurred (see Table 9-2).

Sampling

When a clinician makes an observation on an individual patient they know that they cannot immediately generalize that observation to all of their patients. Likewise, when a scientist performs an experiment, he or she must perform that

TABLE 9-2 Contingency table of hypothesis testing results		
	POPULATION RESULT	
SAMPLE RESULT	H_A true (difference between measures does exist)	H_O true (difference between measures does not exist)
H_A true (difference between measures does exist)	Correct	Incorrect (*Type I error*)
H_O true (difference between measures does not exist)	Incorrect (*Type II error*)	Correct

If the results of the tested sample do not match with what is true in the population at large, either a Type I or a Type II error has occurred.

experiment on a representative *sample* of subjects rather than on the entire *population* of individuals who have the desired characteristics of those to be studied. For example, it would be impractical, if not impossible, to collect data on all patients with hip osteoarthritis in the United States (this would represent the population at large). Instead, a scientist researching hip osteoarthritis must perform studies on a representative sample of the entire population of individuals suffering from hip osteoarthritis. The *sampling frame* represents the group of individuals who have a real chance of being selected for the sample. The sample frame typically does not include the entire population of interest, but instead represents those that have a legitimate opportunity to actually participate in the study.

Selecting an appropriate sample to investigate is a critical step in the design of an experiment. Investigators must set specific inclusion and exclusion criteria for the subjects in their studies. Without the employment of such criteria, there are limits to the generalizability of the study results (this concept is referred to as **external validity** and is discussed in the next chapter). When selecting inclusion and exclusion criteria, it is important that potential confounding factors be controlled for in the study design. For example, if a scientist was performing an experiment to assess the effects of a tai chi exercise program on the balance of older adults, it would be important to somehow control for confounding conditions that may also affect balance such as vertigo or diabetes.

Identifying the appropriate sample size for a study is very important. By testing too few subjects, investigators make the risk of a *Type II error*. A Type II error occurs when difference actually exists in the population at large, but the study results reveal no difference in the study sample. The most common reason for a Type II error is an inadequate sample size. This is also referred to as having low *statistical power* for the study. On the opposite end of the spectrum, having an unnecessarily large sample size can use up limited resources that investigators have to perform research or can subject more individuals than necessary to the risks of study participation.

> ✔ **CONCEPT CHECK**
>
> The most common reason for a Type II error is an inadequate sample size.

Before beginning a study, estimation of an appropriate sample size for a study is done by performing an **a priori power analysis**. The power analysis uses the expected mean differences in measures to be compared, the expected variability in data, and the acceptable amounts of Type I and Type II errors to estimate the projected sample size for a study. The expected mean difference is derived from data from previous studies, pilot data, and investigator intuition. The expected variability in the data is typically in the form of the standard deviation of a specific measure from a previous study or pilot data using a similar sample. *Type I error* occurs when a difference is found in the study sample but there is, in fact, no difference present in the population at large. In most cases, investigators are willing to accept a 5% risk of incurring a Type I error ($\alpha = 0.05$). In contrast, investigators are usually willing to accept a 20% risk of incurring a Type II error ($1 - \beta = 0.80$).

It is worth noting, however, that these values are a bit arbitrary. In some cases a 5% risk of Type I error may be unacceptable because the costs of being wrong are very high. In these cases $\alpha = 0.01$ might be selected. In some circumstances, especially in pilot work where one is trying to decide whether to move forward with a larger study, a more liberal α 5 0.10 might be most appropriate. In selecting a more liberal risk of Type I error the investigators are essentially suggesting that if there is 90% certainty that a difference exists in the population then the question is worth pursuing further. There are many power calculators available online for investigators to use to perform a priori power calculations.

> ✔ **CONCEPT CHECK**
>
> *Type I error* occurs when a difference is found in the study sample but there is, in fact, no difference present in the population at large.

Investigators may employ several types of sampling to determine their potential study participants. *Probability sampling* involves the use of randomization to select individual potential subjects from the sampling frame, whereas with *nonprobability sampling* the selected subjects are not drawn randomly from the sampling frame. With *random sampling*, every potential individual in the sampling frame has an equal chance of being selected for study participation. Computerized random number generators are typically utilized to select potential subjects from the sampling frame when random sampling is employed. *Systematic random sampling* is a method of sampling in which every *x*th individual out of the entire list of potential subjects is selected for participation. For example, out of a list of 200 potential subjects in a sampling frame, every 10th individual on the list might be selected to produce a random sample of 20 subjects.

Stratified random sampling provides a method for dividing the individual members of the sampling frame into groups, or strata, based on specific subject characteristics. For example, members of the sampling frame may be initially grouped into strata by sex (males, females), health status (diagnosed with osteoporosis, not diagnosed with osteoporosis), or some other important characteristic, and then a random sample of potential participants is selected from each stratum. The use of stratified random sampling can be a useful means of preventing potential **confounding variables** from contaminating the results of a study.

Cluster random sampling is a process of dividing the sampling frame into clusters (or groups) based on some common characteristics and then randomly selecting specific clusters to participate in the study out of all possible clusters. All individuals in a selected cluster thus have the opportunity to participate in the study. Performing a study of high-school athletes provides a good example of cluster random sampling. Imagine that a university health system in a large metropolitan area provides outreach athletic training services to 24 different high schools. Researchers at the university want to assess the effectiveness of core stability training on the prevention of lower extremity injuries in high-school basketball players. The researchers could choose to randomly select individual players from each school as potential subjects but this could create several logistical challenges. Alternatively, they could randomly select specific schools (each school is a cluster) to participate. All individual athletes from each selected school are then given the opportunity to enroll in the study.

Random sampling is considered superior to nonrandom sampling because the results of the study are more likely to be representative of the population at large. However, when random sampling is not feasible, nonrandom sampling may be employed. With *convenience sampling*, potential subjects are selected based on the ease of subject recruitment. Studies which seek volunteer participants from the general population is a specific geographic area utilize convenience sampling. Another type of nonrandom sampling is *purposive sampling*. Purposive sampling entails potential subjects from a predetermined group to be sought out and sampled. For example, researchers performing a study of patients with a specific pathology, such as multiple sclerosis, will specifically seek out individuals with this pathology and recruit them to participate in their study. Because of logistical reasons, these two nonrandom sampling techniques are frequently utilized in health care research.

Basic Experimental Research Designs

There are many types of experimental research designs that may be used when constructing an experiment. Each design has pros and cons that must be considered when considering the *internal* and *external validity* of a study (these concepts are discussed in detail in Chapter 10). In general, there are three categories of study designs: pre-experimental, quasi-experimental, and true experimental.

Pre-Experimental Designs

The *one shot posttest* design consists of a single measurement completed after a group of subjects has already received the treatment of interest. In clinical research, this is also referred to as a case series. This type of study design lacks both a baseline measurement (pretest) and a control group for comparison. It is a very primitive study design that has considerable threats to internal validity.

Group 1:   X   O   X = intervention, O = observation

The *one group pretest–posttest* design adds a pretest to the previous design. The inclusion of baseline data and repeated measures is helpful, but the continued lack of control group does not allow the investigator to be confident that any change in measures is strictly due to the intervention. Considerable threats to internal validity remain.

Group 1:   O   X   O

The *static group posttest* design has two groups, one that receives the intervention and one that does not. Both groups are assessed only once. There is no pretest for either group so the investigator cannot be confident that group differences are due exclusively to the interventions. Considerable threats to internal validity remain.

Group 1:   X   O
Group 2:   O

Quasi-Experimental Designs

The *nonrandomized pretest–posttest* design compares two groups before and after intervention. The two groups receive different interventions; however, the assignment of subjects to groups is based on convenience rather than randomization. The lack of randomization limits the internal validity of the study as there may be considerable bias of subject selection into specific groups.

Group 1:   O   X   O
Group 2:   O   X   O

The *time series* design compares a single group at multiple, but regular, time intervals both before and after intervention. This design allows for an understanding of how the intervention affects the course of progression of the dependent variable over time; however, the lack of control group is a threat to the internal validity of the study.

Group 1:　　O　　　O　　　X　　　O　　　O

True Experimental Designs

True experimental designs add the important feature of randomized assignment of subjects to groups. This step alone greatly improves the internal validity of the study design.

In the *randomized posttest* design, subjects are randomly assigned to treatment groups; however, there is no pretest taken before the administration of treatment. While the lack of a pretest may seem like a weakness, it depends on what the outcome measure is. For example, in an injury prevention study assessing the prophylactic effect of a given intervention, there may be no need for a pretest.

R　Group 1:　　　X　　　O　　　R = Randomization
R　Group 2:　　　X　　　0

The *randomized pretest–posttest* design is the gold standard for most experiments. Subjects are pretested, then randomized to assigned groups, and posttested after they receive their assigned intervention. By randomizing subjects after they are baseline tested, it prevents any potential bias on the part of the research team member who is conducting the baseline measures.

Group 1:　　O　　　R　　　X　　　O
Group 2:　　O　　　R　　　X　　　O

✔ CONCEPT CHECK

In general, there are three categories of study designs: pre-experimental, quasi-experimental, and true experimental.

CHAPTER SUMMARY

By following the steps of the scientific method, clinician observations can be translated into hypotheses that can be evaluated via experimental study. The concepts of central tendency, most commonly represented by the mean and standard deviation, are the foundation for inferential statistics. Hypothesis testing allows for the research hypothesis to be confirmed or refuted. The sampling of potential study volunteers is important to the generalizability of the study results. The experimental design of a study forms the infrastructure for the project. Understanding of these issues provides a foundation for performing and interpreting clinically relevant research in the areas of prevention, diagnosis, and treatment.

KEY POINTS

- Clinician observations can be translated into hypotheses that can be evaluated via experimental study by following the steps of the scientific method.
- The concepts of central tendency are the foundation for inferential statistics.
- Hypothesis testing allows for the research hypothesis to be confirmed or refuted.
- Sampling of potential study volunteers is important to the generalizability of the study results.
- Experimental design of a study forms the infrastructure for the project.
- Quantitative inquiry is central to advancing the health sciences.

Critical Thinking Questions

1. What is a null hypothesis and which type of statistic pertains to it?
2. What is Type II error? And, what is the most common reason for it to occur in a research study and how can researchers decrease the risk of it occurring?
3. What does a *sampling frame* represent?

Applying Concepts

1. Using classical test theory:
   a. come up with an idea for a mini-study.
   b. provide an example of a plausible research design for the mini-study you planned.
2. Discuss *how and why* the material presented in this chapter provides an essential foundation for laboratory and clinical research.
   a. Provide current and historical examples from medical research to support your position.

SUGGESTED READING

Greenfield ML, Kuhn JE, Wojtys EM. A statistic primer. Descriptive measures for continuous data. *Am J Sports Med.* 1997;25(5):720–723.

Hopkins WG, Marshall SW, Batterham AM, et al. Progressive statistics for studies in sports medicine and exercise science. *Med Sci Sports Exerc.* 2009; 41(1):3–13.

Tate DG, Findley T Jr, Dijkers M, et al. Randomized clinical trials in medical rehabilitation research. *Am J Phys Med Rehabil.* 1999;78(5):486–499.

CHAPTER 10

VALIDITY AND RELIABILITY

Statistics are like bikinis. What they reveal is suggestive, but what they conceal is vital.

—*Aaron Levenstein, from Quotations About Statistics as quoted in The Quote Garden (www.quotegarden.com/statistics.html)*

CHAPTER OBJECTIVES

After reading this chapter, you will:

- Understand the difference between internal and external validity.
- Be able to discuss participant blinding and explain how it is utilized in experimental design.
- Understand the differences between validity and reliability.
- Understand the different research experimental designs.
- Understand the concept of objective measurement.
- Understand the different types of quantitative data and be able to explain how they are obtained.

KEY TERMS

blinding	limits of agreement (LOA)	standard error of measurement
delimitations	objective measurement	validity
dependent variables	precision	
internal validity	selection bias	

INTRODUCTION

A key to quantitative inquiry is unbiased and **objective measurement** of the **dependent variables**. Measures may be placed on different types of measurement scales and each type of measure is subjected to distinctive forms of statistical analysis. **Validity** is an inherent principle in research design and this important concept has many components. Reliability and agreement of measures are also key components of validity.

TYPES OF QUANTITATIVE DATA

Measures may be obtained via instrumented devices (e.g., electromyography, heart rate monitors, motion analysis systems), clinician measurement (e.g., blood pressure assessed with a standard sphygmomanometer, range of motion assessed with a goniometer), clinician observation (e.g., balance error scoring system, manual muscle testing), or patient self-report (e.g., surveys of health status, functional abilities, pain). Measurement data can usually be classified into one of three types: categorical, ordinal, or continuous. The type of data will influence how the data can be collected and, ultimately, how it can be analyzed statistically.

> ### ✔ CONCEPT CHECK
>
> Measurement data can usually be classified into one of three types: categorical, ordinal, or continuous.

Categorical, or *nominal, data* involve a finite number of classifications for observations. For example, identifying the sex of human subjects provides two possibilities: male and female. For statistical analysis purposes, a numeric value must be assigned to each category; however, the order of numbers assigned to each category is inconsequential. Males could be classified as "1" and females classified as "2" or vice versa, because there are no quantifiable consequences to these assignments. Variables that have more than two categories can also occur. For example, occupational setting may be categorically classified in a manner such as (1) business, (2) manufacturing, (3) health care, (4) education, and so on. Again, the key to categorical data is that the numerical assignment of classifications is not critical to the understanding of the data.

Ordinal data, like categorical data, use categories; however, with ordinal data the order of the numeric classification is of consequence. The most common example of ordinal data is derived from the Likert scale. A survey may ask subjects to respond to how they feel about a certain statement and give five choices: strongly agree, agree, neutral, disagree, and strongly disagree. For statistical analysis, a numeric value will be assigned to each possible response, but in this case the order of the numeric assignment is of consequence. The Likert scale data are likely to be classified as 1=strongly agree, 2=agree, 3=neutral, 4=disagree, and 5=strongly disagree (the order of the numbers could, in theory, be reversed as well). The numbers assigned to each response are of consequence because there is an inherent order to the responses that has a clear meaning. Ordinal data are not strictly limited to Likert scale measures.

Continuous data are measured on a scale that can continuously be broken down into smaller and smaller increments. For example, when measuring the length of a certain object, it could be measured in meters or centimeters or millimeters and so on with each successive measurement unit becoming more and more precise. This property is in stark contrast to categorical or ordinal data. If 1=male and 2=female for categorical data, it is not possible to have a score of 1.6. Likewise with ordinal data on a Likert scale, it is not possible to have a score in between any of the adjacent responses. With continuous data, however, it is always possible to make a measure more precise provided the appropriate measurement tool is available.

VALIDITY

Validity is a concept that is often discussed in experimental design. It is critical to understand that validity has multiple contexts. Validity may be discussed in relation to the structure of the overall design of an experiment, the intervention assessed in an experiment, or the measurements performed in an experiment.

Internal Validity

Internal validity refers to the validity of a study's experimental design. Most experiments are designed to show a causal relationship between an independent variable and a dependent variable. Investigators manipulate an independent variable (e.g., comparing two treatment regimens) to assess its effects on a dependent variable (an outcome measure). If an experiment can conclusively demonstrate that the independent variable has a definite effect on the dependent variable, the study is internally valid. If, however, other factors may influence the dependent variable and these factors are not controlled for in the experimental design, the study's internal validity may be questioned. It is therefore essential for investigators to identify potential threats to internal validity and appropriately control for these threats in the design of the experiment.

Internal validity should be thought of along a continuum rather than as a dichotomous property. In laboratory experiments it is often easier to control for confounding factors, and thus enhance internal validity, than it is in clinical trials.

If all pretest and posttest measures and interventions are performed in a single laboratory session, it is much easier to control extraneous factors that may influence the measures. In contrast, if a clinical trial has measurements taken at time points weeks or months apart, it is much more difficult to control extraneous factors that may influence the follow-up measures. Such extraneous factors are referred to as *confounding variables* and may result in spurious relationships. Brainstorming for potential confounding variables must be done when the experiment is being designed. If extraneous factors may influence measures of the dependent variable over the course of a study, these factors must either be controlled or quantified.

EXAMPLE

Internal Validity

If a study was investigating two physical therapy treatment regimens for hip osteoarthritis and one of the dependent variable was pain, the investigators should realize factors such as analgesic drug use (over the counter and prescription) by the subjects may influence pain measures. The investigators could attempt to control for this confounding factor by instructing subjects to not take any analgesic medications. This stipulation may raise concerns during institutional review of the research protocol and limit the number of patients willing to participate. Alternatively, the investigators could ask subjects to maintain a daily log of analgesic medication use and then use this information as a covariate in their statistical analysis. Either approach is better than not controlling for analgesic drug use at all and thus would improve the internal validity of the study.

Potential threats to internal validity often involve some sort of bias. Bias may be inherent to either the subjects in the study or the experimenters themselves. In terms of the experimental subjects, **selection bias** is an important consideration. The characteristics that subjects have before they enroll in a study may ultimately influence the results of the study. These may include things like age, maturation, sex, medical history, injury or illness severity, and motivation, among many others. Investigators must take such factors into account when establishing their inclusion and exclusion criteria for study participation in an effort to ensure internal validity. Such decisions that investigators make to improve the internal validity of their studies are referred to as **delimitations**.

Likewise, once subjects are enrolled in a study, the formation of study groups (e.g., an intervention group and a control group), care must be taken to make sure that the subjects in different groups have similar characteristics. This is most often accomplished by either randomly assigning subjects to treatment groups or employing some type of matching procedure to make sure that groups are equal in important characteristics at baseline.

The issue of *blinding* is also important to the internal validity of a subject. There are three entities that may be blinded in a study. The subjects may be blinded to whether they are receiving an experimental treatment or a control treatment. This is often accomplished by having a placebo, or sham, treatment that prevents subjects from knowing whether or not they are receiving the active treatment. Blinding of subjects is easier with some interventions such as medication than others such as receiving therapeutic rehabilitation or wearing an external brace. Members of the experimental team who are performing outcome measures should also be blinded to the group assignments of individual subjects and values of previous measurements for individual subjects (this same blinding principle holds true for subjects who are providing self-report information). Lastly, in some instances it is possible to blind clinicians who are treating patients in clinical trials to the group assignments of individual subjects. Again this is easier with some experimental interventions such as medications than with other interventions such as rehabilitation or external appliances. If one of these entities is blinded, a study is referred to as being single-blinded; if two entities are blinded, a study is double-blinded; and if all three are blinded, a study is triple-blinded.

External Validity

While internal validity is related to the design of an experiment, *external validity* relates to how generalizable the results of a study are to the real world. There is a definite trade off between internal validity and external validity. The more tightly controlled a study is in terms of subject selection, administration of interventions, and control of confounding factors, the less generalizable the study results are to the general population. In health care research this is an important issue in terms of translating treatments from controlled laboratory studies to typical clinical practice settings. This concept is also referred to as *ecological validity*. Ultimately, investigators must make decisions that provide the appropriate balance for influencing both the internal and external validity of a study.

✔ **CONCEPT CHECK**

While *internal validity* refers to the validity of a study's experimental design, *external validity* relates to how generalizable the results of a study are to the real world.

Validity of Measures

There are multiple ways of assessing the validity of data and, thus, the measures used in research. Each of the validity characteristics should be considered when assessing the measures utilized in a research study. *Face validity* refers to the property of whether a specific measure actually assesses what it is designed to measure. This is an important issue in the development of "functional tests" for patients in the rehabilitation sciences. For example, it is very important that clinical tests that are part of a functional capacity evaluation to determine if a worker's compensation patient is prepared to return to work actually assess an individual's ability to return to their specific job. Face validity is determined subjectively and most often by expert opinion.

Content validity refers to the amount that a particular measure represents all facets of the construct it is supposed to measure. Content validity is similar to face validity but is more scientifically rigorous because it requires statistical analysis of the opinion of multiple content experts rather than only intuitive judgment.

Accuracy is defined as the closeness of a measured value to the true value of what is being assessed. For example, it is well accepted that a goniometric measure of knee flexion range of motion based on external bony landmarks provides an accurate assessment of the actual motion occurring between the femur and the tibia. Accuracy should not be confused with **precision** of measurement (see discussion in section "Reliability" of this chapter).

Concurrent validity refers to how well one measure is correlated with an existing gold standard measure. This is an important property to be established for new measures aiming to assess the same properties as an existing test. New measures are often developed because existing measures are expensive, or perhaps cumbersome to perform. Measurement of leg length discrepancy is a good example. The gold standard for measuring lower extremity length is via radiographs. A less expensive procedure would be the use of standard tape measures with well-defined procedures. Part of the "validation" of the tape measure technique was to determine concurrent validity with the existing gold standard of radiographic measures. A challenge does exist, however, when there is no gold standard. In this case, the other types of validity must be adequately demonstrated to "validate" a new test.

Construct validity refers to how well a specific measure or scale captures a defined entity. Like many measurement properties, this concept stems from psychology but is applicable to other areas of study such as the health sciences. For example, balance may be considered an important construct of musculoskeletal function. There are, however, many tests to assess the multidimensional constructs of balance. In an elderly population, clinical tests such as the Berg Balance Scale, the Timed Get Up and Go Test, and the Functional Reach Test may be used as part of a comprehensive balance screening protocol. Using specific statistical analysis techniques such as factor analysis, it can be determined whether these three tests all assess the same "construct," or whether in fact they each assess different constructs of balance.

Convergent validity is the measurement property demonstrating whether a given measure is highly correlated with other existing measures of the same construct. Conversely, *discriminative validity* is indicative of a given measure's lack of correlation, or divergence, from existing measures that it should not be related to. When developing new measures it is important that both convergent validity and discriminative validity are assessed against existing measures in related disciplines.

When discussing the "validity" of a measurement, it is critical to understand in what context "validity" is being discussed. Validity of a measurement should not be viewed as an all or nothing phenomenon, but instead the different facets of validity should be viewed on a continuum with each aspect of validity contributing to a comprehensive portfolio of validity.

✔ CONCEPT CHECK

When discussing the "validity" of a measurement, it is critical to understand in what context "validity" is being discussed.

RELIABILITY, AGREEMENT, AND PRECISION OF MEASURES

Reliability of a measure is sometimes discussed as an aspect of validity, but we will discuss it here as a distinct measurement property. *Reliability* refers to the consistency of a specific measurement. The ability of the same tester to produce consistent repeated measures of a test is referred to as *intratester reliability* (also known as *intrarater reliability* and *test–retest reliability*). The ability of different testers to produce consistent repeated measures of a test is referred to as *intertester reliability* (also called *interrater reliability*).

Estimates of reliability for measures of continuous data are often reported as intraclass correlation coefficients (ICC). ICCs are reported on a scale of 0 to 1 with 1 representing perfect reproducibility and 0 representing a complete lack of reproducibility. The ICC should not be confused with Pearson's r which is another type of correlation coefficient but not one that is effective as a reliability estimate. Pearson's r is covered in depth in Chapter 12. Briefly, Pearson's r assesses the association between two continuous measures across a sample of subjects. If as one measure increases in value, the second measure also increases incrementally, the Pearson's r will approach 1. While this would appear to serve as an effective assessment of reliability within measures, the Pearson's r does not assess for systematic error. In other words, if as scores on one measure increase in one unit increments and scores on the second measure increase in two unit increments, the Pearson's r will indicate that scores on the two measures are highly correlated; however, it will not show that the scores of the two measures are systematically diverging from each other. In contrast, the ICC will be lower when systematic error is present.

> ✔ **CONCEPT CHECK**
>
> *Reliability* refers to the consistency of a specific measurement.

Any single observed measure can be thought of as being the true score ± error. For a group of measurements, the total variance can be due to true variance (the variability between subjects) and error variance (the difference between the true score and the observed score). Sources of error may include error or biological variability by the subject, or error by the tester or instrumentation used to take the measure. Recall that, mathematically, variance (s^2) is simply the standard deviation (s) squared. Essentially, reliability may be thought of as the proportion of total variability (s_T^2) that stems from between subject variability (s_t^2). The remainder of the variability is thus attributable to error (s_e^2). This may be expressed with the following formula:

$$\text{Reliability} = \frac{s_t^2}{s_t^2 + s_e^2}$$

The error term can be further divided into systematic error (s_{se}^2) and random error (s_{re}^2). Systematic error may include constant error and bias. Constant error affects all measures in the same manner, whereas bias affects certain types of scores in specific ways (e.g., scores of higher magnitudes may consistently be overestimated while scores of lower magnitudes are underestimated). The reliability formula can thus be expressed more robustly as:

$$\text{Reliability} = \frac{s_t^2}{s_t^2 + s_{se}^2 + s_{re}^2}$$

The calculation of the ICC stems from the parsing of the variability contributions from an analysis of variance (ANOVA). ANOVAs are discussed in detail in Chapter 11. There are several types of ANOVAs but ICC estimates are calculated specifically from the single within factor ANOVA model (also called a repeated measures ANOVA). This analysis is performed to determine if two (or more) sets of measurements are significantly different from each other.

Tables 10-1 through 10-5 illustrate how the results of a repeated measures ANOVA can be used to calculate ICCs from a test–retest study (Weir, 2005). Shrout and Fleiss (1979) presented formulas for six different ICCs. The formula nomenclature includes two terms. The first term may be expressed as either 1, 2, or 3 and the second term as 1 or k. For the first term, in model 1 each subject is assessed by a different set of raters than the other subjects and these raters are randomly selected from all possible raters. In model 2, each subject is assessed by the same group of raters who are randomly selected from all possible raters. In model 3, each subject is assessed by the same group of raters but these raters are the only

TABLE 10-1	Example data set				
TRIAL A1	**TRIAL A2**	**Δ**	**TRIAL B1**	**TRIAL B2**	**Δ**
146	140	−6	166	160	−6
148	152	+4	168	172	+4
170	152	−18	160	142	−18
90	99	+9	150	159	+9
157	145	−12	147	135	−12
156	153	−3	146	143	−3
176	167	−9	156	147	−9
205	218	+13	155	168	+13
156 ± 33	153 ± 33		156 ± 8	153 ± 13	

Reprinted with permission from Weir JP. Quantifying test-retest reliability using the intraclass correlation coefficient and the SEM. *J Strength Cond Res*. 2005;19(1):231–240.

raters of interest (and results thus do not generalize to any other raters). For the second term, 1 indicates that a single observation is being assessed for each trial performed by an individual subject, while *k* indicates that a mean of multiple trials is being assessed for each subject. The six different ICC formulas are shown in Table 10-5. Essentially, each formula estimates the sources of error in the data set.

TABLE 10-2	Two-way analysis of variance summary table for data set A[a]				
SOURCE	**DF**	**SS**	**MEAN SQUARE**	**F**	**P VALUE**
Between subjects	7	14,689.8	2098.4 (MS_B. 1-way) (MS_S. 2-way)	36.8	
Within subjects	8	430	53.75 (MS_W)		
Trials	1	30.2	30.2 (MS_T)	0.53	0.49
Error	7	399.8	57 (MS_E)		
Total	15	15,119.8			

[a]MS_B, between-subjects mean square; MS_E, error mean square; MS_S, subjects mean square; MS_T, trials mean square; MS_W, within-subjects mean square; SS, sum of squares; DF, degrees of freedom; F is calculated value based on MS explained/MS unexplained (error).

Reprinted with permission from Weir JP. Quantifying test-retest reliability using the intraclass correlation coefficient and the SEM. *J Strength Cond Res*. 2005;19(1):231–240.

TABLE 10-3	Analysis of variance summary table for data set B[a]				
SOURCE	DF	SS	MEAN SQUARE	F	P VALUE
Between subjects	7	1330	190 (MS_B: 1-way) (MS_S: 2-way)	3.3	
Within subjects	8	430	53.75 (MS_W)		
Trails	1	30.2	30.2 (MS_T)	0.53	0.49
Error	7	399.9	57 (MS_E)		
Total	15	1760			

[a]MS_B, between-subjects mean square; MS_E, error mean square; MS_S, subjects mean square; MS_T, trials mean square; MS_W, within-subjects mean square; SS, sum of squares.

Reprinted with permission from Weir JP. Quantifying test-retest reliability using the intraclass correlation coefficient and the SEM. *J Strength Cond Res.* 2005;19(1):231–240.

TABLE 10-4	ICC values for data sets A and B[a]	
ICC TYPE	DATA SET A	DATA SET B
1,1	0.95	0.56
1,k	0.97	0.72
2,1	0.95	0.55
2,k	0.97	0.71
3,1	0.95	0.54
3,k	0.97	0.70

[a]ICC, intraclass correlation coefficient.

Reprinted with permission from Weir JP. Quantifying test-retest reliability using the intraclass correlation coefficient and the SEM. *J Strength Cond Res.* 2005;19(1):231–240.

TABLE 10-5	Interclass correlation coefficient model summary table[a]		
SHROUT AND FLEISS	COMPUTATIONAL FORMULA	McGRAW AND WONG	MODEL
1,1	$$\frac{MS_B - MS_W}{MS_B = (k - 1)\ MS_W}$$	1	1-way random
1,k	$$\frac{MS_B - MS_W}{MS_B}$$	k	1-way random

	Use 3,1	C,1	2-way random
	Use 3,k	C,k	2-way random
2,1	$\dfrac{MS_B - MS_E}{MS_S + (k-1)MS_E + k(MS_T - MS_E)/n}$	A,1	2-way random
2,k	$\dfrac{MS_S - MS_E}{MS_S + k(MS_T - MS_E)/n}$	A,k	2-way random
3,1	$\dfrac{MS_S - MS_E}{MS_S + (k-1)MS_E}$	C,1	2-way fixed
3,k	$\dfrac{MS_S - MS_E}{MS_S}$	C,k	2-way fixed
	Use 2,1	A,1	2-way fixed
	Use 2,k	A,k	2-way fixed

[a]Mean square abbreviations are based on the 1-way and 2-way analysis of variance described in Table 10-2. For McGraw and Wong: A, absolute; C, consistency; MS_B, between-subjects mean square; MS_E, error mean square; MS_T, trials mean square; MS_W, within-subjects mean square.

Weir JP. Quantifying test-retest reliability using the intraclass correlation coefficient and the SEM. *J Strength Cond Res.* 2005;19(1):231–240; Shrout PE, Fleiss JL. Intraclass correlations: uses in assessing rater reliability. *Psychol Bull.* 1979;36:420–428; and Mcgraw KO, Wong SP. Forming inferences about some intraclass correlation coefficients. *Psychol Methods.* 1996;1:30–46.

Estimating the Precision of Measures

In addition to estimating reliability with ICC, the *precision* of measurement may be thought of in terms of how confident one is in the reproducibility of a measure. Precision is reported as the **standard error of measurement** (SEM) in the unit of measure and takes into account the ICC of the measure as well as the standard deviation (s) of the data set. The formula is SEM = $s\sqrt{1 - ICC}$. The SEM is expressed in the unit of the measurement of interest. This is in contrast to the ICC which is expressed on a unitless scale ranging from 0 to 1. The SEM may be interpreted as the typical error expected in an individual subject's score.

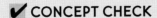 **CONCEPT CHECK**

Precision of measurement may be thought of in terms of how confident one is in the reproducibility of a measure. Precision is reported as the SEM in the unit of measure and takes into account the ICC of the measure as well as the standard deviation.

Limits of Agreement

Bland and Altman (1986) have recommended that the *limits of agreement* **(LOA)** be calculated when two measurement techniques (or two raters) are being compared to each other. This technique compares the absolute differences between two measurement techniques and specifically looks for systematic error. To perform this analysis, data must be on a continuous scale and both techniques must produce the same units of measurement. The arithmetic difference in measures between the two techniques is calculated for each subject. If the difference is zero, the two techniques are identical. The LOA for the entire data set is computed as $LOA = \Sigma(x_1 - x_2)/n \pm 1.96(s_{diff})$, where χ_1 is measurement 1, χ_2 is measurement 2, n is the number of subjects, and s_{diff} is the standard deviation of the difference. The LOA represents a 95% confidence interval of the difference between the two measures.

In addition to calculating the LOA, a Bland–Altman plot should also be constructed and analyzed when comparing two measurement techniques. To do this, for each subject the mean of the two measures is expressed on the x-axis and the arithmetic difference between the measures is expressed on the y-axis. Once the data from all subjects have been plotted, the investigator can observe for systematic error. Figure 10-1 illustrates a Bland–Altman plot using data from data set A in Table 10-6.

Mean difference of measure 1 and measure 2 = 2.75
Standard deviation of difference = 10.0
Limits of agreement = $10.0 + (1.96 \times 10.0) = -16.8, 22.3$

TABLE 10-6   Fictional data of limb girth measures taken two times by the same clinician

MEASURE 1	MEASURE 2	MEASURE 1 – MEASURE 2	MEAN OF 1 AND 2
146	140	6	143
148	152	−4	150
170	152	18	161
90	99	−9	94.5
157	145	12	151
156	153	3	154.5
176	167	9	171.5
205	218	−13	211.5

The arithmetic difference between measures and the mean are calculated for use in the Bland–Altman plot shown in Figure 10-1.

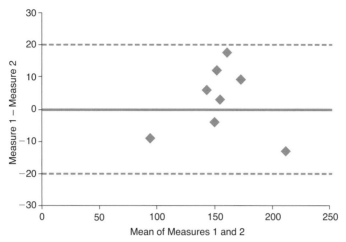

FIGURE 10-1 Bland–Altman plot.

Agreement

Estimates of the consistency or reproducibility of categorical data are called *agreement*. Intrarater and interrater agreement are defined the same as with reliability measures. Estimates of agreement are reported with the kappa (κ) statistic which also ranges from −1 to 1 with 1 indicating perfect agreement, 0 is what would be expected by chance, and negative values indicate agreement occurring less than by chance alone.

Calculation of κ is as follows:

$$\kappa = \frac{p_o - p_e}{1 - p_e}$$

where p_o is the observed agreement and p_e is the expected agreement. p_o and p_e are both derived from a 2 × 2 contingency table of rater agreement.

EXAMPLE

Agreement

Table 10-7 shows data from two clinicians who independently observed the same chronic regional pain syndrome patients for swelling of their involved upper extremities.

(continued)

TABLE 10-7	Fictional data of the agreement of the presence or absence of swelling in 50 patients as assessed by two different conditions		

		CLINICIAN 1		
CLINICIAN 2		**SWELLING PRESENT**	**SWELLING ABSENT**	**TOTAL**
	SWELLING PRESENT	20^a	10^b	30^{m1}
	SWELLING ABSENT	5^c	15^d	20^{m0}
	TOTAL	25^{n1}	25^{n0}	50^n

[a]Both clinicians agree swelling is present, [b]clinicians disagree, [c]clinicians disagree, [d]both clinicians agree swelling in absent.

[n1]Total number of swelling present cases observed by clinician 1, [n0]total number of swelling absent cases observed by clinician 1, [m1]total number of swelling present cases observed by clinician 2, [m0]total number of swelling absent cases observed by clinician 2, [n1]total number of subjects observed by both clinicians.

Calculation of p_o is as follows:

$$p_o = \frac{a + b}{n}$$

$$p_o = \frac{20 + 15}{50} = \frac{35}{50} = 0.70$$

This indicates that the two clinicians both agreed that swelling was present or absent in 70% of the observed patients.

Calculation of p_e is as follows:

$$p_e = ([n^1/n] \times [m^1/n]) + ([n^0/n] \times [m^0/n])$$
$$p_e = ([25/50] \times [30/50]) + ([25/50] \times [20/50])$$
$$p_e = ([0.5 \times 0.6] + [0.5 \times 0.4]) = (0.3) + (0.2) = 0.50$$

This indicates that in this data set the expected agreement between the two clinicians due to chance was 50%.

Thus, κ is calculated as:

$$\kappa = \frac{P_o - P_e}{1 - p_e}$$

$$\kappa = \frac{0.70 - 0.50}{1 - 0.50} = \frac{0.20}{0.50} = 0.40$$

The most common interpretation for κ is as follows:

<0	Agreement is less than by chance
0.01–0.20	Slight agreement
0.21–0.40	Fair agreement

(continued)

0.41–0.60	Moderate agreement
0.61–0.80	Substantial agreement
0.81–0.99	Almost perfect agreement
1.0	Perfect agreement

CHAPTER SUMMARY

Whether a measure is nominal, ordinal, or continuous will dictate how that measure should be analyzed statistically. Validity is an inherent principle in research design and this important concept has many components. Reliability and agreement of measures are also key components of validity.

KEY POINTS

 A key to quantitative inquiry is unbiased and objective measurement of the dependent variables.

 Validity is an inherent principle in research design and this important concept has many components.

 Reliability and agreement of measures are key components of validity.

 To ensure objective results, the design of an experiment to test the hypothesis must be done in an unbiased way.

 Blinding affects and is pertinent to the internal validity of a study.

 Agreement is reported with the kappa statistic that ranges from 0 to 1.

 The randomized pretest–posttest design is the gold standard for most experiments.

 Estimates of the consistency or reproducibility of categorical data are called *agreement*.

Critical Thinking Questions

1. Why is reliability such a pertinent *entity in* any research study and how is this determined?
2. When considering the concept of reliability, what is the difference between *inter-* and *intratester* reliability?
3. Consider the issues of selection bias and delimitations and explain how potential threats to internal validity often involve some sort of bias.

(continued)

Applying Concepts

1. Consider whether a study is valid if it is not reliable or vice versa? Argue your point with examples using contemporary issues from peer-reviewed studies.

2. Design a quantitative study. Include research design, research hypothesis/hypotheses, type of data that will be collected, describe any potential threats to internal validity, external validity of the study, how the study will be determined reliable.

REFERENCES

Bland JM, Altman DG. Statistical methods for assessing agreement between two methods of clinical measurement. *Lancet*. 1986;1:307–310.

Shrout PE, Fleiss JL. Intraclass correlations: uses in assessing rater reliability. *Psychol Bull*. 1979;36:420–428.

Weir JP. Quantifying test-retest reliability using the intraclass correlation coefficient and the SEM. *J Strength Cond Res*. 2005;19(1):231–240.

SUGGESTED READING

Hopkins WG. Measures of reliability in sports medicine and science. *Sports Med*. 2000;30:375–381.

Viera AJ, Garrett JM. Understanding interobserver agreement: the kappa statistic. *Fam Med*. 2005;37:360–363.

CHAPTER 11

TESTS OF COMPARISON

We all know that you can prove anything with statistics.... I recently proved that nobody likes statistics, except for a few professors.... The first person I saw referred to the subject as "sadistics." The second, an old gentleman along the Mississippi River, muttered something about "liars, damned liars and statisticians."

—*Chottiner (1990)*

CHAPTER OBJECTIVES

After reading this chapter, you will:

- Know how estimates of variance are used in testing hypotheses and comparing group values.
- Understand types of data and the differences between parametric and nonparametric statistics.
- Understand the differences between interval and ratio data.
- Learn how to interpret the clinical meaningfulness of data rather than simply focusing on the statistical result.
- Be able to explain issues of statistical significance, clinical meaningfulness, confidence interval analysis, and effect size.
- Understand the importance of context for the critical appraisal of clinical research.
- Know how to consider tests of comparison and the clinical meaningfulness of data rather than simply focusing on the statistical result.
- Understand the need to compile evidence that will assist in making sound decisions about the care of patients and clients.

KEY TERMS

analysis of covariance	parametric and nonparametric statistics	statistical power
null hypothesis	post-hoc comparisons	type I and II errors

INTRODUCTION

This chapter introduces statistical procedures used to test hypotheses and investigate differences between groups or within groups across time. The chapter is an extension of the previous chapter devoted to sampling, probability, and measurement reliability and validity, which are central to the critical appraisal and application of the results of statistical analyses.

The chapter first focuses on types of data and the differences between **parametric and nonparametric statistics**. The primary focus of the discussion of parametric statistics is on analysis of variance (ANOVA) procedures. This section leads the reader through a working example to illustrate how estimates of variance are used in testing hypotheses and comparing group values. This section also introduces concepts of **Type I and II errors**, **statistical power**, and interaction between independent variables and concludes with an introduction to planned and **post-hoc comparisons** and **analysis of covariance**.

The use of *t*-tests and the link between *t*-tests and ANOVA follow the section devoted to ANOVA. In addition to introducing statistical procedures emphasis is placed on the clinical meaningfulness of data rather than simply focusing on the statistical result. An introduction to issues of statistical significance, clinical meaningfulness, confidence interval analysis, and effect size provides a context for the critical appraisal of clinical research.

The chapter concludes with an overview of nonparametric test of comparison and provides a working example of one such statistical procedure, a Mann–Whitney *U* test. Entire texts have been devoted to tests of comparison. It is not the intention here to prepare the reader to perform complex analyses but rather gain an understanding of the basic principles so that the clinical research can be appraised and the results of clinical research applied in a thoughtful process rather than accepted or refuted.

These words offer some insight into the approach to this chapter. First, we do not prove anything with statistics. Proof emerges over time through the accumulation of convincing evidence. Lesson 1 is: do not read to accept the conclusions of a research report as an absolute or final answer. Read to consider and compile evidence that will assist in making a sound decision about the care of patients and clients. Lesson 2: numbers can lie and the misinterpretation of data and statistical analyses can mislead. Intentional misrepresentation and research fraud, while a serious concern and potentially dangerous activity, is thankfully rare. However, the adage "don't believe everything you read" must guide consumption of the clinical literature. This chapter expands on the issue of sampling from populations introduced in the previous chapters. The statistics discussed in this chapter are exercises in probability and there is always the possibility that data drawn from a sample doesn't represent the whole population. Moreover, an inappropriate selection of statistical techniques may also lead to conclusions that are not supported by the data. Careful consideration and critical appraisal informs quality clinical practice. This chapter provides the foundation for critical appraisal of research comparing responses of groups to interventions or treatments used in the care of patients and the prevention of injury and illness.

Lastly, this book in general and this chapter especially was written with the full appreciation that most students preparing for careers in health care are not fond of statistics. Our intent is not to change your mind but to make the medicine as palatable as possible. The practice of evidence-based care depends on consumption (and critical appraisal) of the available evidence (research) so in fact all practitioners claiming to practice from an evidence base must also understand the principles of statistics.

✔ CONCEPT CHECK

It is important to gain an understanding of the basic principles so that the clinical research can be appraised and the results of clinical research applied in a thoughtful process rather than accepted or refuted.

SELECTING STATISTICS AND TYPES OF DATA

There are several statistical procedures that permit analysis of differences between sets of data. These analyses permit comparisons between groups, between measures taken at different times within a group, or a combination of between and within group comparisons. The appropriate statistical procedure is determined by the design of a study and the type of data collected. The first consideration in selecting an analysis is to determine the type or level of the data to be analyzed. Data are categorized as being nominal, ordinal, interval, or ratio.

✔ CONCEPT CHECK

The first consideration in selecting an analysis is to determine the type or level of the data to be analyzed.

Nominal simply means to name. The assignment of numeric values for analysis of nominal (categorical) data is arbitrary. For example, if one were investigating if there is a difference in the prevalence of Carpal tunnel syndrome between left- and right-handed office workers, it would make no difference if left-hand workers were coded as 1s and right-handed workers 2s or vice versa as long as the investigator was clear as to what the 1s and 2s meant while interpreting the results.

Ordinal data, unlike nominal data, are ordered in a particular and meaningful manner. Numeric pain scales represent a common form of ordinal data. We acknowledge that a pain rating of 8 is worse than 5 and 5 is worse than 2. Thus, coding of data is not an arbitrary assignment of numbers. Nominal and ordinal data are analyzed through procedures that differ from those usually appropriate for interval and ratio data.

✔ CONCEPT CHECK

The assignment of numeric values for analysis of nominal data is arbitrary. Ordinal data, unlike nominal data, are ordered in a particular and meaningful manner.

Nonparametric statistical methods of comparison are used to analyze nominal data. Decisions regarding ordinal data are less clear-cut for reasons discussed later but nonparametric procedures can be applied to the analysis of ordinal data without violating assumptions required of parametric statistics. Parametric statistics are appropriate to analyze interval and ratio data under most circumstances.

At this point the type of data has been linked to a type of analysis and the terms "parametric" and "nonparametric" have been introduced. The introduction of these terms has placed the cart ahead of the horse, so let's get the horse back up front and ask: What are the "parameters" that differentiate the type of analysis to be performed? Interval (continuous) and ratio data permit the calculation and useful understanding of a mean or average value and a standard deviation. A mean is a measure of central tendency and a standard deviation is a measure of dispersion. Let's consider the calculation versus interpretation of average values recalling the scenario above with left- and right-handed workers. If right-handed workers were coded as 1s and left-handed workers as 2s, one might find the average of the coding for 40 workers to be 1.2. However, if the left-handed workers were coded as 3s the mean value would be higher. Since the 2s and 3s have the same meaning (identifying left-handed workers) neither average value is meaningful. This is why the mode or most common score is the most useful measure of central tendency when analyzing nominal data.

✔ CONCEPT CHECK

Nonparametric statistical methods of comparison are often used to analyze nominal data. Parametric statistics are appropriate to analyze interval and ratio data under most circumstances.

Ordinal measures are a little more fickle. Some ordinal scales have interval characteristics, an issue discussed later in this chapter. However, let's consider a simple ordinal scale of poor, fair, good, and very good, applied to the rating of videotaped performance of a set of therapeutic exercises incorporated in a home program for patients recovering from rotator cuff tendinopathy. If the values are coded as 0 = poor, 1 = fair, 2 = good, 3 = very good, then, how would one interpret a mean of 1.5? It is not possible for an individual to score 1.5 and we are really not sure if 1.5 is really halfway between fair and good. In this case the appropriate measure of central tendency is the median (score that lies in the middle from high to low when all scores are ranked) while range could be provided as a measure of dispersion.

What are the differences between interval and ratio data? First, let's consider interval data. "Interval" implies that the differences between points of measure are consistent and meaningful. The measurement of elbow flexion range of motion provides an example of interval data. We know that the motion is measured in degrees and the difference between 20 and 30 degrees is the same as the difference between 80 and 90 degrees. A gain or loss of 10 degrees is the same throughout the spectrum of measurement. Contrast range of motion measures to pain scale measures. Is an increase in pain from 1 to 2 the same as an increase from 8 to 9? There is really no way to be sure and this uncertainty affects the ability to interpret average values and variance estimates.

Ratio data are similar to interval data but as the label suggests this level of data can yield meaningful ratio values. Consider measures of force production in comparison to measures of elbow range of motion. If a patient recovering from knee surgery increased their knee extensor force production from 10 to 20 N over a period of time through strength training, we could conclude that their strength has doubled. However, if a patient increased their elbow extension range of motion from 55 to 110 degrees we should not conclude their motion doubled. Why? In the case of the strength measures, which are ratio data, there is an absolute 0 value. It is not possible to have negative strength. However, we know that the extension of the elbow commonly exceeds the 0 value when measured with a standard goniometer. The absence of an absolute 0 precludes the calculation of meaningful ratios. In all other respects interval and ratio data are similar and both types of data are analyzed with the same statistical procedures.

> ✔ CONCEPT CHECK
>
> The absence of an absolute 0 precludes the calculation of meaningful ratios.

Before moving on to ANOVA and further elaborating on the differences between nonparametric and parametric procedures we need to return to measures of dispersion. Variance and standard deviation are measures of dispersion for interval and ratio data while a median and range value are reported for ordinal data respectively and the mode for nominal data. A standard deviation is the square root of variance, and variance is a critical concept in understanding parametric procedures. Parametric statistics *analyze the distribution of variance*, hence the term analysis of variance (ANOVA). But what is variance? Variance is the difference between a score or value and a mean. Thus, for variance or a standard deviation to be of any use the mean must provide useful information. Since the mean score of a set of intervals or ratio data is a very useful measure of central tendency, variance from the mean can be used to compare sets of data.

> ✔ CONCEPT CHECK
>
> Variance and standard deviation are measures of dispersion for interval and ratio data. Variance is the difference between a score or value and a mean; and, a standard deviation is the square root of variance. Parametric statistics analyze the (distribution of) variance.

ANALYSIS OF VARIANCE

ANOVA is at once simplistic and highly complex. The simplicity lies in the calculation of variance. Complexity grows when variance is classified as explained and unexplained and the ratio of explained and unexplained variance is linked to probability. Complexity grows further when more complex research designs are introduced. This section seeks to provide an understanding of variance and ANOVA procedures and interpretation. Issues related to the analysis of data from complex designs are introduced but the reader is referred to texts such as Keppel and Wickens (2004) for further explanation.

To help in understanding variance and therefore ANOVA consider the following scenario (see Box 11-1 to review the steps necessary to complete an analysis): A clinician wants to know if patients recovering from total knee arthroplasty (knee replacement surgery) treated with neuromuscular electrical stimulation (NES) and resistance exercise gain more quadriceps strength in the first 4 weeks than patients who only complete resistance exercise. Sixteen patients consent to participate in the study and are randomly assigned to one of the two groups. Quadriceps strength is measured using a dynamometer on the first day of treatment and after the 4th week of treatment consisting of resistance training on a prescribed schedule. The dependent variable entered into the analysis was the difference between strength measures at the 4th week minus the initial values.

BOX 11.1 | Steps to complete ANOVA

Steps in preparing and completing analysis of variance

1. **Formulate an answerable question that includes identifying independent and dependent variables from a research idea.** For example, "I want to study the effects of electrical stimulation on strength following knee replacement surgery?" is not an answerable question. "Does the addition of neuromuscular electrical stimulation in conjunction with a resistance exercise regimen result in greater improvements in isometric quadriceps strength 6 weeks following knee replacement surgery than an exercise program alone?" is answerable and specific to the scope of the study.

2. **Write the research question in a null form.** The addition of neuromuscular electrical stimulation in conjunction with a resistance exercise regimen does not result in greater improvements in isometric quadriceps strength 6 weeks following knee replacement surgery than an exercise program alone.

   a. Abbreviated, the null is written "NES = no NES"

3. **Collect data.**

4. **Organize data and perform analysis of variance.**

5. **Interpret the results and report findings.**

The results were as follows:

With NES	Without NES
34	20
22	24
28	22
34	24
36	20
32	18
24	26
30	22
Mean = 30	Mean = 22

The mean of all of the scores was 30.

With the data collected it is time to proceed to the analysis, but how does one complete the task? From the outset the question was if the addition of NES-enhanced strength gain in the first 4 weeks of recovery. One look at the data above would lead to the conclusion that indeed it does. However, the process is far more complicated than eyeballing the descriptive statistics (mean and standard deviation). First, it is important to remember the purpose of most research involving comparisons is to infer the results to the population from which the samples were drawn. Thus, the analysis we will undertake with these data will address the question as to whether, if we could study the entire population of knee replacement patients, we would find that NES results in more rapid strength gains in the quadriceps. Since these fictitious data were acquired from small samples of a larger populations (knee replacement patients treated with and without NES) it is possible that subjects in the NES group were inclined to make greater gains for reasons other than NES. The analysis we will perform will estimate the probability that the differences found in our study reflect real population differences.

✔ CONCEPT CHECK

The purpose of most research involving comparisons is to infer the results to the population from which the samples were drawn. The analysis we perform will estimate the probability that the differences found in our study reflect real population differences.

Before we begin performing calculations we need to cover an additional and important concept. While our research question asks if one group differs from another the hypothesis tested in statistics, called the **null hypothesis**, is that there is no difference between groups. The notion of a null hypothesis is a bit counter-intuitive since it is extremely unlikely that two or more sets of scores will be exactly the same. Remember probability; our statistical analysis asks if the data collected provide sufficient evidence that if an entire population could be tested a difference (in this case NES-enhanced strength gains) would be observed. Thus, we perform statistical tests of comparison in an effort to reject a null hypothesis that two sets of data (in this case strength gains in two groups) are drawn from the same population. In rejecting the null the only viable conclusion is that the groups are different. Note that it is not possible to accept a null since two groups will not truly be equal. If we fail to reject a null, we must suspend judgment as to whether groups differ. We will find, however, that the calculation of confidence intervals, to be discussed shortly, helps in interpreting the results of analyses when the null is not rejected as well as when we claim to have found statistically significant differences and reject the null.

✔ CONCEPT CHECK

While our research question asks if one group differs from another the hypothesis tested in statistics, called the null hypothesis, is that there is no difference between groups. In rejecting the null the only viable conclusion is that the groups are different. Note that it is not possible to accept a null since two groups will not truly be equal. If we fail to reject a null, we must suspend judgment as to whether groups differ.

Now let's return to the data and test the null hypothesis that gains in strength through the exercise program alone are equal to those when exercise is supplemented with NES. To do this we will perform ANOVA. Certainly, the use of computer software is recommended for analyzing larger data sets typical of research. However, we will go through the process the old fashion way to illustrate what information obtained through a computerized analysis means. The result of ANOVA is an F value which is a point on an F distribution that permits estimates of probability. However, it is the calculation of an F that really allows for an understanding of the process of ANOVA. The formula for an F is a ratio of variance estimates thus the term analysis of variance. F = mean square explained/mean square unexplained (also sometimes referred to as ms error). What the heck is a mean square? A mean square is essentially the sum of the squared differences from each score and a mean divided by the number of scores minus 1. To calculate a mean square the first step is to calculate the differences between individual scores and a mean score. These values are then squared since the sum of these values always equals zero. The sum of the squared values is then divided by the degrees of freedom to produce a mean square. A more thorough discussion of degrees of freedom (df) is reserved for later but in most cases df = $n - 1$, where n = the number of scores forming the mean. This process is illustrated with our data below.

	With NMS			Without NMS	
Score	d	d^2	Score	d	d^2
34	4	16	20	-2	4
22	-8	64	24	2	4
28	-2	4	22	0	0
34	4	16	24	2	4
36	6	36	20	-2	4
32	2	4	18	-4	16
24	-6	36	26	4	16
30	0	0	22	0	0
Mean = 30	$\Sigma d = 0$	$\Sigma d^2 = 176$	Mean = 22	$\Sigma d = 0$	$\Sigma d^2 = 48$

If we sum the squared values from both groups, the value is 224 and forms the numerator for calculating a mean square. The df in each group equals the number of subjects − 1 or $n − 1$ and since the numerator was derived from both groups the denominator will be equal to $(8 − 1) + (8 − 1) = 14$. The mean square value thus $= 176 + 48/n − 2 = 224/14 = 16$. This mean square represents unexplained variance and will form the denominator of our F ratio.

✔ CONCEPT CHECK

The result of ANOVA is an F value that is a point on an F distribution that permits estimates of probability. F = mean square explained/mean square unexplained. A mean square is essentially the sum of the squared differences from each score and a mean divided by the number of scores minus 1.

What is explained in unexplained variance? This is the heart of the matter of ANOVA. Let's begin with unexplained variance. Take the first score in the group treated with NES, which is 34. The group mean is 30. Why is that 34 not 30? Since our only interest is in our intervention we really have no idea why that 34 is not a 30. It could be related to the subject's age, size, gender, or a number of other factors. The point is that we have not accounted for those factors in the research design and thus can only speculate as to why that score of 34 is not a 30. This variation from the mean is unexplained.

✔ CONCEPT CHECK

Unexplained variance is described as variation from the mean that is attributed to factors beyond the scope of the research design; plausible yet undefined, superfluous factors.

Now we look at the group means. If we were to characterize the average performance of subjects within a group, we could assign each subject the mean value. The value for the group receiving NES differs from the group that did not. These scores differ from the average of all scores or the grand mean. Why are the scores in the group treated with NES different from the grand mean? This can be explained by the treatment received and the sum of the difference between each subject's score, when assigned the group mean score, and the grand mean allows for calculation of explained variance. Now let's complete the process of calculating ms explained. The grand mean (mean of all scores) $= 26$. Thus if each subject in the group receiving NES were given the group mean score, the variance from the grand mean of each subject is 4 and the squared variance is 16. There are 8 subjects in the group and the sum of the squared deviations is $8 \times 16 = 128$. If we move to the group that received exercise alone and assign each subject the group mean of 22, the process repeats and the total ms explained $= 256$. The ms explained $= 256/k$ $- 1$, where $k =$ the number of group means. In this case there are two, so ms explained $= 256$. When a large portion of variance in scores can be explained we are much more likely to conclude that differences observed in a sample reflect real population differences. In this case it appears that a large portion of variance is explained by the treatment rendered since the $F = 256/16 = 16.0$.

INTERPRETING *F*

F, like the normal distribution (see Figures 9-1 and 11-1) is a distribution of values along a continuum. There are, however, an infinite number of *F* distributions that are reflective of the number of df in the numerator and denominator which is determined by the number of variables, the number of levels of those variables, and the number of subjects in a study. In our example there is one variable with two levels (NES vs. no NES). If we added a third group that received a subsensory stimulation, a new level would be added, while if we divided the subjects by gender and then assigned them to treatment, a new variable (gender) would be added. The appropriate *F* distribution is identified by finding the degrees of freedom associated with explained variance and unexplained variance. Fortunately, computer software takes care of selecting the correct reference *F* distribution for an analysis but our simple example allows for a more thorough explanation of degrees of freedom. In this process we assume that the mean value of a group of scores is fixed or not free to vary. Taking the scores in the NES group as an example, the mean $= 30$ is fixed. Given there are 8 scores contributing to that mean 7 could be any value. However, regardless of those 7 scores the 8th would have to result in a group mean of 30 and thus not free to vary or be any value. Thus, 7 scores are free to vary resulting in 7 degrees of freedom.

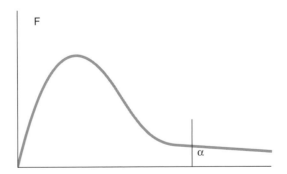

FIGURE 11-1   *F* distribution.

The same case exists for the second group in our analysis thus the degrees of freedom associated with the ms unexplained = 14. Now if we examine the ms explained, we find two group means forming the grand mean. Thus, using the same logic we find that only one of those scores is free to vary since we again assume the grand mean to be a fixed value. Thus the degrees of freedom for explained variance is 1. The F distribution that reflects the probability of the F value = 16 in this analysis is the one associated with 1 df in the numerator and 14 in the denominator.

✔ CONCEPT CHECK

The appropriate F distribution is identified by finding the degrees of freedom associated with explained variance and unexplained variance.

The larger the F (ratio of explained/unexplained variance), the less likely that the differences observed were chance occurrences. In other words, the likelihood of a large F resulting from chance is quite small. By consulting an F distribution table found in many statistics texts (see Table 11-1) we learn that the chances of an $F = 16$ occurring by chance is less than 1 in 100. By convention, researchers are generally willing to accept less than a 5 in 100 risk that an F value obtained is a chance occurrence. The level of risk is known as an alpha value and usually established before the study is begun. When the F value is larger and the probability therefore great that the results reflect real population difference, we reject the null hypothesis and thus conclude that differences observed are due to the effects of our intervention (in this case the introduction of NMS into the treatment). It is important to note that an alpha = 0.05 (acceptance of a 5 in 100 risk of incorrectly concluding that observed differences do not reflect true population differences) is the most common level of risk of being wrong used in research, but it is not an absolute standard. In some cases one might want to be more conservative and accept, for example, a 1 in 100 risk (alpha = 0.01) of being wrong while in exploratory work a more liberal approach might be to accept a 10 in 100 risk (alpha = 0.10).

✔ CONCEPT CHECK

When the F value is larger and the probability therefore great that the results reflect real population difference we reject the null hypothesis and thus conclude that differences observed are due to the effects of our intervention. The alpha value specifies the level of accepted risk of incorrectly concluding that observed differences do not reflect true differences in a population of 100.

TABLE 11-1	Identifying critical values on an *F* distribution with 1 and 14 degrees of freedom												
df2/df1	1	2	3	4	5	10	15	20	30	40	60	120	INF
6	5.987	5.143	4.757	4.533	4.387	4.060	3.938	3.874	3.808	3.774	3.740	3.705	3.669
7	5.591	4.737	4.347	4.120	3.972	3.637	3.511	3.445	3.376	3.340	3.304	3.267	3.230
8	5.318	4.459	4.066	3.838	3.688	3.347	3.218	3.150	3.079	3.043	3.005	2.967	2.928
9	5.117	4.257	3.863	3.633	3.482	3.137	3.006	2.937	2.864	2.826	2.787	2.748	2.707
10	4.965	4.103	3.708	3.478	3.326	2.978	2.845	2.774	2.700	2.661	2.621	2.580	2.538
11	4.844	3.982	3.587	3.357	3.204	2.854	2.719	2.646	2.571	2.531	2.490	2.448	2.405
12	4.747	3.885	3.490	3.259	3.106	2.753	2.617	2.544	2.466	2.426	2.384	2.341	2.296
13	4.667	3.806	3.411	3.179	3.025	2.671	2.533	2.459	2.380	2.339	2.297	2.252	2.206
14	**4.600**	3.739	3.344	3.112	2.958	2.602	2.463	2.388	2.308	2.266	2.223	2.178	2.131
15	4.543	3.682	3.287	3.056	2.901	2.544	2.403	2.328	2.247	2.204	2.160	2.114	2.066
16	4.494	3.634	3.239	3.007	2.852	2.494	2.352	2.276	2.194	2.151	2.106	2.059	2.010
17	4.451	3.592	3.197	2.965	2.810	2.500	2.308	2.230	2.148	2.104	2.058	2.011	1.960

A segment of the full *F* distribution illustrating the critical values with 1 and 14 degrees of freedom (df). The critical value of *F* at an alpha value = 0.05 is 4.600.

Complete *F* distribution tables are available in many statistics books and websites including http://www.statsoft.com/textbook.

ALPHA VALUES AND TYPES OF ERROR

Inferential statistics is truly a game of chance. It is possible that despite a solid research design that the subjects assigned to the NES group simply had a greater capacity to gain strength. However, the probability of this event has been estimated to be less than 1 in 100 and we have rejected the null hypothesis that there is no difference between strength gains in those treated with NES and exercise compared to those who only performed exercise. If indeed further investigation were to reveal that in fact there are not differences in strength gains a Type I error would have occurred. Type I errors occur when a null is rejected when in fact population differences do not exist. The alpha value is really the level of risk of Type I error.

If there is Type I error, it would make sense that there are other types of error. There is, but fortunately the only other known is Type II error. Type II error occurs when a null is not rejected yet a study of the population would reveal differences between groups.

✔ CONCEPT CHECK

Type I errors occur when a null is rejected when in fact population differences do not exist. The alpha value is really the level of risk of Type I error. Type II error occurs when a null is not rejected yet a study of the population would reveal differences between groups.

Again turning to the example above we find the mean differences between groups to be fairly large. Suppose, however, the group means were 24 for the NES group and 22 for the exercise group.

	With NMS				Without NMS		
Score	d	d^2		Score	d	d^2
28	4	16		20	−2	4
16	−8	64		24	2	4
22	−2	4		22	0	0
28	4	16		24	2	4
30	6	36		20	−2	4
26	2	4		18	−4	16
18	−6	36		26	4	16
24	0	0		22	0	0
Mean = 24	$\Sigma d = 0$	$\Sigma d^2 = 176$		Mean = 22	$\Sigma d = 0$	$\Sigma d^2 = 48$

The unexplained variance remains unchanged but the explained variance is now 64 and $F = (64/1)/(224/16) = 4.0$. The degrees of freedom have not changed and a consultation of the F distribution reveals that an $F = 4.0$ will occur by chance more than 5% of the time. We are unwilling to accept this level of Type I error and fail to reject the null hypothesis. The mean differences are nearly 10% and may be of value in clinical practice. Moreover, the collection of additional data likely will reveal that NES results in greater strength gains. A Type II error has likely occurred.

Researchers guard against Type I error by selecting the alpha level. Protection against Type II error is a little more fickle. *Statistical power* is required to decrease the risk of Type II error. Power is influenced by three factors:

- The mean difference between groups
- The variance within groups
- Sample size

In reality, the only factor investigators can control is sample size. Research is costly and time consuming and in some cases poses a risk to participants. Thus, increasing power is not always an easy matter of just adding some subjects. In many cases the variance in a measure can be estimated from previous research and a magnitude of difference between groups that would be of clinical value can be entered into equations to estimate the number of subjects needed to produce an F that would reject a null hypothesis. Such power calculations can be useful but the amount of variance in samples may differ a good bit, especially if the samples are small, and in some cases it is not reasonable to predetermine the size of mean differences that could be deemed important. Moreover, if large samples are studied, it is possible that statistically significant differences (null is rejected) are reported that are of little clinical significance. The issue of magnitude of differences is explored further with the introduction of confidence intervals shortly.

CONCEPT CHECK

Researchers guard against Type I error by selecting the alpha level. *Statistical power* is required to decrease the risk of Type II error.

Our example of ANOVA provides an illustration of the process and introduces some of the challenges of interpreting the results of statistical analyses. Computer technology now allows for the analysis of larger data sets and has fostered more complex research designs. Imagine trying to perform the calculations described above if 100 subjects were enrolled in each group or more variables and levels of variables were introduced. However, while the computer technology will generate the results of an analysis, the interpretation is left to the investigator and consumer. The basic concepts presented here apply to all ANOVA procedures and hopefully lend themselves to enlightening critical appraisal of the clinical research you will read.

COMPLEX DESIGNS AND TERMINOLOGY

The notion that ANOVA has application to a variety of research designs was alluded to earlier in this chapter. For illustrative purposes we introduced and worked through an analysis with the simplest research design with two groups and a single dependent measure recorded once. More complex research designs are common in health care research and this section introduces some of the terminology associated with these designs. In all cases the analysis involves partitioning variance to calculate F ratios but as complexity grows so does the necessity of computer software.

In our example patients were randomly assigned to one of two treatment groups. It was not possible for a patient to be in more than one group so if we label the dependent variable "treatment," the variable is also considered a between-subjects variable. In such research we might be interested in measuring force production at multiple points in time. For example, we might take measurements before surgery, at a point at the beginning of resistance exercise training and at 2 weeks, 4 weeks, and perhaps a few more points for longer-term follow-up. All of the patients would be assessed at each time point regardless of group membership. Thus, in this example, "time" becomes a repeated measure and also considered a within-subjects variable.

When a between-subjects variable and a within-subjects variable exist in a research design the design may be referred to as a "mixed model." Examples of such research designs are very common in health care research. ANOVA is well suited to analyze data generated in mixed model research designs although the process of partitioning variance is beyond the scope of this chapter. The interpretation of F values and probability estimates presented earlier, however, continue to apply to these more complex analyses.

✔ CONCEPT CHECK

When a between-subjects variable and a within-subjects variable exist in a research design the design may be referred to as a "mixed model." Examples of such research designs are very common in health care research.

It is possible to have multiple between-subjects and within-subjects variables within a research design. Perhaps in addition to learning whether NES enhances quadriceps force development following knee surgery, an investigator wants to know whether the responses to treatment differ between men and women. In this case men and women could be randomly assigned to receive or not receive NES creating four groups. Gender is a second between-subjects variable.

An investigator might also be interested in measuring changes in force generation from the nonoperative side to see if the activity during rehabilitation improves strength. Since the operative and nonoperative side measures are derived from the same patient, "side" represents a second repeated measure or within-subjects variable.

INTERACTION

Greater complexity in research designs and thus the data analysis is not necessarily an indicator of better research. In some cases complexity seems to confuse rather than clarify. However, many questions addressed in health care–related research must take into consideration more factors or variables to derive maximum benefit from the work. Consider the example above where gender was added as a second independent, between-subjects variable. The purpose for adding gender to the design is not to determine whether men and women differ in the recovery of strength following knee replacement but rather to investigate whether they differ in response to the intervention being studied. This is a subtle difference in wording but large difference in purpose because the investigator is really seeking to understand the *interaction* between treatment and gender. The concept of studying the interaction between independent variables is important for investigators and research consumers alike.

✔ CONCEPT CHECK

The concept of studying the interaction between independent variables is important for investigators and research consumers alike.

Computer software has made it far easier to analyze data from research where multiple variables are considered in a single analysis and to study the interactions between variables. Unfortunately, the software does not generate results that readily reveal precisely how variables interact. Let's suppose we added gender as a between-subjects variable to our study and the analysis revealed a "significant" interaction between the treatment regimen and gender. What does "significant" interaction really mean? First, recalling our previous discussion "significant" suggests that the finding is unlikely a chance occurrence but rather a reflection of a population phenomenon. Unfortunately, the statistical result tells us little else. To better understand how variables interact we can turn to figures (see Figure 11-2) that include "cell" means and standard deviations as appears below.

✔ CONCEPT CHECK

It is important to remember that "significant" suggests that the finding is unlikely a chance occurrence but rather a reflection of a population phenomenon. Unfortunately, the statistical result tells us little else.

As tables become more complex, however, it becomes more difficult to figure out what these descriptive data mean in terms of understanding interactions between variables. Fortunately, there is a simple solution to a complex issue. The best approach to interpreting and conveying the meaning of interactions between variables is through graphic representation. Consider another example where the interaction of multiple independent variables is of primary interest. In an effort to understand how age effects adaptations to resistance training investigators study younger (<30) and older (>50) year old sedentary adults over 4 sessions of elbow flexion exercises. Consider the table and graph in Figure 11-2. Both demonstrate that gains were made by older subjects over the four exercise sessions. The graphic best calls attention to the interaction that represents the findings of the project.

Change in 6 repetition maximum for elbow curl exercise following 4 sessions of resistance training in younger and older adults.

	Pre	Post
< 30	24.8 ± 2.8	28.1 ± 3.7
> 50	10.9 ± 3.0	18.7 ± 4.0

Assume a significant interaction between age and time (p < .05)

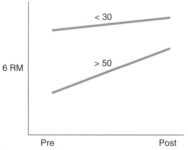

FIGURE 11-2   The significant age by time interaction indicates that the two age groups responded differently over time. There was a slight increase from pre to post 6 RM performance in the <30 age group, but a much larger increase was seen in the >50 age group.

LEVELS OF VARIABLES

In the previous section we explored adding more than one variable into an analysis. It is also possible that there may be multiple levels within a variable. This concept was introduced in the discussion of collecting data at multiple time points with "time" becoming a within-subjects variable. Many variables may include more than two levels. It might be that an investigator wants to study two different forms of NES and thus has three levels of treatment (NES 1, NES 2, and exercise without NES). As with the addition of variables into a research design the addition of levels within a variable adds to the complexity of interpretation. However, the addition of levels of independent variables can maximize efficiencies by allowing completion of one larger study rather than multiple smaller studies and may yield greater insights into the interactions between the variables of interest.

PLANNED COMPARISON AND POST-HOC ANALYSIS

The introduction of multiple levels of an independent variable introduces additional elements into the analysis and interpretation of data. Let's consider a study as described in the previous section with three levels within the variable treatment. We will assume that the dependent measure is change in force production so we have a single between-subjects variable with three levels. Assume further that ANOVA reveals a statistically significant difference. This finding allows us to reject the null that $mean_a = mean_b = mean_c$ but does not reveal where significant differences between the mean value lie. It could be that $mean_a > mean_b$ but $mean_b$ is not different from $mean_c$ or the difference could lie between $mean_b$ and $mean_c$ or perhaps each of the means differs from the other two. In order to learn where differences lie additional analysis is required.

Investigators may plan to perform comparisons between pairs of means (preplanned pairwise comparison) or perform a post-hoc test. There are multiple approaches to post-hoc testing including Tukey, Scheffe, and Bonferroni procedures. Each has advantages and applications but for our purpose it is simply necessary to understand that when one encounters reference to one of these procedures that the investigator/author is conveying that additional analyses were performed to isolate the sources of significant (likely not due to chance) differences between sets of scores.

CONCEPT CHECK

For our purpose, it is simply necessary to understand that when one encounters reference to procedures of post-hoc testing the investigator/author is conveying that additional analyses were performed to isolate the sources of significant (likely not due to chance) differences between sets of scores.

At this point one may ask why, in the scenario described, an investigator would not simply use the procedures previously described and simply perform three comparisons, A to B, A to C, and B to C, to identify where differences between groups might be. The problem with this approach, and the necessity of planned comparison and post-hoc analyses is that the risk of Type I error exists with each analysis performed. Thus, if three analyses are performed with an alpha = 0.05, the potential for Type I error occurring somewhere is 15%. Thus, the conventional approach is to see if any difference exists between means (or in other words a portion of a null hypothesis can be rejected) with a known and reasonable risk of Type I error and finding the sources of the differences once it is known that at least a portion of the null can be rejected.

CONCEPT CHECK

The risk of Type I error exists with each analysis performed. Stated differently, with each additional analysis there is an added possible risk for Type I error.

ANALYSIS OF COVARIANCE

Before moving on to other topics two matters related to ANOVA warrant a brief mention. The research consumer will occasionally encounter ANCOVA that signifies analysis of covariance. ANCOVA is a special case of ANOVA where a variable is introduced for the purpose of accounting for unexplained variance. When used appropriately, which is not always the case, ANCOVA increases statistical power (chance of rejecting the null hypothesis). The introduction of a covariant, however, must be planned and readily justified. From the perspective of the research consumer ANCOVA has little impact on the process of critical appraisal and interpretation of data assuming the introduction of a covariate is based on sound rationale. If the rationale does not appear to justify the analysis, move on, the data may not support the conclusions drawn by the investigator.

✔ CONCEPT CHECK

ANCOVA is a special case of ANOVA where a variable is introduced for the purpose of accounting for unexplained variance.

MANOVA refers to multivariate analysis of variance or case where more than one dependent measure is analyzed simultaneously. MANOVA, as the label might suggest, is a complex subject and not appropriate for all situations where more than one dependent variable is measured. It is best applied when the investigator is interested in the affect of the independent variable(s) on the collection of dependent variables. For example, if an investigator was interested in the response to a specific exercise regimen on function in patients recovering from a lateral ankle sprain, one might include single leg stance on foam surface, single leg hop for distance, and a timed running and cutting drill as dependent measures. Since all relate to the construct of function MANOVA would be appropriate. If a significant difference was observed between function of patients undergoing the specific exercise and a general recommendation for progression to walking and running, follow-up analyses would be needed to determine on which, if any, functional tests patients differed. It is possible that differences only emerge when the combination of dependent measures is analyzed. This issue is addressed in greater detail by Pedhazur (1997).

✔ CONCEPT CHECK

MANOVA refers to multivariate analysis of variance or case where more than one dependent measure is analyzed simultaneously. It is best applied when the investigator is interested in the affect of the independent variable(s) on the collection of dependent variables.

The performance of a MANOVA also allows for the analysis to be completed with a prescribed alpha level (e.g., $P = 0.05$) rather than partitioning the risk of Type I error over multiple analyses. MANOVA is not, however, appropriate in all cases where there are multiple dependent measures of interest. Take, for example, a study comparing repeated cold applications and medication versus medication alone in patients recovering from knee surgery. An investigator might assess reports of pain and measure knee range of motion, isometric knee extension force, and gait speed. Each dependent measure is of unique interest and those data should be analyzed separately. If those data were entered into MANOVA, it is possible that statistically significant and important differences in one dependent measure would not be identified. Thus, although MANOVA might protect against Type I error the loss of potentially important findings should preclude performing the analysis. The decision to perform MANOVA must be made in full consideration of whether the investigators are interested in changes in a construct represented through multiple dependent variables or if the variables are each of unique interest.

T-TESTS

Before exploring confidence intervals a brief discussion of *t*-tests is warranted. Some readers might have expected this discussion earlier since *t*-tests are often introduced before ANOVA. *t*-tests, however, are really a special case of ANOVA where there are only two sets of data in the comparison. However, $t^2 = F$ so it is equally permissible to perform ANOVA as was done above. Like F, t values are points on a curve and there are an infinite number of t distributions, each corresponding to the degrees of freedom associated with unexplained variance. The degrees of freedom associated with explained variance is always 1 since there are only two sets of data.

t- tests and ANOVA are also similar in that between and within subject data can be analyzed. A dependent *t*-test is used to analyze within subject data. For example, if a cohort were tested for gains on a timed test of stair climbing before and after a 3 week lower extremity exercise program a dependent *t*-test would be used to test the null hypothesis the stair climbing speed before and after the exercise program were equal.

An independent *t*-test is appropriate for between subjects analyses. The formulae for dependent and independent *t*-tests differ. Statistical software used in these analyses will guide the selection of the appropriate calculations. To illustrate the process, the formula for an independent *t*-test is presented below and the process of performing the analysis is described using the data from the study of NES described previously. To illustrate the process, the formula for an independent *t*-test is presented below and the process of performing the analysis is described using the data from the study of NES described previously. The independent *t*-test formula is:

$$t = \frac{mean_A - mean_B}{S_{pool}\sqrt{\dfrac{1}{n_A} + \dfrac{1}{n_B}}}$$

where:

$$S_{pool} = \sqrt{\frac{S_A + S_B}{2}}$$

Note that in this example the group sizes are equal and an assumption of equal within group variance is made. Large differences in group size and variance affect the outcome of *t*-test analyses and must be accounted for through the use of modified formulas. This work is typically done with commercially available software but the investigator must recognize the potential problems as well as the available solutions under special circumstances.

Recall that SD is the square root of variance and thus the link between the simple formula for *t* and ANOVA. If the values from our example are entered into the equation we find, with a bit of compensation for rounding error that $t = 30 - 22/2 = 4$ or $t = $ square root of *F* (16). When we compare the calculated value for *t* (4.0) with the critical value (see Table 11-2) we again find (as we did when performing ANOVA on these data) the calculated value exceeds the critical value and thus the null hypothesis is rejected.

A quick glance at an *F* and a *t* distribution reveals that all *F* values are positive while *t* values may be positive or negative (see Figure 11.3). This leads to one other issue associated with *t*, directional hypotheses. The null associated with ANOVA is that two groups are equal (A = B) while with *t* we have a choice of a null of A ≥ B or vice versa A ≤ B.

Again let's return to our example of the study of NES. If we assign A to the NES group and B to the exercise group, we could write a null hypothesis A ≤ B. If the null is rejected, then A must be greater than B or NES more effective than exercise alone. We really do not care if exercise alone is better than NES or equal to NES because if NES is not greater then we would not use the treatment. In this case the point

TABLE 11-2	Identifying critical values on a *t* distribution with 14 degrees of freedom			
df \P	0.05	0.025	0.01	0.005
6	1.943	2.446	3.142	3.707
7	1.894	2.365	2.998	3.499
8	1.860	2.306	2.896	3.355
9	1.833	2.262	2.821	3.250
10	1.812	2.228	2.764	3.169
11	1.796	2.201	2.718	3.106
12	1.782	2.179	2.681	3.055
13	1.771	2.160	2.650	3.012
14	**1.761**	**2.145**	2.625	2.977
15	1.753	2.131	2.602	2.947
16	1.746	2.120	2.583	2.921
17	1.740	2.110	2.567	2.898

A segment of the full *t* distribution illustrating the critical values with 14 degrees of freedom (df). Note that the numerator df of *t* is always = 1. The critical value of a one-tailed test = 1.761, while that of the two-tailed test is 2.145.

Complete *t* distribution tables are available in many statistics books and websites including http://www.statsoft.com/textbook.

associated with a 5 in 100 error would be found on the right side of the distribution and the *t* required to reject the null a bit smaller (creating greater statistical power) than if we had to account for error on both sides of the distribution. When we consider only one side of the distribution we are performing a one-tailed *t*-test. If both A>B and B>A would be of interest then a two-tailed *t*-test is performed. In fact, it is unusual to be interested in both alternatives and thus one-tailed tests are most commonly performed. Thus, when performing a one-tailed *t*-test there is a greater chance of rejecting the null than when performing a two-tailed test or ANOVA.

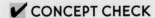 **CONCEPT CHECK**

t-tests are really a special case of ANOVA where there are only two sets of data in the comparison. Like *F*, *t* values are points on a curve and there are an infinite number of *t* distributions, each corresponding to the degrees of freedom associated with unexplained variance.

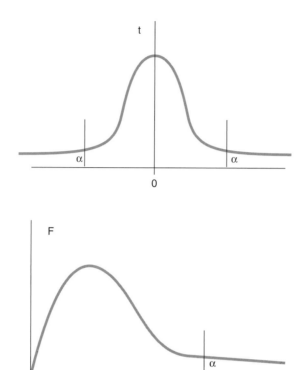

FIGURE 11-3   *F* and *t* distributions.

SIGNIFICANCE AND CONFIDENCE INTERVALS

The foregoing discussion on testing of hypotheses is highly reflective of research in health care in prior decades. However, there has been a gradual realization of the limitations of ANOVA, and *t*-tests for that matter, in the analysis of between group or within group (repeated measures taken from the same subjects across specific time points) differences. The roots of the problem were introduced in conjunction with Type II error and statistical power. ANOVA, *t*-tests, and the nonparametric procedures introduced at the close of this chapter address the probability that differences observed reflect population differences but do not address the magnitude of differences. Thus, it is possible to reject a null hypothesis and conclude, for example, that NES improves strength gains, when the magnitude of the strength improvement is of little clinical consequence, or conversely fail to reject a null when the possibility of clinically meaningful differences exists.

> ### ✔ CONCEPT CHECK
>
> It is possible to reject a null hypothesis and conclude little clinical consequence or conversely fail to reject a null when the possibility of clinically meaningful differences exists.

The solution to this problem, championed by Altman et al. (2000), is the reporting of confidence intervals. As with ANOVA, computer software can perform the calculations easily. Our purpose is to focus on the interpretation of confidence intervals and provide only one example of the calculation process. We recommend *Statistics with Confidence* (Altman et al., 2000) for a thorough explanation of the calculation and interpretation of confidence intervals across a spectrum of applications.

Using the data from our hypothetic NES study entered into analysis with Confidence Interval Analysis software the following result was obtained:

95% CI = 3.7 − 12.3.

This result could be obtained by hand using the following formulas. The first step in calculating CI is to calculate a pooled standard deviation using the formula:

$$S_{pool} = \sqrt{\frac{(n_1 - 1)S_1^2 + (n_2 - 1)S_2^2}{n_1 + n_2 - k}}$$

where k equals the number of samples, which in this case is 2.

The next step is to calculate the standard error of the difference SE(d) as follows:

$$SE(d) = S_{pool} \cdot \left(\frac{1}{n_1} + \frac{1}{n_2} \right)$$

And lastly, the confidence interval is calculated by adding and subtracting from the difference between means observed in the study, the product of the t value associated with the selected alpha level and the degrees of freedom, and the SE(d) as follows:

$$CI = d - t \times SE(d) \text{ to } d + t \times SE(d)$$

How does this result compare to that obtained by ANOVA or *t*-test analysis? In all cases the null that improvements in quadriceps force generation following NES and exercise is equal the improvements with exercise alone is rejected. The reporting of this result with a CI requires more explanation. The 95% CI in this case does not include 0 as the lower limit is 3.7. Thus, we can conclude with 95% certainty that population differences exist. Moreover, we now have a sense of the magnitude of the differences that would be observed if the whole population could be studied. In other words, we are 95% certain that the true population difference would lie between 3.7 and 12.3 Nm. Now we can ask if these differences are clinically meaningful.

It is likely that most clinicians would agree that a 12-Nm greater improvement in force production would warrant the use of NES. However, a 4-Nm difference is a little less convincing and thus one may hesitate to apply these results in clinical practice. Is the extra time and effort warranted for this level of improvement? Of course, this is a judgment call but now a decision that can be better informed than if we were to rely solely on the mean differences observed in our study of samples and the knowledge that there is 95% certainty that some real population difference exists.

In our case the 95% CI is wide given the nature of the data. A statistically meaningful difference may not reflect clinically meaningful differences and the clinician may await more information before including NES into a plan of care. How would more information affect the 95% CI and the clinical decision process? Similar to our discussion regarding Type II error and statistical power, a larger sample will increase power and narrow the 95% CI. Sometimes data from multiple studies can be pooled in a process known as meta-analysis to provide more refined estimates of CIs. Meta-analysis is discussed in greater detail in Chapter 18. It is also important to note the relationship between an alpha value and a CI. A 95% CI implies an alpha value = 0.05. If a more conservative alpha of, for example, $P = 0.01$ were selected then the 99% CI would be calculated.

✔ CONCEPT CHECK

A statistically meaningful difference may not reflect clinically meaningful differences; thus, additional information may be needed before deciding on a plan of care.

Now consider the case where a null is not rejected or, in other words, statistically significant differences were not found. Recall the scenario in this chapter where the mean of the participants receiving NES was reduced to 24. Entering these data into the CIA software we obtain the following 95% CI: −2.3−6.3. Since the 95% CI includes 0 we are not certain that, in fact, the population difference is not 0. However, we might believe that a difference of 4 or more units would be clinically meaningful. Thus, rather than rejecting the notion the NES improves strength gains we again await more information and a narrower confidence interval before including NES in the routine care of knee replacement patients, but we do not fully reject the possibility that the treatment might yield benefit as the true population mean may lie within the range we believe clinically important.

The fundamental problem of relying on the probability that differences observed in a sample reflect population differences is that the magnitude of a difference is not considered. As noted, statistical power increases the likelihood of finding "statistically significant" differences or in other words rejecting the null hypothesis. The addition of more subjects without a change in group differences will ultimately lead to the rejection of a null hypothesis regardless of the size of the differences. Conversely, it is possible that important differences are not "statistically significant" because of a lack of statistical power.

While it behooves an investigator to perform a power analysis before beginning a study so that sufficient power exists this is not always a simple matter. First, in some cases there is a lack of existing data to allow for the precise estimation of sample variance that is required for power analysis. Moreover, power calculations performed to select sample size are usually based on the variable of primary interest. If important findings emerge regarding other measures a lack of power may preclude rejecting a null hypothesis despite differences between groups that are of clinical interest. In summary, the reliance on probability estimates alone in the consideration of research findings may result in dismissing differences that require further investigation or accepting as important or "significant" differences that are of such magnitude that they are of little clinical importance.

✔ CONCEPT CHECK

The fundamental problem of relying on the probability that differences observed in a sample reflect population differences is that the magnitude of a difference is not considered. The reliance on probability estimates alone in the consideration of research findings may result in dismissing differences that require further investigation or accepting as important or "significant" differences that are of such magnitude that they are of little clinical importance.

To review, consider the result of our ANOVA ($F = 16$, $P < 0.05$) and the 95% CI = $3.7-12.3$ reported previously. The CI does not include 0 and thus we are 95% certain that a true population difference exists. This conclusion is the same as rejecting a null hypothesis when the selected alpha level = 0.05. In other words, if the 95% CI does not include "0," the null hypothesis can be rejected with the same level of certainty as was done through ANOVA or completion of a t-test. Moreover, the research consumer now has a clearer understanding of the magnitude of the effect. If only the statistical result and mean differences and variance estimates are reported, as was once common, the reader is left either to conclude that a difference exists and the point estimate of the difference is the mean value, calculate the CI on their own or to calculate and interpret effect size. The latter two options are possible but require additional work

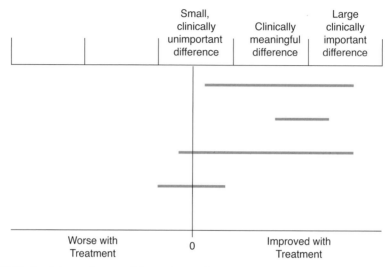

FIGURE 11-4   Interpreting confidence intervals.

and understanding on the part of the consumer. It is better for all when investigators simply provide the CI associated with the preselected alpha value ($P = 0.05$ corresponds to a 95% CI, $P = 0.01$ to a 99% CI, etc.) because the consumer has more work to do.

Take, for example, the four bars on the graph representing CIs in Figure 11-4. The first represents a situation where the null is rejected but the CI approaches 0 and is very large. The consumer is left with a great degree of uncertainty regarding the true magnitude of treatment effect. In this case more data are needed to narrow the CI, an issue of power to be discussed shortly, before being convinced that the treatment will generate, on average, a clinically beneficial effect.

In the second bar the CI is narrow and regardless of where the true population effect lies within the CI the intervention is of clinical importance. This is the best-case scenario in data reporting. The third bar includes "0" so we cannot be certain that a difference between treatments truly exists. However, the interval is also large and if the true population difference falls toward the right side of the bar, the intervention might help a lot of patients. Lastly, we have an interval that includes "0" and does not include differences that are of clinical interest. Thus, even if this result represents a Type II error the small magnitude of the difference would lead us to conclude that the treatment is of little value. These examples hopefully convey the value to the consumer when CIs are reported. In some cases the CI can confuse rather than clarify when limits approach "0" and intervals are very large but it is likely better to be a bit confused and reserve judgment than accepting an outcome as important simply because a null hypothesis was rejected.

EFFECT SIZES

Another useful approach to understanding what the observed differences between groups mean in terms of magnitude of effect, or in other words the typical response to intervention, is through the calculation of effect size. Like other aspects of statistics, the subject of effect size is broader than our focus here. There are multiple approaches to effect size depending on the purpose of the research and the nature of the data. However, when we consider differences between groups, effect size calculations place the magnitude of differences between groups in the context of group variance.

✔ CONCEPT CHECK

When we consider differences between groups, effect size calculations place the magnitude of differences between groups in the context of group variance.

Jacob Cohen (1988) contributed greatly to the use and interpretation of effects size and Cohen's d is one of the most commonly referenced methods of calculating effect size as follows:

$$d = \frac{mean_a - mean_b}{s_{pool}}$$

where s is the pooled variance estimate calculated as follows:

$$S_{pool} = \sqrt{\frac{(n_1 - 1)S_1^2 + (n_2 - 1)S_2^2}{n_1 + n_2}}$$

Hedges (1981) offers a similar formula; however, the denominator was based on the degrees of freedom as follows:

$$S_{pool} = \sqrt{\frac{(n_1 - 1)S_1^2 + (n_2 - 1)S_2^2}{n_1 + n_2 - k}}$$

and yields somewhat higher effect size estimates.

Using the data from our working example of the effects of NES on force production we find using Cohen's formula that:

$$s = \sqrt{(7 \times 5.01)} + \frac{(7 \times 2.62)}{8 + 8} = \frac{53.35}{16} = 3.33$$

Thus $d = (30 - 22)/3.33 = 2.4$.

What does an effect size of 2.4 mean? First, the difference between groups is 2.4 times larger than the standard deviation, which represents a large shift across a normal distribution. However, is there a standard to assist in interpreting effect size? Returning to the work of Cohen we find he suggested that an effect size of 0.2 represents a small effect, 0.5 a moderate effect, and >0.8 a large effect. These values provide some guidance but are based in social science rather than biomedical research. There is no substitute for knowledge of the nature of data and clinical populations when considering the magnitude of effect. Certainly, large effects are more likely of clinical importance than small effects. Moreover, an effect that is not considered of consequence by the patient and/or clinician is too small to guide a plan of care regardless of the probability of Type I error. The research consumer should use effect size estimates as one element of critical appraisal of research reporting group comparisons. If effect size is not reported, the value can often be estimated from the descriptive (mean and standard deviation) data reported. Much like an over reliance on probability of Type I error (P values) one can rely on effect size estimates alone to guide clinical decisions based on the research literature.

✔ CONCEPT CHECK

There is no substitute for knowledge of the nature of data and clinical populations when considering the magnitude of effect. The research consumer should use effect size estimates as one element of critical appraisal of research reporting group comparisons.

NONPARAMETRIC STATISTICS

In the introduction of this chapter the type of data or level of measurement was linked to the selection of the appropriate analysis. The notion of population parameters of mean and standard deviation was introduced in preparation of our discussion of parametric statistics in general and ANOVA in particular. It is time to turn attention to nonparametric statistics but before doing so a couple of points of clarification are warranted.

First, the terms nonparametric and distribution-free are sometimes used interchangeably. It is important to note that when parametric analyses are completed it is assumed that the data are based on observations of a normally distributed population with similar variance and samples are drawn at random. These assumptions can be tested (histogram or box plot allows for assessment of distribution while Levene's test tests a null that population variances are equal). If these assumptions are not met, nonparametric procedures may be the appropriate analytical methods. Such circumstances may occur with small samples and one may see a nonparametric analysis of interval or ratio data from a small sample. These issues, however, rarely impact the analysis of data in the clinical research literature and the use of nonparametric procedures is generally reserved for ordinal and nominal data. Moreover, violation of the assumptions is unlikely to have a substantial impact on the statistical outcome as procedures such as ANOVA are robust and not highly sensitive to departures from these assumptions nor the conclusions drawn from research if one considers the magnitude of effect in conjunction with the probability that differences observed represent a true population difference. Keppel and Wickens (2004) offer a more complete discussion of the issues related to violating the assumptions underlying ANOVA.

✔ **CONCEPT CHECK**

It is important to note that when parametric analyses are completed it is assumed that the data are based on observations of a normally distributed population with similar variance and samples are drawn at random.

It is also worth noting that nonparametric statistics test hypotheses about medians or in the case of nominal data, distribution. Knowledge of population variance is necessary to generate confidence intervals. Thus these procedures are somewhat more difficult to interpret in the context of clinically meaningful differences and the magnitude of effect of health care intervention.

There are multiple nonparametric procedures described in statistics texts. The most appropriate nonparametric test in a particular circumstance depends on the nature of the data and research method of the study. We will discuss three of the most common nonparametric procedures; Mann−Whitney U, Kruskal−Wallis one-way analysis of variance by ranks, and Friedman two-way analysis of variance by ranks. Information on other tests of group comparison can be found in texts by Daniel (see section "Suggested Reading" at the end of this chapter).

✔ **CONCEPT CHECK**

Nonparametric statistics test hypotheses about medians or in the case of nominal data, distribution. The most appropriate nonparametric test in a particular circumstance depends on the nature of the data and research method of the study.

Mann—Whitney *U* Test

The Mann—Whitney *U* test is analogous to the paired *t*-test discussed and the ANOVA performed for illustration earlier in this chapter. The analysis tests the null hypothesis that the median score in one group (A) is < or = to the median score of a second group (B) (A ≤ B). If the analysis reveals the median of B > A, we might reject the null hypothesis. However, we would want to know the probability that the result was a chance finding. As with parametric tests reference tables allow us to know the probability of a test result occurring by chance (see Table 11-3). Recall that the parametric statistics discussed previously result in *F* and *t* values. The Mann—Whitney *U* result is designated as a *T* (capital vs. *t* used to designate a parametric test). As with parametric tests the null hypothesis (A ≤ B) is only rejected if the probability of obtaining a *T*-value is sufficiently small (e.g., less than 5%). The process of performing a Mann—Whitney *U* is described by Daniel (see section "Suggested Reading" at the end of this chapter).

Kruskal—Wallis One-way Analysis of Variance by Ranks

A Kruskal—Wallis one-way analysis of variance by ranks is similar but appropriate when there are more than two groups. The result of a Kruskal—Wallis one-way analysis of variance by Ranks is a *H*-value and the probability of *H* can be found by consulting with a table specific to this analysis.

Friedman Two-Way Analysis of Variance by Ranks

A Friedman two-way analysis of variance by ranks is appropriate for analyses where there are repeated measures within one group. For example, patients

TABLE 11-3 Contingency table for Mann–Whitney *U*					
N1>	**6**	**7**	**8**	**9**	**10**
N2					
6	31	36	40	44	49
7	36	41	46	51	56
8	40	46	**51**	57	63
9	44	51	57	64	70
10	49	56	63	70	77

A segment of the full Mann–Whitney distribution illustrating the critical value with eight participants (N1 and N2) in each of the groups at an alpha value = 0.05.

Complete Mann–Whitney *U* contingency tables are available in many statistics books and websites including http://www.zoology.ubc.ca/~bio300/StatTables.pdf.

suffering from chronic ankle instability might be asked to rank four commercial ankle stabilizers for comfort and effectiveness. Freidman labeled the test statistic for this test an X^2_r and the probability of a result can be determined by referring to a reference table specific to the Friedman analysis. The reference tables for these nonparametric procedures can be found in statistics texts devoted to, at least in part, nonparametric procedures. These sources are noted because these analyses are relatively easily completed by hand with small data sets. The formulas for these analyses are also found in these texts. The formulas differ from one another and might appear a little strange as illustrated in the Mann–Whitney U analysis but all are similarly easy to negotiate.

Note that none of these nonparametric tests allow for the analysis of repeated measures from multiple groups known as a mixed model design. This represents one of the major limitations of these statistical tests in clinical research since change across time with different interventions is often the purpose of an investigation. This reality has led to the analysis of ordinal data such as pain ratings with parametric statistics. In these cases the data are assumed to possess interval properties. In many cases this may be a reasonable assumption but the research consumer should be aware of the assumptions made and be provided with reasonable justification for the analyses performed.

MANN–WHITNEY *U* EXAMPLE SCENARIO

The Mann–Whitney U is the appropriate statistic for the scenario described in the following text. Like other nonparametric procedures we must consult statistics texts for the appropriate formula and contingency (probability) references. It is our intent to illustrate the process rather than devote extensive time and resources teaching a statistical technique that many research consumers will encounter but that few clinicians will ever be asked to execute. We again recommend Daniel (see section "Suggested Reading" at the end of this chapter) for a more detailed discussion of the Mann–Whitney U and other nonparametric tests.

Does NES cause more discomfort than exercise alone in patients recovering from knee replacement surgery? Let's assume that the participants in the study of NMS also rated their level of discomfort during their treatment session. Discomfort was measured on a 0 to 10 scale with 0 representing no discomfort and 10 representing discomfort that resulted in discontinuing the treatment session. We want to know if the application of NES increased their discomfort but recognize that these data are ordinal. Thus we turn to the Mann–Whitney U and generate a null hypothesis that the discomfort with NES is $\leq$ exercise without NMS.

The data are as follows:

With NES	Without NES
7	5
4	4
3	4
5	3
6	5
6	4
3	4
4	2

The first step in completing the analysis is to rank the scores across both groups from the lowest to the highest. Tie scores are given the average rank. As you will see, for example, a score of 3 then occupies 2nd, 3rd, and 4th rank. The middle value is 3 so all scores of 3 are given a rank of 3. Scores of 5 occupied the 10th, 11th, 12th, and 13th ranks and the middle value = 11.5, so all scores of 5 were ranked 11.5. The ranked data were as follows:

NMS		Without NMS	
Score	Rank	Score	Rank
		2	1
3	3		
3	3		
		3	3
4	7		
4	7		
		4	7
		4	7
		4	7
5	11.5		
		5	11.5
		5	11.5
		5	11.5
6	14.5		
6	14.5		
7	16		
Sum of ranks	76.5		59.5

Formula:

$$T = S \times \frac{n(n + 1)}{2}$$

where S is the sum of the ranks in group X and n the number of participants in group X. The assignment of X is arbitrary but in this case we are interested in X > Y and/or discomfort with NES > exercise without NES so NES was assigned as X.

Continuing:

$$T = 76.5 \times \frac{8(9)}{2} \text{ or } 76.5 - 36 = 40.5$$

As with ANOVA and t-tests we need to know what is the probability of obtaining a $T = 40.5$ by chance and consult a contingency table for the Mann–Whitney U. Figure 11.2 displays a section of the table for the sample size in the example and an alpha level of 0.05. With an alpha level of 0.05 the value located on the contingency table is 51. Since our calculated T (40.5) is less than 51 we cannot be 95% confident that the median discomfort reported with the use of NES is greater than with exercise alone. The raw data suggest this is a possibility but we must suspend judgment until more data are available.

A NOTE ON PARAMETRIC ANALYSIS OF ORDINAL DATA

On occasion, one may encounter research where a parametric statistical test (e.g., ANOVA) is used to analyze ordinal data. Based on our discussion thus far such a procedure would seem inappropriate. This may be the case or the analysis may represent a compromise between the desire to answer a question of interest and the absence of a wholly appropriate statistical technique. For example, assume that we want to know if a thrust manipulation is more effective than a muscle energy technique for relieving pain in patients with mechanical low back pain. We elect to measure pain with a 0 = no, 10 = worst pain possible anchored in a 0 to 10 scale. From our previous discussion the resulting data are ordinal. However, the study design calls for randomly assigning patients to one of two treatment groups (treatment is the variable and there are two levels: thrust manipulation and muscle energy) and measuring pain before treatment, immediately after treatment, and every 6 hours thereafter for 2 days. Time becomes a second variable in this case with 10 levels. The design is an example of a mixed model with patients separated into groups while the measure of pain perception is repeated within each group. None of the nonparametric procedures noted previously will permit analysis of these data and allow the investigators to investigate the *interaction* between the variables. The investigator may assume the pain data possess interval properties and perform ANOVA. Will this assumption affect the analysis and thus the conclusions drawn from the investigation? The answer lies in the degree to which the assumption is valid and it is incumbent on the investigator to argue their case. The research consumer can then weigh the argument as they appraise the work. There is no black and white answer but like many compromises in research has shades of gray.

CHAPTER SUMMARY

This chapter is devoted to examining differences between groups. The selection of the appropriate test requires a determination as to the nature of the data. Ratio and interval data are associated with parametric procedures while ordinal and nominal data are managed using nonparametric methods. ANOVA is the most common parametric procedure used in analyzing data related to group comparisons and the chapter devotes considerable attention to the basic components of such an analysis.

Attention is briefly turned to *t*-tests before examining the issues of magnitude of effect and clinical meaningfulness. Advances in statistics and the evolution of evidence-based practice as well as the field of clinical epidemiology have altered the perspective as to how research data are best interpreted and applied in clinical practice. We are in fact living in an era of change, which, while a step forward in health care, adds another layer of uncertainty as to what the research we read really means in the context of caring for our patients. Many investigators and clinicians received instruction in statistics at a time where the risk of Type I error was the dominant concern and nonsignificant differences (in which the calculated F or t values could occur by chance >5 in 100 times) were rarely reported in the clinical literature because such reports were rejected by editors.

The fundamental problem of relying on the probability that differences observed in a sample reflect population differences is that the magnitude of a difference is not considered. The reliance on probability estimates alone in the consideration of research findings may result in dismissing differences that require further investigation or accepting as important or "significant" differences that are of such magnitude that they are of little clinical importance. The reporting of confidence intervals addresses the issues of probability while providing an interval in which true population differences lie. Effect size reporting provides the consumer with a sense of the magnitude of the difference between group mean values in relation to the variance among subjects. Each has the potential to assist the research consumer appraise clinical research that is the overarching mission of this book.

Nonparametric statistics is a broad topic well beyond the scope of this chapter. The limited coverage here is not to imply that these analyses are of less importance. There are, however, multiple nonparametric techniques. We chose to perform one such technique to illustrate the process and discuss the interpretation of findings. It is hoped that this offers a foundation for exploration of research related to diagnostic procedures, prevention, prognosis, and intervention found in the next section.

See Table 11-4 for a summary of the tests of comparison covered in this chapter.

TABLE 11-4 Summary of tests of comparison	
Parametric tests of comparison	
Analysis of variance (ANOVA)	Calculation of F value
	One or more independent variables with two or more levels
	Analysis of interaction between variables
	Independent variables may be between subjects or within subject (repeated measure)
t-test	Special case of ANOVA involving one independent variable with two levels
	Independent variable may be between subjects or within subject which is referred to as a dependent t-test
Analysis of covariance (ANCOVA)	ANOVA with the introduction of a variable that is not a part of the null hypothesis that explains a portion of otherwise unexplained variance
Multivariant analysis of variance	Similar to ANOVA except that multiple dependent measures are analyzed simultaneously
Nonparametric tests of comparison	
Mann–Whitney U	Analysis of ordinal data from two groups
Kruskal–Wallis one-way analysis of variance by ranks	Similar to Mann–Whitney U but used for analysis when there are more than two groups
Friedman one-way analysis of variance by ranks	Analogous to repeated measures ANOVA where subjects are measured two or more times

KEY POINTS

☞ Statistics do not prove anything.

☞ Do not read to accept the conclusions of a research report as an absolute or final answer.

Numbers can lie and the misinterpretation of data and statistical analyses can mislead.

 Most students preparing for careers in health care are not fond of statistics.

 Careful consideration and critical appraisal informs quality clinical practice; thus, it is necessary to understand the principles of statistics.

Critical Thinking Questions

1. Why do we not prove anything with statistics?
2. How should we read scientific writing, data, and statistical results?
3. Why is an understanding of statistics important to the practice of evidence-based care?
4. Why is it important to remember the adage "don't believe everything you read" must guide consumption of the clinical literature?

 ## Applying Concepts

1. Discuss the various factors that influence statistical power.
   a. Consider the role and responsibility of a research in controlling these factors.
2. What are the "parameters" that differentiate the type of analysis to be performed?
   a. Discuss examples of clinical relevance.
   b. Consider methodical *and* practical implications of exploring the same clinic question from more than one research perspective, using different types of analyses to test the same or different hypotheses in order to compare findings.
   c. Consider the possible clinical implications that might result from such an approach.
3. Consider the implications of the following scenarios, and discuss plausible clinical examples:
   a. A research study where misinterpretation of data and statistical analyses can mislead.
   b. A clinical study in which the results do not match the conclusion(s).
   c. Manipulating the findings of a study to justify a desired clinical effect or outcome.
   d. Critical appraisal of research comparing responses of groups to interventions or treatments used in the care of patients and the prevention of injury and illness.

REFERENCES

Altman DG, Machin D, Bryant TN, et al. *Statistics with Confidence*. 2nd ed. London, UK: BMJ Books; 2000.

Chottiner S. Statistics: towards a kinder, gentler subject. *Journal of Irreproducible Results*. 1990;35(6):13–15.

Cohen J. *Statistical Power Analysis for the Behavioral Sciences*. 2nd ed. Mahwah, NJ: Lawrence Erlbaum Associates; 1988.

Hedges LV. Distribution theory for Glass's estimator of effect size and related estimators. *J Educ Stat*. 1981;6:107–128.

Keppel G, Wickens TD. *Design and Analysis: A Researcher's Handbook*. 4th ed. Upper Saddle River, NJ Prentice-Hall; 2004.

Pedhazur EJ. *Multiple Regression in Behavior Research*. New York: Holt, Rinehart and Winston; 1997.

SUGGESTED READING

Daniel WW. *Biostatistics: A Foundation for Analysis in the Health Sciences*. 9th ed. New York: John Wiley & Sons; 2008.

Glass GV, Peckham PD, Sanders JR. Consequences of failure to meet assumptions underlying fixed effects analysis of variance and covariance. *Rev Educ Res*. 1972;42:237–288. Available at: http://www.basic.northwestern.edu/statguidefiles/levene.html.

CHAPTER 12

MEASURES OF ASSOCIATION

Do not put your faith in what statistics say until you have carefully considered what they do not say.

—William W. Watt (as quoted in
www.quotegarden.com/statistics.html)

CHAPTER OBJECTIVES

After reading this chapter, you will:

* Understand that the purpose of research can be to investigate relationships between variables rather than compare group differences.
* Learn how to introduce the methods and statistical analysis of research into relationships or correlations between variables.
* Understand that the type of data dictates the appropriate statistical approach and the statistical approach affects how results are interpreted.
* Learn to recognize and understand the relationships between variables.
* Understand that there are limitations to the conclusions that can be appropriately drawn from statistical results.
* Learn that probability estimates can be, and often are, provided in association with point estimates of association.
* Know that the interpretation of the *P*-values requires some elaboration.

KEY TERMS

conclusions	interpretations	predictor variables
correlations between variables	limitations	probability estimates
criterion variable	*P*-values	results
data	point estimates of association	variables

INTRODUCTION

In many circumstances the purpose of research is to investigate relationships between **variables** rather than compare group differences. This chapter introduces the methods and statistical analysis of research into the relationships or **correlations between variables**. As with research into group comparisons, the type of **data** dictates the appropriate statistical approach and the statistical approach affects how **results** are interpreted. While understanding the relationships between variables can be highly informative, there are **limitations** to the **conclusions** that can be appropriately drawn. Moreover, while **probability estimates** can be, and often are, provided in association with **point estimates of association**, the **interpretation** of the *P*-**values** requires some elaboration. These issues are discussed in more detail at the end of the chapter.

✔ CONCEPT CHECK

In many circumstances the purpose of research is to investigate relationships between variables rather than compare group differences.

PURPOSE AND METHODS

There are numerous circumstances where knowledge of the association between variables can inform health care practice. Sometimes we want to know more about the association between characteristics that individuals possess such as, for example, the relationship between body mass index (BMI) and systolic blood pressure. We also might want to know about the association between external events and individual characteristics such as barometric pressure and pain and stiffness in patients with rheumatoid arthritis. The relationship between events and population values may also be of interest. For example, the relationship between weather and the incidence of some diseases such as influenza has been investigated, and such information is useful in planning public health responses and immunization strategies. In each of these examples data are collected that allow the estimation of the strength of the relationships between variables.

The methods employed vary between investigations. This is not to imply that any research method is appropriate. There are several considerations related to the research methods investigating association. The first of these considerations parallels that of studies of comparison, namely measurement error and data validity. The less precise a measurement is, the lower the association between that variable and any other variable unless the direction and magnitude of error is similar for each of the variables being studied. Thus, it is possible that a strong relationship exists between two variables but the strength of the relationship is underestimated due to measurement imprecision. Validity of data may or may not affect the strength of the relationship between two measurements. If a measurement is reliable and fairly precise, a strong association may be found; however, the interpretation of the association may be misleading since the data from one or more measurements may not reflect the underlying construct that the investigator was intending to measure.

✔ CONCEPT CHECK

When investigating association (between variables), data are collected that allow the estimation of the strength of the relationships between variables.

Beyond consideration of reliability and validity the researcher and research consumer must consider additional issues including the timing of measurements and the sample being studied. Some variables are fairly stable over time, others change predictably over time, while others change rapidly and less predictably. If one were to investigate the association between bone mineral density in the hip and leg press strength, one might perform densitometry one day and strength measures the next. Neither strength nor bone mineral density is likely to change greatly in the span of a few days. If, however, one were to investigate the relationship between serum cortisol levels and BMI the time of day when serum samples were drawn must be controlled due to the known diurnal variation in serum cortisol concentrations. If one wanted to investigate the association between catecholamine levels and blood pressure following a bout of resistance exercise, the measures must be taken concurrently as soon after exercise as possible. While these examples are simplistic the take-home point is that the investigator and research consumer must consider timing when interpreting and applying the results of research into the association between variables.

✔ CONCEPT CHECK

The researcher and research consumer must consider the timing of measurements and the sample being studied.

In addition to, and perhaps more important, the critical appraisal of research into the associations between variables is a complete description and careful consideration of the sample tested. The more homogeneous a sample, the more likely the strength of the association between variables will be underestimated. Take, for example, the association between undergraduate grade point average (GPA) and performance (graduate GPA) in a highly competitive graduate program. Since the only students accepted into the program had a very high GPA as an undergraduate (let's say 3.5 or better) there is very little variance between them (homogeneity). Moreover, since acceptable grades in the graduate school are A and B there is limited variance between students in graduate school grades. In other words, the sample has resulted in a restricted range of values from a larger scale (e.g., 0 to 4.0 GPA). An analysis of these data is likely to lead to the conclusion that there is little association between undergraduate achievement and graduate school performance. If, however, all students across the spectrum of undergraduate GPA were enrolled in the graduate program and a full spectrum of grades (A to F) awarded, a much stronger association between undergraduate and graduate achievement would likely emerge. The research consumer should consider whether the sample studied truly represents the range of the population of interest and, from a clinical perspective, whether the sample is similar to patients in their practice. Generalization of results into clinical practice is a judgment of the clinician but the investigator/author must provide sufficient description to allow a thoughtful decision on the part of the clinician.

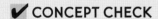 **CONCEPT CHECK**

The more homogeneous a sample, the more likely the strength of the association between variables will be underestimated.

DATA ANALYSIS

As with the statistical methods used for comparisons between groups described in the previous chapter, the first consideration when analyzing data to estimate the strength of an association between variables is to determine the type of data at hand. Recall that interval and ratio data can be analyzed with analysis of variance (ANOVA) because variance estimates can be calculated. Variance estimates are also central to estimating the strength of a relationship between variables that are interval or ratio data. Ordinal and nominal data are analyzed through nonparametric procedures. We will begin with the analysis and interpretation of measures of association involving interval and ratio data and then address nonparametric procedures.

> ✔ CONCEPT CHECK
>
> The first consideration when analyzing data to estimate the strength of an association between variables is to determine the type of data at hand.

REGRESSION

The fundamental statistic for the analysis of interval and ratio data to estimate the strength of the association between variables is regression analysis, which is also the foundation for ANOVA. In fact, ANOVA is really a special case of regression. As with ANOVA, the more the variables under consideration, the more complex the analysis. Similar to the analyses for comparisons between groups where t-tests were identified as the simplest form of ANOVA and used when only pairs of data were being considered, simple linear regression is the simplest form of regression. Simple linear regression, often identified as a Pearson product moment correlation (PPMC) and designated as a Pearson ρ or simply an ρ value, is used to measure the strength of the association between pairs of data that are interval or ordinal.

> ✔ CONCEPT CHECK
>
> Simple linear regression is often identified as a Pearson product moment correlation (PPMC) and is designated as a Pearson ρ or simply an ρ value.

Although correlation coefficients can be quickly calculated with commercial software, the formula is straightforward and hand calculation is fairly easy:

$$r = \frac{n(\Sigma xy) - (\Sigma x)(\Sigma y)}{\sqrt{(n(\Sigma x^2) - (\Sigma x^2))(n(\Sigma y^2) - (\Sigma y^2))}}$$

where N is the number of pairs of data, X is the values of one variable, and Y is the values of the second.

The resulting ρ value will range from -1.0 to 1.0 with -1.0 reflective of a perfect inverse relationship (one variable [e.g., X] increases in magnitude while the second [e.g., Y] decreases) and 1.0 a perfect direct relationship (when the magnitude of X increases there is a corresponding increase in Y). The interpretation of values between -1.0 and 1.0 is discussed later.

> ## EXAMPLE

Regression

Zhou et al. (2009) explored the relationships between obesity indices and blood pressure in a large sample of Chinese adults. Each of the measures of obesity (e.g., BMI, waist circumference) and blood pressure are interval data. Thus, PPMC coefficients were calculated to estimate the strength of the relationships of interest. Of course, computer software was used as there were data from more than 29,000 people. However, a small subset of the data might have generated the table below that will allow illustration of the calculation of a PPMC.

SUBJECT	BMI	SYSTOLIC BLOOD PRESSURE	X^2	Y^2	XY
1	28.0	128	784	16,384	3,584
2	31.0	145	961	21,025	4,495
3	24.0	115	576	13,225	2,760
4	29.0	140	841	19,600	4,060
5	32.0	160	1,024	25,600	5,120
6	22.0	120	484	14,400	2,640
7	23.0	115	529	13,225	2,645
8	33.0	150	1,089	22,500	4,950
Sum	222	1,073	6,288	145,959	30,154

$r = N\Sigma XY - (\Sigma X)(\Sigma Y)/\sqrt{N\Sigma X^2 - (\Sigma X)^2} \sqrt{N\Sigma Y^2 - (\Sigma Y)^2}$

$r = 8(30,154) - 23,8206/(\sqrt{8(6,288) - 222^2}) (\sqrt{(8)14,5959 - 1,073^2})$

$r = 3,026/(31.9) (127.8) = 0.74$

In this very small sample a strong relationship was observed between BMIs. Zhou reported the association between BMI and systolic blood pressure to be 0.43 for men and 0.51 for women. Although fictitious our data illustrate two points. First, small samples, even in real settings, may yield estimates well above true population values. Second, even with a very small data set calculations are cumbersome and time consuming. Computer software is really essential for managing data that is informative to clinical practice; however, the interpretation of the results continues to require an understanding of the analytical procedures used for analysis.

It is also possible to estimate the association between multiple variables through multiple regression, which is conceptually similar to adding variables or levels of variables and performing ANOVA rather than a *t*-test. Multiple regression is an important but also extensive statistical topic. Indeed, entire texts have been devoted to the subject, and we recommend those by Pedhazur (1997) or Cohen et al. (2002) for more information.

For our purposes let's consider a simple case where the association between two variables, labeled **predictor variables**, and a third **criterion variable** is estimated.

Even in this simple case there are multiple approaches to the question. One could only be interested in the association between the predictor variables combined, as illustrated in Figure 12-1, or perhaps identifying the variable with the strongest association with the criterion variable and then determining how much the addition of the second variable adds to the picture, as illustrated in Figure 12-2.

Let's consider the second approach using the data set above. When multiple regression is performed the process yields an R^2 value that can be defined as the variance in the criterion variable (Y) explained by a predictor variable (X) or predictor variables ($X1$, $X2$, etc.). Note that with multiple regression R^2 values are generated while the PPMC yields ρ values. The product of $(r)^2 = R^2$ or, in other words, when the PPMC is squared the value is equal to that that would have been obtained through multiple regression. We will learn that it is often helpful to square a PPMC ρ value to enhance the interpretation of the results of an analysis that will be discussed later. The relationship between ρ and R^2 also confirms that the PPMC is really just a special case of multiple regression.

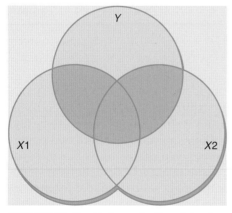

FIGURE 12-1 Variance in *Y* explained by the combination of *X*1 and *X*2.

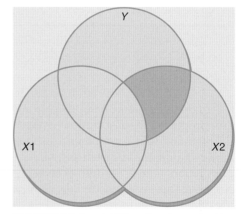

FIGURE 12-2 Additional variance in *Y* explained by the addition of *X*2.

Before discussing the interpretation of ρ and R^2 let's return to our example and consider what happen when $X2$ was added to the analysis. Note that the R^2 when $X1$ and $X2$ were entered is not the sum of the variance in Y explained by $X1$ plus the variance in Y explained by $X2$, but rather the variance explained in Y by $X1$ plus any additional variance in Y explained by the addition of $X2$ as illustrated below. The only exception to this rule is when there is no association between $X1$ and $X2$ in which case both variables explain completely unique portions of variance in Y.

It is possible to explore the relationships between variables while controlling for the influence of other variables through the calculation of partial and semipartial correlations. While beyond the scope of this discussion you may refer to Pedhazur for a detailed explanation.

EXAMPLE

Multiple Regression (Study and Data Set are Fictitious)

A group of clinicians wanted to study the relationships between strength, stair climbing function, and patient self-report of community mobility in community dwelling women between 75 and 85 years of age. Fourteen participants consented to participate and were familiarized with the study protocol consisting of maximum leg press strength, time to climb 12 stairs, and completion of a 100-point community mobility scale. Three trials of leg press performed on a dynamometer and three stair climbing trials were completed. The community mobility assessment (CMA) is anchored by 100 = no mobility limitations and 0 = unable to access the community independently.

Assuming data from the participants were as follows:

SUBJECT	STRENGTH (N/KG)	STAIR CLIMBING TIME (SEC)	COMMUNITY MOBILITY ASSESSMENT
1	10.8	18	72
2	9.5	27	64
3	11.4	23	85

(continued)

4	9.8	34	70
5	7.8	38	50
6	10.2	20	88
7	8.0	25	75
8	12.0	15	90
9	8.6	17	77
10	13.0	12	95
11	8.8	14	88
12	9.0	17	80
13	8.2	28	60
14	10.5	17	75

Data were analyzed through regression analysis and the calculation of PPMCs between individual variables with SPSS Version 16.0 software.

Model Summary

MODEL	R	R^2	ADJUSTED R^2	STD. ERROR OF THE ESTIMATE
1	0.869[a]	0.754	0.710	6.79904

[a]Predictors: (Constant), Stair climbing (sec), Strength (N/kg).

Analysis of Variance[b]

MODEL		SUM OF SQUARES	DF	MEAN SQUARE	F	SIGNIFICANCE
1	Regression	1562.718	2	781.359	16.903	0.000[a]
	Residual	508.496	11	46.227		
	Total	2071.214	13			

[a]Predictors: (Constant), Stair climbing (sec), Strength (N/kg).
[b]Dependent variable: Community mobility assessment.

Coefficients[a]

Multiple regression analysis revealed a statistically significant (very low probability that a relationship = 0) and strong association between strength, stair climbing time, and self-reported community mobility with approximately 75% of variance in community mobility explained by these two predictor variables. This

(continued)

finding does not identify the strength of the individual contributions to community ambulation. Examining the correlation between the individual factors yields further clarity.

Stair Climbing versus Community Mobility Assessment: Correlations

		COMMUNITY MOBILITY ASSESSMENT	STAIR CLIMBING (SEC)
Community mobility assessment	Pearson correlation	1	−0.826[a]
	Significance (two-tailed)		0.000
	N	14	14
Stair climbing (sec)	Pearson correlation	−0.826[a]	1
	Significance (two-tailed)	0.000	
	N	14	14

[a]Correlation is significant at the 0.01 level (two-tailed).

The analysis reveals a strong correlation between stair climbing ability and self-reported community ambulation. The correlation of $\rho = -0.826$ reveals that as time to climb stairs decreases, self-reported community mobility increases (hence the negative value), and the stair climbing ability explains 68% (-0.826^2) of the variance in community ambulation. The results of the regression analysis and this finding mean that strength only added an additional 7% of explained variance in community mobility scores when combined with stair climbing ability and there is not 95% certainty that strength added any explained variance. (Note $t = 1.796$, $P = 0.100$.) This means that the addition of strength data to the model did not significantly (null $\rho = 0$) improve the explanation of variance in community mobility.

Coefficients[a]

MODEL		UNSTANDARDIZED COEFFICIENTS		STANDARDIZED COEFFICIENTS	T	SIG.
		β	Std. error	β		
1	(Constant)	74.711	18.150		4.116	0.002
	Strength (N/kg)	2.543	1.415	0.317	**1.796**	**0.100**
	Stair climbing (sec)	−1.072	0.288	−0.657	−3.719	0.003

[a]Dependent variable: Community mobility assessment.

(continued)

Does that mean that strength is unimportant to community mobility?

Further investigation reveals that strength is also significantly and strongly correlated with community mobility scores ($\rho = 0.668$, or explaining approximately 45% of variance in community mobility). How can two predictor variables each explain large portions of variance in a third criterion variable?

Strength versus Community Mobility Assessment: Correlations

		STRENGTH (N/KG)	COMMUNITY MOBILITY ASSESSMENT
Strength (N/kg)	Pearson correlation	1	0.668[a]
	Significance (two-tailed)		0.009
	N	14	14
Community mobility assessment	Pearson correlation	0.668[a]	1
	Significance (two-tailed)	0.009	
	N	14	14

[a]Correlation is significant at the 0.01 level (two-tailed).

The answer lies in the strong correlation between the predictor variables. The analysis reveals a fairly strong link ($\rho = -0.533$) between leg press strength and stair climbing time, and examination of the scores confirms greater strength is associated with faster climbing.

Strength versus Stair Climb: Correlations

		STRENGTH (N/KG)	STAIR CLIMBING (SEC)
Strength (N/kg)	Pearson correlation	1	−0.533[a]
	Significance (two-tailed)		0.049
	N	14	14
Stair climbing (sec)	Pearson correlation	−0.533[a]	1
	Significance (two-tailed)	0.049	
	N	14	14

[a]Correlation is significant at the 0.05 level (two-tailed).

(continued)

The assessment of these associations does not imply cause and effect. However, a logical argument could be made for exercises to promote strength and stair climbing repetitions in an effort to improve reported community mobility. This would provide the foundation for clinical research into these questions.

INTERPRETING ρ AND R^2

The first consideration when interpreting estimates of association has yet to be introduced. *P*-values or probability values were discussed in the preceding chapter in the context of hypothesis testing. When exploring differences between groups the *P*-value is an indication that the differences observed when studying a sample are reflective of true population differences. *P*-values relate to statistical differences but as noted in the preceding chapter offer little to understanding clinical meaningfulness. The *P*-values found in association with ρ and R^2 also relate to hypothesis testing and also generally are of little value when considering the meaningfulness of an association between variables. While it is possible to test the hypothesis that the association between variables exceeds any value (e.g., $\rho \geq 0.50$), by far the most common use tests the hypothesis that the association between X and Y does not equal 0 ($rXY \neq 0$). Thus, the fact that a "significant" relationship has been identified is nearly useless when considering the meaningfulness of the analysis.

> ✔ **CONCEPT CHECK**
>
> When exploring differences between groups the *P*-value is an indication that the differences observed when studying a sample are reflective of true population differences.

If a *P*-value is not informative, then what statistic should the research consumer be most concerned with? The answer is the R^2 value (with a confidence interval) or the portion of variance in Y explained by the predictor variable(s). This is also why it is important to recognize the relationship between PPMC and multiple regression. The usefulness of the R^2 value is revealed when one considers interpretation of ρ values although interpretation of R^2 is far from straightforward. Investigators and statisticians have provided some guidelines for interpreting ρ values (Note: table values are for interpreting ρ, not ρ-square) such as:

Interpretation of pearson product moment correlation (ρ values)

0.00 to 0.25	0.00 to −0.25	Little, if any correlation
0.26 to 0.49	−0.26 to −0.49	Low correlation
0.50 to 0.69	−0.50 to −0.69	Moderate correlation

(continued)

| 0.70 to 0.89 | −0.70 to −0.89 | High correlation |
| 0.90 to 1.0 | −0.90 to −1.0 | Very high correlation |

Domholdt E. *Rehabilitation Research: Principles and Applications*. 3rd ed. St. Louis, MO: Elsevier Saunders; 2005.

However, the application of these guidelines may prove misleading. Let's assume, for example, that investigators found that the correlation between BMI and serum cholesterol in men over 40 years of age was $\rho = 0.49$. Such a finding could be interpreted as a low correlation and therefore unimportant. However, many factors may influence serum cholesterol and an $R^2 = 0.24$ (0.49^2) indicates that 24% of the variance in serum cholesterol is explained by BMI. Such a finding might suggest a strategy for reducing serum cholesterol and thus quite important.

✔ CONCEPT CHECK

The usefulness of the R^2 value is revealed when one considers interpretation of ρ values.

There are two important points to be made here. The first is that measures of association do not imply cause and effect. It is possible that reducing BMI would have no effect on serum cholesterol. Additional clinical research would be needed to determine if lowering BMI would affect serum cholesterol. If the issue of cause and effect is still puzzling since it seems reasonable that lowering BMI would be associated with reduced serum cholesterol across a sample of older men, consider the converse. It would be unlikely that lowering serum cholesterol through medication would impact BMI. The issue of cause and effect will be discussed further near the end of the chapter but the introduction here leads to a second key point; investigators and research consumers really need to understand the nature of the data at hand to interpret measures of association and comparison. As noted in the previous chapter statistically significant differences may be of little clinical meaning and thus misinterpreted. Interpreting the strength and importance of measures of association and teasing out cause and effect relationships requires knowledge of the subject matter and careful critical appraisal rather than reference to a published scale that, while well intended and applicable in some circumstances, can potentially mislead.

✔ CONCEPT CHECK

Measures of association do not imply cause and effect.

The second point to be made is that while measures of association cannot confirm cause and effect, these analyses can build useful predictive models. Recall that in the discussion of multiple regression the terms predictor and criterion variables were introduced. These terms imply that the values of the predictor variables, in fact, predict the value of the criterion variable. Take, for example, the use of skin-fold measures to estimate body composition. These formulas are derived from regression analyses where the variance in body composition as measured from a standard (e.g., underwater weighing) explained by skin-fold measures was identified. Since a large portion of the variance in the criterion variable body composition (as measured through underwater weighing) was explained by the predictor variables (skin-folds) the use of skin-fold measures is an acceptable (although not perfect) and more easily performed means of estimating body composition. Note that the prediction model does not imply cause and effect, but rather a means of predicting an outcome in one measure, based on the values of predictor measures.

✔ CONCEPT CHECK

While measures of association cannot confirm cause and effect, these analyses can build useful predictive models. Note that the prediction model does not imply cause and effect, but rather a means of predicting an outcome in one measure, based on the values of predictor measures.

MANAGING ORDINAL AND NOMINAL DATA

The analysis of ordinal data is straightforward. The analysis used most often is a Spearman rank order correlation and the result designated as a Spearman ρ. The process of calculating a Spearman ρ is illustrated in the following example.

EXAMPLE

Calculating a Spearman ρ

A clinician wants to learn about the association between perceived pain and changes in systolic blood pressure in patients suffering from tension headaches. To investigate the question a small pilot study is conducted where blood pressure is recorded on three occasions when patients are free of pain. Patients are then instructed to contact the investigators when a headache develops and blood pressure

(continued)

is again recorded and perceived pain is recorded on a 10-cm visual analog scale. Since the pain measures are deemed to be ordinal data the investigator selects a nonparameter Spearman rank order correlation for data analysis.

The formula for a Spearman rank order correlation is as follows:

$$\text{Spearman } (\rho) = 1 - ((6\Sigma d^2)/n(n^2 - 1))$$

where d is the difference in ranks between pairs of data and n is the number of subjects.

The pilot study yielded the following data set:

SUBJECT	CHANGE IN SYSTOLIC BLOOD PRESSURE	RANK	PAIN SCORE	RANK	d	d^2
1	10	47	5	−1	1	
2	−5	1	5	1	0	0
3	15	6	5.5	2	4	16
4	0	2	9	7	−5	25
5	5	3	6	3	0	0
6	20	7	8	6	1	1
7	12	5	6.5	4	1	1
Sum						44

Spearman $\rho = 1 - ((6(44))/7(49 - 1)) = 1 - 0.79 = 0.21$.

The pilot study suggests there is a small relationship between changes in systolic blood pressure and perceived pain with a tension headache. Such a result may cause investigators to question whether the expense of conducting a larger clinical trial can be justified.

The result is similar to that of a PPMC, with values ranging from −1.0 to 1.0, negative and positive values reflecting the direction of the relationship.

The analysis of the association between ordinal values is more complicated than those for ordinal, interval, or ratio data. The most common approach is a Cramer's V correlation that is based on chi square (χ^2) values. One application of an χ^2 analysis is to test the hypothesis that two nominal variables are independent. The text by Daniel (see section "Suggested Reading" at the end of this chapter) provides a detailed discussion of χ^2 including tests of independence. If the null hypothesis that two variables are independent is rejected, a Cramer's V can be calculated to measure the strength of the relationship.

The following example illustrates this process.

EXAMPLE

Calculating a Cramer's *V*

An investigator sought to determine if there is a relationship between living environment and activity level. Participants in the study were classified as living in a rural, suburban, or urban environment based on population density and classified as being sedentary, moderately active, or active based on scores on an International Physical Activity Questionnaire Short Form (IPAQ-SF). Note that the data related to the community in which individuals lived is nominal while the activity level data is ordinal. As with other analyses the appropriate statistic is based on the lowest level of data. Thus a χ^2 analysis was performed on the data set found below to determine if activity level is independent of where people live.

The sample consisted of 800 urban dwellers, 845 suburban dwellers, and 680 rural dwellers with activity profiles described below.

	ACTIVE	MODERATELY ACTIVE	SEDENTARY	TOTAL
Urban	280	400	120	800
	(222)	(378.5)	(206.5)	
Suburban	150	325	390	845
	(234.4)	(400)	(218)	
Rural	215	375	90	680
	(186.6)	(321.7)	(175.5)	
Total	645	1,100	600	2,325

Actual and expected (in parentheses) values.

$\chi^2 = 175.6$, $P < 0.01$.

Thus the hypothesis that living environment and activity level are independent is rejected. What is the strength of the association between living environment and activity level observed in this sample? The Cramer's *V* is calculated as follows:

$$V = \sqrt{\frac{\chi^2}{nt}}$$ where *n* is the sample size and *t* is the smallest number of rows or columns minus 1. In this case there are 2325 participants and 3 rows and columns, so $t = 2$.

The result is Cramer's $V = 19.4$. One might conclude that there is a rather modest association between living environment as defined for the study and activity level measured in the study with urban and rural dwelling people less likely to be sedentary.

ASSOCIATION VERSUS CAUSE

The results of the Cramer's *V* analysis in the previous section bring back to issues of interpretation and cause and effect. While this analysis identified a relationship, there is no suggestion of cause and effect. One may speculate that urban dwellers tend to walk more often to complete daily tasks including commuting to work and shopping and rural dwellers spend more time on tasks requiring physical labor but such speculation would require more investigation to confirm or refute.

In some cases two variables may appear highly associated due to correlation with a third variable. A statistics professor once observed that there was a correlation between the number of drunks and the number of churches in communities. He observed that a small nearby town had very few drunks and five churches. The modest size university had many more drunks and nearly 20 churches. The capital city had still more drunks and about 100 churches while New York City had even more drunks and hundreds of churches. One could speculate that frequent drunkenness caused people to repent and attend church, requiring more churches to be built or perhaps that lengthy sermons caused folks to drink more. Of course, what the professor was commenting on was the spurious or incidental association between two variables associated with the population of the communities.

✔ CONCEPT CHECK

In some cases two variables may appear highly associated due to correlation with a third variable.

It requires more than measures of association to establish cause and effect. In some cases experimental designs can test hypotheses of cause and effect derived from studies of association. In other cases cause and effect is established through a preponderance of evidence. The link between cigarette smoking and many diseases offers one example. Research ethics would preclude randomly assigning some people to regular cigarette smoking while forcing others to refrain. Thus, a randomized trial on the effects of smoking in humans is not feasible. However, I doubt the readers of this book would argue that cigarette smoking is harmless. It has only been through extensive retrospective study that the body of evidence grew to an extent where it is not possible that smoking is unrelated to the incidence of disease.

✔ CONCEPT CHECK

It requires more than measures of association to establish cause and effect.

The discussion above and the previous introduction to the interpretation of ρ and R^2 values identified the difficulties and limitations of interpreting measures of association. In that discussion the value of R^2 as a proportion of explained variance was introduced. In closing it is important to note that because Spearman ρ and Cramer's V are nonparametric statistics the square of these values is meaningless. The interpretation of these statistics truly requires knowledge of the literature on the question being addressed and the nature of the data in making informed decision regarding studies that address the association between variables.

CHAPTER SUMMARY

This chapter provides an introduction to the research and statistical methods used to investigate the association between variables. Consideration for critically appraising and generalizing research that provides estimates of association as well as the most common analyses are reviewed. Although the calculation of estimates of association is fairly easy, interpretation of estimates of association for clinical applications is often less straightforward. Some investigators have relied on P-values to make a case for the clinical meaningfulness of their findings210 ather than considering the magnitude of an observed association in the context of multifactorial relationships. In some instances inferences of cause and effect have evolved from studies of association. The knowledge of the associations between variables can inform clinical decisions and generate new research questions. The consumer-clinician, however, must consider the magnitude and clinical meaningfulness of estimates of association in the context of the complexity of interrelated variables rather than accepting, at face value, that reported relationships are of importance.

KEY POINTS

- Knowledge of the association between variables can inform health care practice.
- The less precise a measurement is, the lower the association between that variable and any other variable unless the direction and magnitude of error is similar for each of the variables being studied.
- Validity of data may or may not affect the strength of the relationship between two measurements.
- Generalization of results into clinical practice is a judgment of the clinician and requires thoughtful decision on the part of the clinician.
- The fundamental statistic for the analysis of interval and ratio data to estimate the strength of the association between variables is regression analysis.

- *P*-values relate to statistical differences but offer little to understanding clinical meaningfulness.
- Because Spearman ρ and Cramer's V are nonparametric statistics the square of these values is meaningless.

Critical Thinking Questions

1. Why is it important to be cautious about measurement error and data validity in measurements of association?
2. What is the first consideration when analyzing data to estimate the strength of an association between variables?
3. Why can interval and ratio data be analyzed with analysis of variance?
4. If a *P*-value is not informative, then what statistic should the research consumer be most concerned with?

Applying Concepts

1. Discuss considerations related to the research methods investigating association.
2. Consider why the answer to question #2 above is important to measures of association; and, provide a clinical example to illustrate and support your opinion.

REFERENCES

Cohen P, Cohen J, West SG, et al. *Applied Multiple Regression/Correlation Analysis for the Behavioral Sciences.* 3rd ed. Marwah, NJ: Lawrence Erlbaum; 2002.

Domholdt E. *Rehabilitation Research: Principles and Applications.* 3rd ed. St. Louis, MO: Elsevier Saunders; 2005.

Pedhazur EJ. *Multiple Regression in Behavior Research.* New York: Holt, Rinehart and Winston; 1997.

Zhou Z, Hu D, Chen J. Association between obesity indices and blood pressure or hypertension: which index is the best? *Public Health Nutr.* 2009;12(8):1061–1071.

SUGGESTED READING

1. Daniel WW. *Biostatistics: A Foundation for Analysis in the Health Sciences.* 9th ed. New York: John Wiley & Sons; 2008.

PART III

CLINICAL RESEARCH: DIAGNOSIS, PREVENTION, AND TREATMENT

CHAPTER 13

EVALUATION AND DIAGNOSIS: RESEARCH METHODS AND DATA ANALYSIS

*No amount of experimentation can ever prove me right; a
single experiment can prove me wrong.*

—*Albert Einstein, MD (1879–1955), from Poor Man's College,
as quoted in The Quotations Page (www.quotationspage.com)*

CHAPTER OBJECTIVES

After reading this chapter, you will:

- Understand and explain the purpose of patient interview and observation.
- Be able to explain and describe the importance of physical examination procedures.
- Be able to explain why observations are a key part in the evaluation process.
- Be able to explain the purpose and process of clinical research.
- Be able to define and decrease investigational bias.
- Understand the concepts of sensitivity and specificity.
- Be able to calculate sensitivity and specificity values.
- Understand and calculate likelihood ratios.
- Understand positive and negative prediction values.
- Understand and interpret receiver operator characteristic (ROC) curves.

KEY TERMS

blinding

clinical trials

control biases

diagnostic continuum

estimates of sensitivity
   and specificity

false negative results

false positive

generalizability of research findings

methodologic flaws

methodologic quality in research

nonclinical research

positive and negative likelihood
   ratios or receiver operator
   characteristic curves

positive and negative
   prediction values

special tests

therapeutic intervention

validity

INTRODUCTION

The ability to identify tissue damage or disease that is responsible for a patient's symptoms is the foundation of **therapeutic intervention**. The clinician needs to know what is wrong before it can be made right. Health care providers use a variety of diagnostic procedures including laboratory testing, diagnostic imaging, physical examination, interviewing, and observation. Decisions regarding return to work or sports participation, referral for emergent and nonemergent care, as well as the development of rehabilitation plans of care, stem from the evaluation process.

Patient interviews and the performance of physical examination procedures, often referred to as **special tests**, are the primary tools available to the physical therapists, occupational therapists, and athletic trainers evaluating an individual seeking care. Unfortunately, not everyone with a particular condition will report the same symptoms. Moreover, many of the physical examination procedures used by these clinicians may fail to detect the condition that the procedure is intended to identify or render positive findings in the absence of the condition.

The limitations related to diagnostic testing are not exclusive to the patient interview and physical examination procedures. Diagnostic imaging and laboratory procedures may also lead to incorrect conclusions. For example, magnetic resonance imaging (MRI) without contrast may fail to detect glenoid labrum pathology (Volpi et al., 2003) or identify damage to the intervertebral discs unrelated to the pain generator in a patient complaining of low back pain (Ernst et al., 2005; Grane, 1998).

The limitations associated with diagnostic testing should not dissuade the clinician from performing these assessments. Despite the inherent flaws most diagnostic tests do provide the clinician with useful information. What is needed is an understanding of how well the diagnostic procedures employed perform in routine practice so that the results can be interpreted in the context of other information and examination results.

An understanding of the performance of diagnostic procedures is derived from clinical research. This chapter provides an overview of the **diagnostic continuum** and addresses the differences between research into diagnostic testing and prevention or treatment strategies. Issues of **methodologic quality in research** of diagnostic testing are reviewed so that the clinician can identify **methodologic flaws** that threaten the **validity** of data reported in such studies. Lastly, the statistical procedures used to generate estimates of the value of diagnostic testing are presented.

PHYSICAL EXAMINATION PROCEDURES

Observation, interview, and the performance of physical examination procedures are the primary methods available to the physical therapists, practitioners in allied health care professions, and athletic trainers during the injury evaluation process. Ordering for diagnostic imaging and laboratory studies is outside their scope of practice. The continuum from observation to the use of sometimes costly medical technology is, however, important for all who practice in health care to understand. First, it is truly a continuum of decision making. The first clues as to the underlying problem are often obtained through simple observation. A patient who is unable to bear weight on a recently injured ankle is more likely to have sustained a fracture than the one who can walk (Bachmann et al., 2003). A patient with back pain that cannot tolerate sitting in a waiting area is likely to have pathology involving the intervertebral discs. Observation often guides the opening questions in an interview with a patient. Through observation and interview the list of diagnostic possibilities shrinks and one or two conditions emerge as the most likely culprits of the patient's complaints.

✔ CONCEPT CHECK

The purpose of clinical observation is to guide the opening questions in an interview with a patient. Through observation and interview the list of diagnostic possibilities shrinks and one or two conditions emerge as the most likely culprits of the patient's complaints.

The clinician can then select physical examination procedures that will help confirm or refute the existence of the suspect conditions. This process then guides decisions related to returning to work or sport participation making a referral to a physician or, if indicated, an other care provider. In many cases the ultimate diagnosis has been established prior to referral only to be confirmed through reevaluation and additional diagnostic testing.

Advances in health care have greatly expanded the diagnostic tools available to physicians and other providers. MRI, for example, was not available 40 years ago. Such technology offers greater diagnostic accuracy in many situations but at a greater cost. MRI has not replaced observation, interview, and physical examination. In fact these assessment techniques are necessary to identify patients likely to benefit from MRI. The Ottawa Ankle Rules (Stiell et al., 1992) provide an excellent example of observation and physical examination guiding the decision as to whether a radiographic assessment of the injured ankle is warranted. Research reveals that when the Ottawa Ankle Rules are applied and radiographs are not warranted the risk of not identifying a fracture is very low (Bachmann et al., 2003). Through the application of the Ottawa Rules unwarranted exposure to radiation and the costs associated with radiographic studies are reduced.

Unfortunately, not all assessment techniques perform as well as the Ottawa Ankle Rules nor have most been as extensively studied. There are, however, a lot of reports related to diagnostic testing that are of importance to the clinician. Research into the performance of diagnostic tests differs from research into, for example, prevention efforts and treatment outcomes. The results of research into the outcomes of treatments and prevention efforts are far more convincing when the responses to particular intervention are compared with the outcome following another treatment, a placebo treatment, or a no treatment control. The key point is that the outcomes in a group of subjects receiving a treatment of interest need to be compared to some other group. The details of methods of controlling investigational bias in these types of studies are presented in preceding chapters. In studies of diagnostic procedures comparison to another group of patients or subjects is unnecessary. As we shall see these studies require that the results of the diagnostic test of interest are compared to the results of an established standard. Investigational methods, and therefore sources of investigational bias, differ substantially and are the subject of this chapter.

HOW CAN CLINICAL RESEARCH IMPROVE PATIENT EVALUATION?

The examination of injured and ill patients is common to many medical and allied medical disciplines. One challenge in health care lies in maximizing benefit to the patient without squandering talent, time, and money on procedures that are of little benefit or pose more risk than can be justified by the likely benefit. How can a clinician select the best diagnostic tests?

The only way to find answers to clinical questions is through **clinical trials**. This does not imply that **nonclinical research** is not valuable. Many advances in health care have resulted from research and development of new diagnostic technologies. However, not until a diagnostic test is studied in the population it is intended to benefit can the true magnitude of benefit and risk be elucidated.

The process of searching for clinical studies and an overview of clinical research was provided in earlier chapters. It will take only a few attempts at reviewing the literature on specific topics to find disagreement in the conclusions drawn by researchers based upon the data they have collected and analyzed. Sorting through clinical research to find "truth" is a real challenge. Differing results can be due to differences in sample sizes between studies. Large samples are more likely to reflect the true state of a population than smaller samples. Differences may result from subtle variations in the populations from which samples were drawn. Differences may even result from chance where, through random selection, an investigator enrolls individuals who are more or less likely to benefit from a particular procedure. Lastly, differences in study outcomes may be due to a failure to **control biases** that threaten the validity of data.

The clinician–consumer of clinical research must understand the relationship between study methods and threats to the validity of data. The methods of studies of prevention, treatment, and diagnostic procedures, and therefore the steps that minimize investigational bias, differ. Issues related to diagnostic studies are discussed here, while those related to prevention and treatment are found in Chapters 14–16 of Part III.

DESIGN OF STUDIES OF DIAGNOSTIC TESTING

Estimating the usefulness of any diagnostic procedure involves comparing the results of a diagnostic test to the results of an established, often termed "gold," standard. In a study of diagnostic test performance of, as an example, a Lachman test (Torg, Conrad, & Kalen, 1976) of the integrity of the anterior cruciate ligament (ACL), the results of the Lachman test might be compared to the results from MRI or operative findings. In such a study one could determine how often a positive Lachman test was found in patients with a torn ACL, how often the test was not positive in those with an intact ACL, as well as how often a Lachman test was interpreted as positive in those with an intact ligament or negative in patients ultimately found to have torn their ACL. The preceding sentence describes the formation of four subgroups—correct interpretation in patients with and without a torn ACL and incorrect interpretation representing **false positive** and **false negative results**. These four mutually exclusive groupings are the foundation of statistical analysis for studies involving tests with dichotomous outcomes (positive or negative result) such as a Lachman test. If a test is on a continuous scale (i.e., such as creatine kinase levels in individuals being evaluated for myocardial infarction), then a somewhat different analysis is required to assess diagnostic test performance (Sackett et al., 1992). However, a gold standard identifying those with and without the diagnosis of interest is still needed to estimate the usefulness of the test of interest.

Aside from identifying a diagnostic test of interest and an appropriate gold standard, there are other methodologic issues that may affect the conclusions drawn by investigators regarding particular tests and the value of the findings of a published study to individual clinicians. Before addressing these issues, however, we will digress briefly and return to the diagnostic continuum.

As noted in the beginning of this chapter the procedures used to establish diagnoses are imperfect. Test results may fail to detect pathology when it is present (false negative results) or suggest pathology is present when it is not (false positive). It was further noted that studies of diagnostic testing assess the performance of diagnostic tests with a gold standard measure. One may ask why, if a gold standard test is available this procedure is not just applied to all those for whom a particular diagnosis is in question? The answers to this question are found in the setting, timing, scope, costs, and risks associated with the diagnostic process. These issues often overlap. When someone is injured and becomes ill, health care providers may be called upon to make care decisions in settings where some technologies are not available. Upon presentation there may also be a broad spectrum of diagnostic possibilities. Ascertaining the medical history of the patient and their current complaints the clinician can probably narrow the field of likely diagnoses. In order to confirm or refute the presence of the most likely conditions the clinician can then proceed to the physical examination of the patient. An effectively structured physical examination will substantially increase or decrease the clinician's suspicion regarding the presence of one or more specific condition.

EXAMPLE

Physical Examination used to Narrow Down Diagnostic Possibilities

Take for example the examination of a patient presenting following an acute onset of knee pain. From a history the clinician must learn about previous episodes of knee and lower extremity injuries and about the events preceding the onset of the current symptoms. Assuming that the patient has never sustained an injury before, and experienced an acute onset of pain when their knee struck the dashboard of a car during a front end collision, the diagnostic possibilities narrow. Certainly injury to the posterior cruciate ligament, fracture, and contusion is possible. A patient who bears weight comfortably, has little effusion, but is tender on the anterior proximal tibia with well localized ecchymosis, has more likely sustained a contusion than a fracture. This diagnosis becomes more likely if the examination of the knee reveals normal ligamentous integrity. In this case the evaluation has been timely, can be completed almost anywhere, and has narrowed the scope of diagnostic possibilities with a high degree of certainty.

(continued)

Two issues, at a minimum, emerge from this example. First, how much confidence should the examiner place in the results of the assessment of the ligamentous integrity of the knee and how should one proceed if multiple diagnoses remain highly plausible? The first issue leads to the central issue in this chapter. Studies of diagnostic procedures are needed to guide clinicians as they ponder the certainty of their diagnosis. The less certain one is of a particular diagnosis the greater the likelihood that something else is wrong. When this is the case the use of advanced medical technologies may be warranted. The use of advanced diagnostic procedures (e.g., MRI) comes at a cost and in some cases (e.g., spinal tap to work up a patient who may have meningitis) with a risk. The more that is known about how well a structured interview, observation, and when indicated, physical examination procedures perform in establishing specific diagnoses, the more selective the use of higher cost and riskier procedures can become. Thus, studies of the diagnostic accuracy of responses to specific questions and the finding of studies of diagnostic procedures are important to the advancement of health care.

Research into the performance of diagnostic procedures provides the clinician with information as to the likelihood of false positive and false negative results or conversely the degree of confidence one can place on positive and negative test results in the care of individual patients. Applying research results to the care of individual patients raises two important issues that the research consumer must consider before becoming concerned over the influence research methods on the data derived and conclusions drawn from an investigation. The research consumer must decide if the subjects enrolled in a study of diagnostic tests were sufficiently similar to patients in their care to support the generalization of the results. If for example a physical examination procedure was found useful in detecting rotator cuff disease in older men, would the same procedure be equally useful in the evaluation of young throwing athletes? Often the answers to such questions are not available and the research consumer is left to make such a judgment. In a similar vein the research consumer must ask if their training and preparation is sufficiently similar to those performing a diagnostic test in a research study. A physical examination procedure performed by a board certified orthopaedic surgeon may yield different results than the same test performed by a clinician without the specialized preparation of the surgeon (Cooperman, Riddle, & Rothstein, 1990). Once again, the answer to such a question is unlikely to be found in the research literature and it is left up to the research consumer to pass judgment on the question. If after considering the **generalizability of research findings** into one's practice the results of the paper remain of interest, the research consumer must consider the validity of the data reported. Essentially the reader must assess whether the investigators used research methods that minimized potential bias and maximized data validity.

✔ **CONCEPT CHECK**

An effectively structured physical examination will substantially increase or decrease the clinician's suspicion regarding the presence of one or more specific condition.

ASSESSING RESEARCH OF DIAGNOSTIC INSTRUMENTS

Once a sufficiently established reference standard has been identified investigational bias can be minimized through a few important, but fairly simple steps. Consumers of research into diagnostic techniques should also be familiar with the research methodology to identify when data are threatened by bias due to investigational methods.

EXAMPLE

14-Item Assessment Tool

Whiting et al. developed a 14-item assessment tool (see Table 13-1) to assist consumers in evaluating the methodologic quality of research into diagnostic tests. Scores of 10 or more are considered to reflect sound research methods.

TABLE 13-1 The QUADAS tool			
ITEM	YES	NO	UNCLEAR
1. Was the spectrum of patients representative of the patients who will receive the test in practice?	( )	( )	( )
2. Were selection criteria clearly described?	( )	( )	( )
3. Is the reference standard likely to correctly classify the target condition?	( )	( )	( )
4. Is the time period between reference standard and index test short enough to be reasonably sure that the target condition did not change between the two tests?	( )	( )	( )
5. Did the whole sample or a random selection of the sample, receive verification using a reference standard of diagnosis?	( )	( )	( )

(continued)

6. Did patients receive the same reference standard regardless of the index test result?	( )	( )	( )
7. Was the reference standard independent of the index test (i.e., the index test did not form part of the reference standard)?	( )	( )	( )
8. Was the execution of the index test described in sufficient detail to permit replication of the test?	( )	( )	( )
9. Was the execution of the reference standard described in sufficient detail to permit its replication?	( )	( )	( )
10. Were the index test results interpreted without knowledge of the results of the reference standard?	( )	( )	( )
11. Were the reference standard results interpreted without knowledge of the results of the index test?	( )	( )	( )
12. Were the same clinical data available when test results were interpreted as would be available when the test is used in practice?	( )	( )	( )
13. Were uninterpretable/intermediate test results reported?	( )	( )	( )
14. Were withdrawals from the study explained?	( )	( )	( )

Reprinted with permission from Whiting P, et al. *BMC Med Res Meth.* 2003;3:25.

Of these 14 items some assist in addressing the issue of generalization to one's practice, the quality of the reference standard, and the ability to reproduce the diagnostic test in question (items 1, 2, 3, 8, 9, and 12). Subject selection has the potential to bias results as well as influence the generalization of research findings into individual settings as discussed previously. Studies should include a spectrum of patients to whom the test in question would typically be applied in a clinical setting. Spectrum bias is introduced when only patients very likely (based on history or other criteria) to be suffering from the condition of interest are studied or when patients that clearly do not have a condition are included (Katz, 2001; Sackett et al., 1992).

Items 10 and 11 address the issue of **blinding** of assessors. Blinding of investigators performing, or interpreting, the results of the diagnostic test being investigated as well as those responsible for the results of "gold standard" assessment to each others finding is essential. If, for example, clinicians performing a drop arm test (Magee, 1997) are aware of MRI findings, their interpretation of the drop test may be biased and improve estimates of the value of the test.

(continued)

It is also important that all subjects of a research study into diagnostic tests receive all testing (items 5 to 11). If only those believed to have rotator cuff pathology, perhaps based on a drop arm test, are evaluated by MRI. The true number of false negative results will be reduced due to the study methods employed. Thus, the data are biased toward underreporting of false negative results. This form of bias is referred to as "work-up" bias. It is also important that the diagnostic test is studied and the reference test is administered in a manner that it is unlikely the condition changes between examinations (item 4).

Lastly, it is important to note that some tests may not yield useful data and not all subjects can complete all testing (items 11 and 12). Those that have struggled with integrating data acquisition systems such as electromyography, motion analysis, and force plates know that some trials do not yield useful data. Furthermore, those who suffer from claustrophobia may not tolerate being confined in an MRI unit. While generally less critical to making decisions about the use of a diagnostic procedure in one's practice, these issues become important when repeated testing may be necessary and to help identify those patients for whom a diagnostic test may be contraindicated or poorly tolerated.

✔ CONCEPT CHECK

To decrease investigational bias, blinding of investigators performing, or interpreting, the results of the diagnostic test being investigated as well as those responsible for the results of "gold standard" assessment to each others finding is essential.

STATISTICS AND INTERPRETATIONS

Research reports from studies of the performance of diagnostic tests will describe how the data were analyzed and provide estimate of the diagnostic test performance. To understand and apply the results from such studies the research consumer needs to understand the basics of the data analysis and the meaning of the values reported. The results from studies of diagnostic tests may be reported in several forms including **estimates of sensitivity and specificity, positive and negative prediction values, positive and negative likelihood ratios, or receiver operator characteristic curves**.

At first glance these terms may be new and the statistics associated with studies of diagnostic tests difficult. At this point it is important to address two issues. The first is simply that each of the above noted statistics emerge from the same foundation and require nothing more than simple multiplication and division. The second is to emphasize that the values derived are estimates of test performance. It is not possible to study the administration of a diagnostic test in all patients for whom such testing would be appropriate. Thus, researchers study samples from a population and the diagnostic testing is typically completed by one or a few clinicians. Thus, one can search the literature and find varying estimates of test performance. Larger samples are more likely to offer more accurate estimates and in some cases there are a sufficient number of studies to permit a meta-analysis (described in Chapter 18) that will yield even more precise estimates of test performance.

The foundation of the above noted statistical values was actually presented in the previous chapter. When one compares the results from a diagnostic test with a dichotomous result (positive or negative) of interest to the results of a "gold standard" diagnostic test, four subgroups or cells are formed. Table 13-2 illustrates the four cells. The values included will be used in an upcoming example so that the calculation process can be followed. From such a table sensitivity and specificity, positive and negative prediction values, and positive and negative likelihood ratios can be calculated. An expansion of the table vertically is needed to generate receiver operator characteristic curves; a topic reserved for the end of this chapter.

TABLE 13-2   Contingency table of test results used to calculate sensitivity and specificity

	GOLD STANDARD RESULT		
	POSITIVE (CONDITION PRESENT)	NEGATIVE (CONDITION ABSENT)	TOTAL
Positive examination using test under study	Cell A True positive $n = 18$	Cell B False positive $n = 3$	21
Negative examination using test under study	Cell C False negative $n = 5$	Cell D True negative $n = 12$	14
Total	23	15	35

Sensitivity $= 18/23 = 0.78$.
Specificity $= 12/15 = 0.80$.

THE BASICS—SENSITIVITY AND SPECIFICITY

Sensitivity and specificity are central concepts to understanding test performance characteristics. Sensitivity and specificity are related to the ability of a test to identify those with and without a condition and are needed to calculate likelihood ratios.

Sensitivity addresses the ability to detect an illness or specific injury confirmed (via the gold standard) to exist. In other words sensitivity is the number of illnesses or injuries that are correctly diagnosed by the clinical examination procedure being investigated (cell A) and divided by the true number of illnesses/injuries (cells A + C) (based on the criterion or gold standard measure) and is calculated as follows (Sackett et al., 1992; Fritz & Wainner, 2001):

$$\frac{\text{No. diagnosed as having a condition by clinical examination prodedure}}{\text{No. diagnosed as having a condition based upon gold standard}} = \frac{A}{A + C}$$

Consider 35 patients with knee injuries. Following assessment via an anterior drawer test 18 are correctly diagnosed as being ACL deficient. All 35 undergo arthroscopic surgery and 20 are found to have torn their ACL. From the formula above 18/23 yields a sensitivity of 0.78.

Specificity is calculated from the right side of the table and addresses the potential to rule out the presence of a condition when it is truly absent. Thus, specificity is the number of individuals correctly classified as not having the condition of concern based on the test being investigated (cell D) and divided by the true number of negative cases (cells B + D) (based on the criterion or gold standard measure).

$$\frac{\text{No. diagnosed as having a condition by clinical examination prodedure}}{\text{No. diagnosed as not having a condition by gold standard}} = \frac{D}{B + D}$$

From the previous example 15 patients did not have an ACL tear. Let's assume however, that 3 of these patients were judged to have positive anterior drawer tests, thus only 12 were correctly classified as not having injured their ACL. Thus the specificity is 12/15 or 0.8.

Ideally a diagnostic procedure would have high specificity and high sensitivity. Unfortunately many diagnostic tests lack sensitivity or specificity or both. What impact do the estimates of sensitivity and specificity have on clinical practice? The acronyms SnNOUT, a sensitive test with a negative result rules out, and SpPIN, a specific test with a positive result rules in, introduced by Sackett el al. (1992), offer the answer. SnNOUT reminds us that tests with high sensitivity are good at ruling out a condition. SpPIN is the reminder that tests with high specificity are good at ruling in a condition. At first consideration these acronyms may appear counterintuitive. However, recall that sensitivity is calculated from the left column of the table. A sensitive test is the one with relatively few false negative findings; thus, a negative examination finding effectively rules out the condition of interest. Conversely, tests with high specificity will have few false positives; thus, a positive result using a diagnostic test with high specificity has identified the target disorder.

The calculation and interpretation of sensitivity and specificity are predicated on the effort to identify individuals with and without a target disorder of interest. These values are calculated "vertically" using cells A and C or B and D, respectively. Positive and negative prediction values offer a different approach to assessing the usefulness of diagnostic tests. A positive prediction value addresses the question: if a diagnostic test is positive, what is the probability the target condition is present? Conversely, a negative prediction value provides an estimate that the target condition is not present when the diagnostic test is negative.

Since the positive and negative prediction values address the meaning of a positive or negative exam finding rather than the presence or absence of the target condition the cells used to calculate these values differ. Positive predictive values are calculated by:

$$PPV = \frac{A}{A + B}$$

Using the data from Table 13-2, PPV = 18/18 + 3 = 0.86. Thus, when an anterior draw test is positive there is an 86% chance that the ACL is torn.

Negative prediction values are calculated by:

$$NPV = \frac{D}{D + C}$$

Again using the data in Table 13-2 and referring to the previous example, NPV = 12/12 + 5 = 0.70. Thus, a negative anterior drawer test may occur in 30% of individuals with torn ACL.

A few questions and issues are starting to arise. First, it is important to point out that the data used in this example is fictitious. The sensitivity and specificity of the anterior drawer test have been estimated to be 0.62 and 0.88, respectively. Second, and more importantly, sensitivity and specificity are calculated differently than PPV and NPV. Which values are most useful to the clinician?

The answers to this question are found when one considers the prevalence of the target disorder and the application of the values into the examination of individual patients. Sackett et al. (1992) illustrated the relationship between prevalence and PPV and NPV. The PPV associated with a condition with lower prevalence will be less than the PPV of a condition with a higher prevalence. The converse is true regarding NPV: a condition with a lower prevalence will yield a higher NPV than the one with a higher prevalence. In summary as prevalence falls, PPV also fall and NPV rise (Sackett et al., 1992).

In the example above 23 of 35 patients entering the study had torn their ACL. This represents 66% of the enrolled patients, a rather high prevalence. However, if the selection criteria were athletic individuals who experienced an acute, disabling

TABLE 13-3	Contingency table of test results used to calculate sensitivity and specificity		
	GOLD STANDARD RESULT		
	POSITIVE (CONDITION PRESENT)	**NEGATIVE (CONDITION ABSENT)**	**TOTAL**
Positive examination using test under study	*Cell A* True positive $n = 18$	*Cell B* False positive $n = 30$	38
Negative examination using test under study	*Cell C* False negative $n = 5$	*Cell D* True negative $n = 120$	125
Total	23	150	153

knee injury while playing contact sports and presented with hemarthrosis, such a prevalence rate might not be surprising. To examine the effect of prevalence on the values we have calculated let's assume a prevalence rate of 6.6% instead of 66%. The values in cells A and C can remain the same, 23 ACL injured patients are included in the study. The low prevalence rate translated into many more (10 times as many in this example) patients without ACL injury. If the rate of false positive findings remains the same, a reasonable assumption, then the table would appear as Table 13-3.

The calculation of sensitivity and specificity yield the same values as before because the values are calculated vertically. (Sensitivity = $18/23$ = 0.78, Specificity = $120/150$ = 0.80.) However, the PPV = $18/(18 + 30)$ = 0.47 has fallen dramatically; NPV = $120/(120 + 5)$ = 0.96 has risen. It is difficult to interpret PPV and NPV unless the prevalence of the target condition is known or to compare values from studies with differing prevalence rates. Sensitivity and specificity values are relatively stable across a spectrum of prevalence values, one reason that they are of more use to the clinician.

While more stable estimates than PPV and NPV, values related to sensitivity and specificity are still difficult to apply in clinical practice. What does a sensitivity estimate really mean when a clinician examines a patient with an injured knee? The answer unfortunately is, not too much. Now you are left wondering why you have spent the time to read this far. PPV and NPV estimates are unstable across varying prevalence rate and sensitivity and specificity are difficult to apply. Be patient, help is on the way in the form of likelihood ratios.

> ✔ **CONCEPT CHECK**
>
> Sensitivity and specificity are related to the ability of a test to identify those with and without a condition and are needed to calculate likelihood ratios.

LIKELIHOOD RATIOS

Likelihood ratios (LRs) are values derived from estimates of sensitivity and specificity. Like sensitivity and specificity LRs offer insight into those diagnostic procedures that are generally more and less useful. However, unlike sensitivity and specificity LRs can be applied by the clinician to the examination of individual patients. Knowledge of the LRs associated with the diagnostic procedures a clinician employs will influence the level of certainty that a condition does or doesn't exist at the end of the examination.

A positive likelihood (+LR) ratio is indicative of the impact of a positive examination finding on the probability that the target condition exists. For tests with dichotomous results a +LR is calculated as follows:

$$(+)LR = \frac{Sensitivity}{1 - Specificity}$$

Using the examples above the +LR would equal $0.90/(1 - 0.8) = 3.9$ (95% CI = 1.4 − 11.0). This means that, based upon our hypothetical numbers, a positive anterior drawer is 3.9 times more likely to occur in a patient with a torn anterior cruciate than the one with an intact ligament. Further applications of LRs in the context of clinical practice will be developed later.

A negative LR addresses the impact of a negative examination on the probability that the condition in question is present. A negative result of a diagnostic test with a small likelihood ratio suggests that the chance that the target condition exists is very low. Negative likelihood is calculated as follows:

$$(-)LR = \frac{1 - Sensitivity}{Specificity}$$

Again using the values from the preceding tables the negative likelihood ratio would equal $(1 - 0.90)/0.8 = 0.28$ (95% CI = 0.12 − 0.64). In this test the examiner would find a positive anterior drawer 28/100th as often in uninjured knees as compared to injured knees. Jaeschke et al. (1994) summarized likelihood ratios (positive and negative) into broader categories of clinical value as follows:

(+LR > 10 or −LR < 0.1)	Large, often conclusive shift in probability that a condition is present
(+LR of 5–10 or −LR 0.1–0.2)	Moderate, but usually important shifts in probability that a condition is present

| (+LR of 2–5 or −LR 0.2–0.5) | Small, sometimes important shifts in probability that a condition is present |
| (+LR of 1–2 or −LR 0.5–1) | Very small, usually unimportant shifts in probability that a condition is present |

From our examples above one could conclude that for an anterior drawer test the +LR of 3.9 suggests that a positive test results in a small to moderate, but likely important, shift in the probability of a torn ACL. The −LR of 0.28 suggests that a negative test results in a small to moderate shift in probability favoring an intact ACL.

✔ CONCEPT CHECK

A positive likelihood (+LR) ratio is indicative of the impact of a positive examination finding on the probability that the target condition exists. A negative likelihood ratio addresses the impact of a negative examination on the probability that the condition in question is present.

Applications

The diagnostic test used in the examples above, like all other diagnostic procedures, is not conducted in isolation. Diagnosis is a process during which information is gathered to narrow the range of diagnostic possibilities. A carefully conducted interview and observation form the foundation of a physical examination. As the examination proceeds, a level of suspicion that a narrowing list of diagnostic possibilities is developed. Certainly one is more reporting an acute injury and presenting on crutches with a very swollen knee has torn the ACL than the one who reports a gradual onset of anterior knee pain that is made worse by prolonged sitting. Once the clinician has narrowed the diagnostic possibilities consideration is turned to the physical examination and other diagnostic assessment that may confirm or rule out specific diagnoses. Thus, the clinician has some level of concern that a specific condition exists before proceeding with additional testing.

This pretest level of suspicion can be quantified as pretest probability. Pretest probability values will vary between clinicians and the circumstances of the individual patient. The key is to recognize that a level of suspicion regarding diagnostic possibilities exists before the examination procedure of interest (e.g., anterior test) is performed. The results of diagnostic tests will change the level of suspicion of a diagnosis, but how much?

Fritz and Wainner (2001) described the relationship between "pretest probability" and likelihood ratios. Understanding this link is prerequisite to understanding the impact of diagnostic test results on "posttest probability" or the degree of certainty a condition does, or does not exist, after a clinical examination is completed.

Before demonstrating the impact of diagnostic tests with higher and lower LRs, stop and consider probability. Probability implies uncertainty. Consider how often you are absolutely, positively, certain of a diagnosis at the end of a physical examination. These events happen, of course, but not as often as most of us would like. Uncertainty is inherent in the clinical practice of athletic training. However, decisions regarding referral, plans of treatment, and a physician's use of additional diagnostic studies revolve around the level of certainty (probability) that a condition does or does not exist. The value of specific examination procedures may be best viewed in the context of their impact upon patient care decisions based on a positive or negative result.

EXAMPLE

Application of LRs on Posttest Probability of a Condition Being Present or Absent

Using the values derived above, consider the examination of a 32-year-old patient who reports "twisting their knee" while playing volleyball at a company picnic 3 days ago. The patient denies a history of injury to either knee and reports that after the injury they quit playing but were able to walk with mild discomfort. They awoke the following morning with a swollen painful knee and were evaluated in an emergency department. No fracture was identified and they were provided crutches, analgesic medications, and referred for further evaluation. From this history injury to the ACL cannot be ruled out. Let's suppose that the clinician's observation and experience suggest that 33% of the patients with similar presentation are ultimately found to have a torn ACL. The pretest probability is 33%. Probability can be converted into an odds ratio using the formula:

$$\text{Odds} = \frac{\text{Probability}}{1 - \text{Probability}}$$

Thus, in this case odds = $0.33/(1 - 0.33) = 0.33/0.66 = $ ½. Thus, the odds of the patients having a torn ACL are 2 to 1 against. Suppose when the knee is examined with an anterior drawer the result is positive. What impact does that finding have on the probability that the ACL is torn, knowing that false positive tests are possible? Posttest probability is calculated by first multiplying the pretest odds by the LR+ to yield posttest odds. Thus, the posttest odds in this case are $0.5 \times 3.9 = 1.95$. The conversion to posttest probability is made using the formula posttest probability = posttest odds/(posttest odds + 1). Continuing our example yields a posttest double of pretest probability ($1.95/2.95 = 0.66$). The result of this physical examination procedure has raised the concern that the patient has suffered an ACL tear.

The clinician has more information, but what should be done to manage the patient? The clinician has three options. The first is to abandon the target disorder as the cause of the signs and symptoms that the patient presents with and search for

(continued)

alternative answers. The second option is to pursue additional testing. Lastly, the clinician can accept the diagnosis of the target disorder and address treatment options with the patient. The first option is selected when the likelihood of the target disorder is very low. Take for example an athlete complaining of ankle pain following an inversion mechanism injury. The athlete is able to weight bear into the clinic although there is a noticeable limp. Upon palpation there is no tenderness in the distal 6 cm of the lateral malleolus, nor tenderness over the tarsal navicular or base of the fifth metatarsal. The literature suggests that the prevalence of fractures following inversion ankle injuries is about 15%. The – LR of the Ottawa Ankle Rules has been estimated at 0.08. If the 15% prevalence is used as the pretest odds $(0.015/1 - 0.015 = 0.176)$ the odds following application of the Ottawa Ankle Rules $= 0.176 \times 0.08 = 0.014$. Thus, there is only a 1.4% (posttest probability $= 0.014/1.014$) chance of a fracture of clinical significance. In this case the clinician abandons the target disorder of fracture as the problem and seeks alternative diagnoses.

At the other end of the spectrum let's consider a truck driver who landed awkwardly when he slipped while exiting the truck cab. He states his knee twisted and he heard a loud pop. On initial evaluation a Lachman test was positive and a large hemarthrosis developed within a few hours. The history and the development of the hemarthrosis causes the clinician to estimate a 70% probability (pretest odds $0.7/1 - 0.7 = 2.33$) of a tear of the anterior cruciate. Using a +LR of 9.6 for the Lachman Test, posttest odds $= 2.33 \times 9.6 = 22.4$. Thus, the posttest probability $= 22.4/23.4 = 96\%$. While further diagnostic testing may be warranted to identify collateral damage to the menisci and other structures, a plan of care should be developed for this ACL deficient knee.

The preceding examples lie at the comfortable end of the diagnostic spectrum, first because of the high degree of certainty that exists and second because the consequences of the rare missed diagnoses (a treatable fracture of the ankle and an intact ACL) are likely fairly minor. A treatable ankle fracture will likely be detected upon follow-up and the intact ACL will likely be confirmed before beginning a surgical procedure. How does the clinician manage the patient in the middle where after a diagnostic work-up a fair degree of uncertainty remains?

This is a difficult decision. To begin with what is a "fair degree" of uncertainty? In general the more serious the consequences of being wrong the broader our definition of uncertainty. At this point the clinician really has only two options, perform additional testing or refer to a provider better prepared to evaluate the patient. Additional testing (e.g., MRI) is indicated when a "fair degree" of uncertainty exists. Such additional assessment should be taken in the context of the diagnostic process. For example, the posttest probability of 75%, following a Lachman test, is really the pretest probability for MRI. The LR+ for MRI assessment of anterior cruciate tears has been estimated at 21.5 (Vaz et al., 2005). These values (pretest odds $= 0.75/1 - 0.75 = 3$) yield posttest odds of 64.5/1 or a probability of 98%. Once again the probability of an ACL tear leaves the clinician in a position to accept the diagnosis and move on to discussion of treatment option. Before we move forward, however, please appreciate even with advanced technology such as MRI complete certainty is not achieved.

✔ CONCEPT CHECK

Pretest probability, LR and test result will yield a posttest probability. Posttets probability can be quickly estimated with a nomogram.
NOTE: Refer to suggested readings for example illustrations of the nomogram.

Receiver Operator Characteristic Curves

Receiver-operator characteristic curves (ROCcs) have multiple applications in data management including the assessment of diagnostic procedures where data from a procedure of interest are on a continuum rather than dichotomous (positive or negative). Laboratory testing often involves such diagnostic measures and Sackett et al. (1992) offer an excellent explanation of the use of ROCc using serum creatine kinase measures in patients with chest pain to identify those with myocardial infarction.

While ROCcs look different they are really an extension of the sensitivity, specificity, and likelihood ratios. The following example illustrates the process with a small twist. Ruotolo et al. reported that a loss of internal glenohumeral rotation poses a risk of shoulder pain in college baseball pitchers. At what point does the degree of loss of motion become a concern? Or in other words, at what point does the diagnosis of restricted internal rotation warrantintervention? The answers to this question are found when one considers the prevalence of the target disorder and the application of the values into the examination of individual patients. Sackett et al. (1992) illustrated the relationship between prevalence and PPV and NPV. The PPV associated with a condition with lower prevalence will be less than the PPV of a condition with a higher prevalence. The converse is true regarding NPV: a condition with a lower prevalence will yield a higher NPV than the one with a higher prevalence. In summary as prevalence falls, PPV also fall and NPV rise (Sackett et al., 1992). In the example above 23 of 35 patients entering the study had torn their ACL.

EXAMPLE

ROCcs

To illustrate the process a fictitious data set (Table 13-4) has been developed to consider. Preseason evaluation of 200 college pitchers reveals the following about the differences in internal rotation between the dominant and nondominant arms.

(continued)

TABLE 13-4	Table of fictitious data set		
NUMBER OF PLAYERS	MOTION RESTRICTION	INCIDENCE RATE OF SHOULDER PAIN	NUMBER WITH SHOULDER PAIN
45	<5 degrees	11%	5
40	5–10 degrees	17.5%	7
55	10.1–15 degrees	49.1%	27
40	15.1–20 degrees	67.5%	27
20	>20 degrees	90%	18

The ROCc (Table 13-5) is developed from the sensitivity and specificity estimates at each "level" by creating five A, B, C and, D plots. Plotting sensitivity and specificity reveals the associated ROCc Figure 13-1. In general the point nearest the upper left corner "northwest is best" identifies the best balance between sensitivity and specificity. In this case intervening to improve internal shoulder rotation in players with greater than 10 degree side-to-side differences offers the best opportunity to reduce risk (LR+ = 2.3 for 10+ degrees or more loss). Those with less than a 10 degree side-to-side difference are lower risk (LR+ = 1.4) which may allow for attention to be directed at those with high risk.

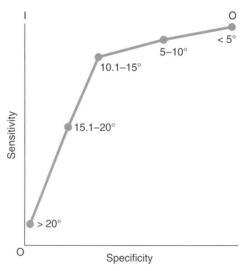

FIGURE 13-1 Receiver operator characteristic curve identifying 10 degrees (northwest corner) as a cutoff where intervention to improve internal shoulder range of motion is most likely to benefit.

(continued)

Table 13-5   Table of ROCcs developed from sensitivity and specificity estimates for shoulder pain

		SHOULDER PAIN	
		PRESENT	**ABSENT**
≳ Motion Restriction	≥20 degrees	18	2
	15.1–20 degrees	27	13
	10.1–15 degrees	27	28
	5–10 degrees	7	33
	<5 degrees	5	40
>20 degrees	18 a	2 c	
	66 b	114 d	

Sensitivity = a/a + c = 18/84   Specificity = d/b + d = 144/116 = 0.98
= 0.21
a, b, c, and d cells identified—same structure is used for all calculations

15.1–20 degrees	45	15
	59	91

Sensitivity = a/a + c = 45/84   Specificity = d/b + d = 91/116 = 0.78
= 0.54

10.1–15 degrees	72	43
	12	73

Sensitivity = a/a + c = 72/84   Specificity = d/b + d = 73/116 = 0.63
= 0.86

5–10 degrees	79	76
	5	40

Sensitivity = a/a + c = 79/84   Specificity = d/b + d = 40/116 = 0.34
= 0.94

<5 degrees	84	116
	0	0

Sensitivity = a/a + c = 84/84   Specificity = d/b + d = 0/116 = 0.0
= 1.00

Although less commonly cited in the clinical literature than measures of specificity, sensitivity, or likelihood ratios, ROCcs allow for the identification of critical points along continuous measures to guide clinical practice. ROCcs can also be applied to the analysis of clusters of diagnostic or prognostic criteria. These applications were discussed in detail in previous chapters in Part II.

CHAPTER SUMMARY

The principal purpose of this chapter was to provide the reader with an understanding of the research methods and statistical techniques used to assess how well diagnostic tests perform in clinical practice. Investigators need to strive to implement research methods that minimize the risk of biasing their data. Consumers of the research literature must be able to assess the quality of the research methods employed in the studies they read to permit critical analysis prior to applying research findings to their clinical practices.

There are multiple measures of diagnostic performance including sensitivity and specificity, positive and negative prediction values, positive and negative likelihood ratios, and receiver operator characteristic curves. For the reasons discussed in the chapter likelihood ratios provide the most stable and clinically useful estimates of a performance of tests with dichotomous outcomes. A receiver operator characteristic curve provides clinicians information about tests that generate measures on a continuous scale such as blood pressure, range of motion, and serum enzyme levels. There are multiple applications of receiver operator characteristic curves beyond investigation of diagnostic techniques. However, the basic principles of curve generation always apply and thus can be generalized across research disciplines.

KEY POINTS

- Diagnostic testing should be used as an aid instead of a crutch for a clinician.
- History and observation should help greatly in narrowing the scope of possible injuries during the evaluation process.
- Diagnostic tests have limitations.
- An effectively structured physical examination will substantially increase or decrease the clinician's suspicion regarding the presences of one or more specific conditions.
- The only way to find answers to clinical questions is through clinical trials.
- Special tests will not always deliver a clear-cut decision.
- The amount of confidence a clinician has in assessment results determines the likelihood of a correct diagnosis.
- Clinical research must be sorted through because of all the varying results in the data.
- Comparing the clinical study with the current standard is important in research.
- Statistics are crucial to research methods because they provide numerical evidence that can be ranked to form valid conclusions.

Critical Thinking Questions

1. Why are the Ottawa Ankle Rules beneficial?
2. How can a clinician select the best diagnostic tests?
3. How are results from diagnostic tests reported?
4. What are two negatives to diagnostic testing?
5. Which are more valid and reliable, sensitivity and specificity values or PPV and NPV?

Applying Concepts

1. Is it possible to have a positive test in someone without the target condition?
2. How can this information be applied in my practice and teaching?

REFERENCES

Bachmann LM, Kolb E, Koller MT, et al. Accuracy of Ottawa Ankle rules to exclude fractures of the ankle and mid-foot: systematic review. *BMJ* 2003;326:417.

Cooperman JM, Riddle DL, Rothstein JM. Reliability and validity of judgments of the integrity of the anterior cruciate ligament of the knee using the Lachman test. *Phys Ther.* 1990;70:225–233,

Ernst CW, Stadnik TW, Peeters E, et al. Prevalence of annular tears and disc herniations on MR images of the cervical spine in symptom free volunteers. *Eur J Radiol.* 2005;55:409–414. Epub 2005 Jan 1.

Fritz JM, Wainner RS. Examining diagnostic tests: an evidence based perspective. *Phys Ther.* 2001;81:1546–1564.

Grane P. The postoperative lumbar spine. A radiological investigation of the lumbar spine after discectomy using MR imaging and CT. *Acta Radiol Suppl.* 1998;414:1–23.

Jaeschke R, Guyatt JH, Sackett DL. User's guide to the medical literature, III: how to use an article about a diagnostic test. B: what are the results and will they help me in caring for my patients? The Evidence-Based Medicine Working Group. *JAMA.* 1994;271:703–707.

Katz DL. *Clinical Epidemiology and Evidence-Based Medicine.* Thousand Oaks, CA: Sage Publications; 2001:41.

Magee DJ. *Orthopedic Physical Assessment.* 3rd ed. Philadelphia, PA: W.B Saunders; 1997:560–572.

Sackett DL, Haynes RB, Guyatt GH, et al. *Clinical Epidemiology: A Basic Science for Clinical Medicine.* 2nd ed. Boston MA: Little, Brown & Co; 1992.

Stiell IG, Greenberg GH, McKnight RD, et al. A study to develop clinical decision rules for the use of radiography in acute ankle injuries. *Ann Emerg Med.* 1992;21:384–390.

Torg JS, Conrad W, Kalen V. Clinical diagnosis of anterior cruciate ligament instability in the athlete. *Am J Sports Med.* 1976;4:84–93.

Vaz CE, Camargo OP, Santiago PJ, et al. Accuracy of magnetic resonance in identifying traumatic intraarticular knee lesions. *Clinics.* 2005;60:445–450.

Volpi D, Olivetti L, Budassi P, et al. Capsulo-labro-ligamentous lesions of the shoulder: evaluation with MR arthrography. *Radiol Med (Torino).* 2003;105:162–170.

Whiting P, Rutjes AW, Reitsma JB, et al. The development of QUADAS: A tool for the quality assessment of studies of diagnositc accuracy included in systematic review. *BMC Med Res Meth.* 2003;3:25.

SUGGESTED READING

Myers JB, Laudner KG, Pasquale MR, et al. Glenohumeral range of motion deficits and posterior shoulder tightness in throwers with pathologic internal impingement. *Am J Sports Med.* 2006;34:385–391.

Ruotolo C, Price E, Panchal A. Loss of total arc of motion in collegiate baseball players. *J Shoulder Elbow Surg.* 2006;15:67–71.

CHAPTER 14

SCREENING AND PREVENTION OF ILLNESS AND INJURIES: RESEARCH METHODS AND DATA ANALYSIS

It's clear that prevention will never be sufficient.

—*Luc Montagnier, from Luc Montagnier*
Quotes as quoted in BrainyQuote
(www.brainyquote.com/quotes/l/lucmontagn339337.html)

CHAPTER OBJECTIVES

After reading this chapter, you will:

- Understand the concept of injury prevention.
- Be able to discuss the principles of injury risk identification and prevention research design based on the tenets of clinical epidemiology.
- Be able to explain why risk identification and injury prevention are concepts often linked to each other.
- Understand why prospective study designs yield much more robust information about injury risk factors than retrospective study designs.
- Understand that randomized-controlled trials are the hallmark of injury prevention research design.
- Explain how randomized-controlled trials provide higher levels of evidence than retrospective or nonrandomized designs.

- Understand that the limitations of case control designs must be emphasized when discussing the results of case control studies.
- Understand that risk factor studies and screening studies share similar characteristics.
- Explain why the issue of injury definition can be more problematic in retrospective studies as opposed to prospective studies.

KEY TERMS

etiology	prevalence	prospective
incidence	prevalence ratio	relative risk
injury rate	prevention	retrospective

INTRODUCTION

Injury **prevention** is often touted as one of the hallmarks of the clinical practice of sports medicine and occupational medicine; however, there is a remarkable dearth of research literature in this area. Risk identification and injury prevention are concepts that are often linked to each other. It is logical to assume that before injury prevention initiatives are implemented, the factors most likely to predict specific injuries in particular populations should first be well understood. Unfortunately, this is not often the case as injury prevention initiatives are often initiated before proven risks and predispositions are identified in a scientific fashion.

The principles of injury risk identification and prevention research design are based on the tenets of clinical epidemiology. **Prospective** study designs yield much more robust information about injury risk factors than **retrospective** study designs. Similarly, randomized-controlled trials are the hallmark of injury prevention research design providing higher levels of evidence than retrospective or nonrandomized designs.

MODEL OF INJURY PREVENTION

Participation in exercise and sports yields considerable physical and mental health benefits for individuals of all ages. Unfortunately, the risk of musculoskeletal injury and to a lesser extent other medical conditions is inherent to participation in exercise and sport. Bahr and colleagues have established a four-stage injury prevention paradigm that is useful from both theoretical and practical perspectives (see Figure 14-1).

The first step in this paradigm is to establish the extent of the injury problem. While this step often comes from anecdotal observations (i.e., a coach noting an increase in hamstring strains during the current season), establishing the extent of

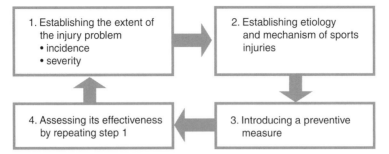

FIGURE 14-1 Framework of risk identification and injury prevention. (Reprinted with permission from Bahr R, Kannus P, van Mechelen W. Epidemiology and sports injury prevention. In: Kjaer M, Krogsgaard M, Magnusson P, et al., eds. *Textbook of Sports Medicine: Basic Science and Clinical Aspects of Sports Injury and Physical Activity.* Malden, MA: Blackwell Science Ltd; 2003.)

an injury is ideally done through prospective injury surveillance. The best example of this is the Injury Surveillance System utilized by the National Collegiate Athletic Association (Agel et al., 2007). In this system, certified athletic trainers from representative schools that offer each sport report the details of all sports-related injuries as well as the number of athletes participating in all practices in games. The tracking of injuries as well as exposures (participation in practices or games) allows for the estimation of not only the number of injuries incurred by athletes participating in a particular sport but also the rate of injuries per unit of exposure and the overall risk of participating athletes of being injured.

The second step in this paradigm is to establish the **etiology** and mechanisms of the sports-related injuries. The cause of a sports injury may be traumatic or atraumatic. In the case of traumatic injuries documenting the source of trauma is important. For example, determining whether a particular traumatic injury is typically caused by an athlete being struck with a ball, with an implement such as a bat, or from contact (legal or illegal) with an opposing player will provide considerably different potential injury prevention solutions. Identifying the mechanism of injury is normally done through purely observational research. In contrast, identifying risk factors that may be involved in the etiology of a specific injury may require the collection of baseline data as an assessment of potential risk factors followed by a prolonged period of injury surveillance. An example of this is that high-school soccer and basketball players who have poor balance are at an increased risk of suffering acute ankle sprains (McGuine & Keene, 2006).

The third step in the injury prevention paradigm is to introduce a preventative measure. Care must be taken when selecting the preventative measures to be implemented. The intervention should be based on the information gained in the first two steps of the paradigm. For example, if a large number of field hockey players were observed to be suffering eye injuries due to being struck in the face with the ball, an intervention of mandatory eye protection may be an appropriate injury prevention initiative to attempt. Conversely, if numerous soccer players were suffering leg and knee injuries due to hard tackles from behind by their opponents, an intervention of more strict enforcement of penalties for illegal tackles may be appropriate. Lastly, if specific biomechanical or physiological factors have been shown to increase injury risk (i.e., poor balance), injury prevention that addresses such deficits (i.e., balance training) may be warranted. One of the biggest challenges in injury prevention research is to avoid the use of the "shotgun approach" of injury prevention. For example, if an experimental injury prevention program is implemented that includes numerous interventions (i.e., dynamic warm-up, flexibility exercises, balance training, strength training, and plyometrics) and that program is shown to prevent injuries, researchers and clinicians are left not knowing which aspect(s) of the intervention actually caused the reduction in injuries. For this reason, the implementation of injury prevention programs that contain single intervention strategies (i.e., flexibility exercises) is strongly encouraged.

The fourth and final step of the injury prevention paradigm is to reassess the extent of the injury problem after the implementation of the injury prevention intervention. If the **incidence** and severity of injuries has been substantially reduced, the permanent implementation of the intervention is likely warranted. In contrast, if the intervention is unsuccessful, then its use should not be retained.

CONCEPT CHECK

The steps in the Bahr et al. (2002) paradigm are:

1. To establish the extent of the injury problem;
2. To establish the etiology and mechanisms of the sports-related injuries;
3. To introduce a preventative measure; and
4. To reassess the extent of the injury problem after the implementation of the injury prevention intervention.

By repeating the steps of the paradigm, it may become apparent that particular athletes (either certain position players or those who have specific physiological or biomechanical profiles) are, in fact, at greater risk of certain injuries and that they would benefit most from targeted injury prevention programs.

RISK IDENTIFICATION: RESEARCH DESIGN ISSUES

The design of studies of injury risk factors may be of either a prospective or retrospective nature with prospective designs being preferred. There are several factors that are important to designing these types of studies including, but not limited

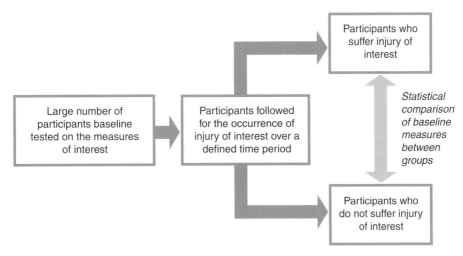

FIGURE 14-2   Flow chart of the design of a prospective study of injury risk factors.

to, adequate sample size, clear definition of injury with specific diagnostic criteria, and the determination of a representative comparison group.

Prospective Designs

A prospective cohort design is the gold standard for studies of injury risk factors (see Figure 14-2). A large group of participants who are potentially "at risk" for suffering the injury of interest are baseline tested on a number of measures that represent potential risk factors. These participants are subsequently followed over time to determine whether or not they go on to suffer the injury of interest. Statistical comparisons of the potential risk factors are then made between participants who were injured and those who did not suffer injury. These results allow for the most robust determination of injury risk factors.

Determining an appropriate sample size is a critical step in designing a prospective study of injury risk factors. The use of injury surveillance data is very useful in determining sample size. Please refer to the following examples.

EXAMPLE

ACL Injuries

While considerable attention is paid to anterior cruciate ligament (ACL) injuries in female athletes participating in sports such as basketball, the incidence rate of these injuries has been reported as 0.23 per 1000 athlete-exposures (one athlete-

(continued)

exposure equals participation in one practice or game) (Agel et al., 2007). Thus, we could expect an ACL injury to occur in a female collegiate basketball player for every 4000 athlete-exposures. To put this into perspective, consider that the typical NCAA division I women's basketball player participates in an average of 27 games and 89 practices per year for a total of 116 athlete-exposures per year. Assuming that each team has 12 players in each game or practice, a team can expect to generate 1392 athlete-exposures per year. Accordingly, at least three teams would have to be followed during a single season to expect one ACL injury. Alternatively, the same team could be followed for 3 years with the expectation of a single ACL injury occurring.

It becomes obvious that in order to generate a substantial number of women's basketball players who sustain ACL injuries, a very large number of participants would need to be baseline tested and followed for subsequent injuries. For example, if an a priori power analysis indicated that 30 injured subjects were required, an estimated total of 130,435 athlete-exposures would be required to obtain 30 ACL injuries at the reported rate of 0.23 injuries per 1000 athlete-exposures. With each team having an average of 1392 athlete-exposures per season, in order to obtain a total of 130,435 athlete-exposures, researchers would need to baseline test and follow 93.7 teams in a single season if they hoped to have 30 ACL-injured participants. Alternatively, they could test and follow 46.9 teams over 2 years, 31.2 teams over 3 years, or 18.7 teams over 5 years. These calculations are designed to put the large scale of prospective risk factor studies into focus.

Ankle Sprains

As another example of sample size estimation for prospective risk factor studies, let's use ankle sprains, a more commonly occurring injury in women's basketball. The incidence rate for ankle sprains has been reported to be 1.89 per 1000 athlete-exposures (Agel et al., 2007). Again, assume that an a priori power analysis estimates that 30 participants suffering ankle sprains are necessary to adequately power the study. An estimated total of 15,873 athlete-exposures would be required to obtain 30 ankle sprains at the reported rate of 1.89 injuries per 1000 athlete-exposures. With each team having an average of 1392 athlete-exposures per season, in order to obtain a total of 15,873 athlete-exposures, researchers would need to baseline test and follow 11.4 teams in a single season if they hoped to have 30 ankle sprain–injured participants. Alternatively, they could test and follow 5.7 teams over 2 years, 3.8 teams over 3 years, or 2.3 teams over 5 years.

As these examples show, the incidence rate of the injury being studied greatly influences the estimation of the number of participants that need to be baseline tested in prospective studies of injury risk.

With a prospective study of injury risk, the definition of the injury of interest can be tightly controlled. For example, confirmation of injuries such as fractures or ligament sprains can be performed using diagnostic imaging such as x-ray or MRI, respectively. Alternatively, specific criteria can be established for physical examination criteria to be used by all participating clinicians. These are issues that must be established during the design of the study rather than during the injury surveillance period of the study.

Choosing the representative comparison group for those subjects who suffer injuries is an important consideration in the design of prospective injury risk factor studies. The preferred method is to compare the baseline measures of the injured cohort to the uninjured cohort (all of the subjects who did not suffer injuries). Alternatively, some researchers will "match" each subject in the injured cohort with a comparable subject from the uninjured cohort. The matching is typically made on anthropomorphic characteristics such as sex, age, height, and mass, but will often include sport-specific factors such as position and participation time as well. The use of "matched" controls is open to the bias of the investigators in making these decisions. The comparison of the injured cohort to the entire uninjured cohort is thus the preferred method.

✔ CONCEPT CHECK

The incidence rate of the injury being studied greatly influences the estimation of the number of participants that need to be baseline tested in prospective studies of injury risk.

Screening Studies

Prospective studies for risk factors may also be described as "screening" studies. In sports medicine and occupational medicine it is very common for athletes and workers to receive a physical exam before they are allowed to participate in organized athletics or before they are hired for specific jobs. Essentially, clinicians are trying to identify risk factors or "screen" these individuals for particular injuries or diseases. Risk factor studies and screening studies share similar characteristics.

EXAMPLE

Sudden Cardiac Death

An example of a common screening procedure in sports medicine is risk of sudden cardiac death. Obviously, sudden cardiac death in any athlete is a catastrophic event and whenever a young, seemingly healthy individual dies during exercise it is

(continued)

typically seen as a preventable event. In an effort to identify potential athletes who may be at risk of sudden cardiac death, preparticipation physicals often involve electrocardiography (EKC) and echocardiography in addition to physical examination by a physician. The efficacy of the more expensive echocardiography testing, however, has been questioned through controlled study (Basavarajaiah et al., 2008).

In a study of over 3500 elite athletes in the United Kingdom, the **prevalence** of hypertrophic cardiomyopathy, the most common cause of sudden cardiac death, was found to be only 1.5% ($n = 53$) (Basavarajaiah et al., 2008). Of these 53 athletes identified with hypertrophic cardiomyopathy (HMC) via echocardiography, only 3 were found to be at greater risk of sudden cardiac death with more intensive testing. The authors conclude that echocardiography is thus not a cost-effective screening procedure for risk of sudden cardiac death because the prevalence of the most common predisposing condition is so low. While this clinical issue continues to be under debate by clinicians and scientists, this example illustrates the challenges associated with the magnitude of screening studies.

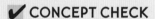

✔ CONCEPT CHECK

Prospective studies for risk factors may also be described as "screening" studies.

Retrospective Designs

Studies of injury risk factors are sometimes performed using a case control design (see Figure 14-3). Case control studies are by definition retrospective in nature and are sometimes called ex post facto (literally, after the fact) designs. In this case,

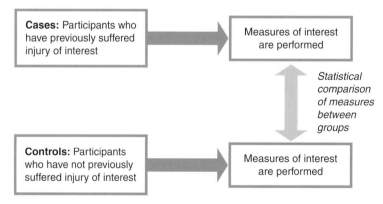

FIGURE 14-3   Flow chart of a case control study. By definition, all case control studies utilize a retrospective design.

individuals who already have suffered the injury of interest are compared to a control group that has not suffered the injury of interest. Each "case" subject who has suffered the injury of interest is assigned a matched "control" subject who has not suffered the injury of interest, hence the use of the term "case control" study design.

✔ CONCEPT CHECK

Studies of injury risk factors are sometimes performed using a case control design. Case control studies are by definition retrospective in nature and are sometimes called ex post facto (literally, after the fact) designs.

The most obvious advantage of the case control design over the prospective cohort design is that the number of subjects required for testing is dramatically lower. If we again use our example of risk factors to ACL injuries among women's collegiate basketball players and assume that our power analysis provides a recommended sample size estimate of 30 subjects per group, we find that in order to obtain our 30 ACL-injured players we simply have to recruit 30 female collegiate basketball players who have previously injured their ACL and 30 matched controls who have not injured their ACL; this is in comparison to the prospect of having to baseline test and follow all of the participants of over 90 women's basketball players over a single season in order to generate 30 ACL-injured participants using the prospective design. The retrospective design does, however, have a serious limitation in comparison to the prospective design. Because the measures of "risk factors" are being taken after the injury of interest has occurred, there is no way to know if these measures were present before the injury occurred (truly being a risk factor) or if the current measure is a result of being an adaptation to the injury that developed after the onset of injury. The importance of this limitation has led some to recommend that the term "injury risk factor" should never be used when describing the results of a study that utilized a case control design.

This limitation, however, does not mean that case control designs should never be used. First, the results of a case control study of potential risk factors to the injury of interest can provide pilot data that is very helpful in identifying what potential risk factors should be measured when designing a prospective study. Second, some injuries are very rare (i.e., they have a very low incidence rate) and performing a prospective study of risk factors to this injury may not be feasible. Even in such situations, however, the limitations of case control designs must be emphasized when discussing the results of case control studies; and, thus, the results must be put into their proper context.

The issue of injury definition can be more problematic in retrospective studies as opposed to prospective studies. Ideally, injury confirmation can be obtained using imaging methods or strict diagnostic criteria that can be derived from participants' medical records. The reality is, however, that many case control studies rely on patient self-report for their injury history. This may work for some major injuries, such as an ACL tear, where individuals are likely to truly know whether or not they have been diagnosed with this injury; but may be more problematic for an injury such as an ankle sprain that may be quite difficult to operationally define for a lay person. Care must be taken in the design of case control studies to assure tight control over inclusion criteria for the "case" group.

✔ CONCEPT CHECK

The issue of injury definition can be more problematic in retrospective studies as opposed to prospective studies.

The matching of "control" subjects to the "case" subjects is another important consideration in the study design. The matching is typically made on anthropomorphic characteristics such as sex, age, height, and mass, but will often include sport-specific factors such as position and participation time as well. The limitation of this method is that the choice of "matched" controls is open to the bias of the investigators in making these decisions. Care must be taken to avoid any bias when determining subject selection.

ESTIMATING INJURY RATES AND RISKS

The estimation of **injury rates** and risks is accomplished through injury surveillance systems. Doing this, however, is not as simple as just counting the number of injuries that occur or the number of injured people. There are several important nuances to understand in the determination of the number of injuries or injured people within a given sample of interest. These include understanding the difference between injury incidence and prevalence, injury rates and risks, and specifications of how injuries are defined.

The *prevalence* of an injury or illness is defined as the proportion of a sample that has a given injury or illness at a single time point. The prevalence may be presented as either a proportion or a percentage. The prevalence expressed as a percentage may be expressed by the formula:

$$\text{Prevalence} = \left(\frac{\text{No. of injured subjects}}{\text{No. of total subjects}} \right) \times 100$$

For example, if there are 100 athletes on a middle school girls track team and 15 of these athletes are currently injured, the prevalence of injury is 15%. Note that prevalence provides estimates of injury or illness occurrence at one snapshot in time. It does not provide any indication to how many injuries have previously occurred or how many injuries will occur in the future. The prevalence of an injury or illness may fluctuate at different time points. With some occupations or athletes, more individuals may suffer injuries during different seasons of the year or points in an athletic season. For example, in northern climates work-related injuries may increase for laborers who work outdoors during the winter because of the increased likelihood of injury causing falls due to ice-covered ground or sidewalks. Likewise in competitive athletes, overuse injuries may be more common early in competitive seasons when the greatest change in training volume is likely to have occurred. Prevalence is an estimate of the number of injured or ill individuals in comparison to the entire sample at risk at a given time point.

The *incidence* of an injury or illness refers to the number of new cases of the pathology in a given period of time. To establish the incidence of pathology, a surveillance system must be in place to record the number of new cases. This requires a prospective study design. For example in sports medicine, the number of athletes who suffer ankle sprains during a full season of competitive basketball may be of interest. To calculate the incidence of ankle sprains during a season, participating athletes must be monitored for the occurrence of new ankle sprains for the entire length of the season. If in one collegiate conference there are 10 basketball teams each with 15 players, and 8 of them suffer new ankle sprains during the course of a season, the incidence may be calculated as 15 newly injured players out of a population at risk of 150 players, or 10%.

✔ CONCEPT CHECK

Prevalence is an estimate of the number of injured or ill individuals in comparison to the entire sample at risk at a given time point. Incidence refers to the number of new cases of the pathology in a given period of time.

The incidence of an injury or illness may be expressed in several different manners. The *incidence proportion* represents the number of newly injured individuals in a defined population over a given period of time. This is expressed with the formula:

$$\text{Incidence Proportion} = \left(\frac{\text{No. of newly injured subjects}}{\text{No. of total subjects participating}} \right)$$

The number of athletes suffering ankle sprains during a basketball season described in the previous paragraph is an example of an incidence proportion. With incidence proportion, an individual either sustains an injury or illness or they do not. There is no way of accounting for multiple injuries in the same individual over the course of time when using incidence proportion.

Incidence rate is defined as the number of new cases that occur per unit of person-time at risk. In order to calculate incidence rate, the amount of time that each individual is exposed to injury or illness risk must be calculated. For example in sports, this may be determined by quantifying the number of hours (or games or practices) that an individual athlete participates during a defined period of time. In occupational medicine, the total number of days (or hours) worked during a defined period of time may be quantified. Importantly, the use of incidence rate also allows for the tabulation of multiple new injuries or illnesses among the same individual over the defined time period. For example, a basketball player may suffer an ankle sprain to their right limb in the first week of the season and a sprain to their left ankle in the last week of the season. When using incidence proportion, this individual would only be counted once; however, with incidence rate, both new injuries could be expressed. Incidence rate can be expressed with the formula:

$$\text{Incidence Rate} = \left(\frac{\text{No. of new injuries}}{\text{Total exposure time}} \right)$$

While the terms "injury risk" and "injury rate" may seem interchangeable, understanding the difference between injury *risk* and *rate* is a very important concept. *Injury risk* refers specifically to the probability of new injury per individual. The numerator of injury risk is the number of individuals suffering a new injury in a given period of time, while the denominator is the total number of individual exposed to risk of injury over that given period of time. The incidence proportion described above is an example of injury risk.

Alternatively, *injury rate* specifically refers to the number of new injuries per unit of exposure time. The numerator for injury rate is the number of new injuries and the denominator is the total number of person-time at risk of all individuals at risk. The *incidence rate* described above is an example of injury rate.

The estimation of the amount of exposure to risk of injury or illness that each individual has is very important. For risk of chronic diseases such as pancreatic cancer, the amount of exposure would typically be expressed as person-years. Because each individual is under constant, albeit relatively low, risk for developing this disease over their lifespan every year they live is considered a unit of exposure. In occupational medicine, every day (or hour) that a worker performs their job is considered a unit of exposure. In athletics, the unit of exposure may be defined in ways such as player-seasons, hours (or minutes) of sport participation, or most commonly as an "athlete-exposure." An athlete-exposure refers to one athlete participating in one practice or game.

Lastly, the definition of an injury or illness to be counted must be clearly defined. In diseases such as type II diabetes or emphysema, specific diagnostic criteria are typically clearly established in the medical literature. Definitions of some musculoskeletal injuries, however, may not be so easily defined. In sports medicine and occupational medicine, the definition of "time loss" and "non–time loss" injuries must be considered. A *time loss injury* refers to an injury that forces a worker to miss work or an athlete to not participate in their sport, whereas a *non–time loss injury* refers to an injury requiring medical care but the worker or athlete is able to continue with their regular participation in work or sport.

✔ **CONCEPT CHECK**

With incidence proportion, an individual either sustains an injury or illness or they do not. There is no way of accounting for multiple injuries in the same individual over the course of time when using incidence proportion.

STATISTICAL ANALYSIS

There are several statistical analyses that are important to understand when designing, executing, and interpreting screening and prevention studies. These include concepts such as risk ratios, rate ratios, **relative risk** reduction, absolute risk reduction, numbers needed to treat, and odds ratios.

The simplest comparison between two measures of injury incidence is to calculate the ratio of the injury incidence between two groups. If the ratio of the injury prevalence estimates between two groups is taken, this is referred to as the *prevalence ratio*. If the ratio of injury risk estimates between two groups is calculated, this is referred to as the *risk ratio*. Lastly, if the ratio of the injury rate estimates between two groups is determined, this is termed the *rate ratio*. As with most epidemiologic statistics, the point estimate must be evaluated along with its 95% confidence interval. The key cutline for determining the efficacy of treatment (or increased risk) for ratio estimates is whether or not the confidence interval crosses the 1.0 line on the log scale (see Figure 14-4).

When assessing injury risks or rates between two groups, another simple method of comparison is the calculation of the relative risk of injury between the two groups. *Relative risk* (RR) is simply calculated by dividing the injury rate in the intervention group by the injury rate in the control group. (It must be noted that either injury rates or injury risks may be used to calculate relative risk and the other statistics in this chapter.) *Relative risk* simply provides a proportion of injury incidence between two groups and is identical to the calculation of risk ratio (or rate ratio).

Unfortunately, comprehension of this calculation is not necessarily intuitive.

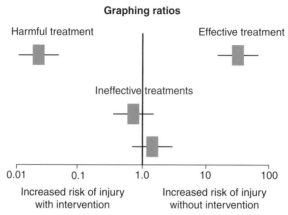

FIGURE 14-4   Interpretation of odds ratio point estimates and confidence intervals. Note the log scale.

A statistic that is more easily understood is the *relative risk reduction* (RRR). This is calculated by simply taking 1 minus the relative risk and multiplying by 100. Relative risk reduction represents the percentage that the experimental condition reduces injury risk compared to the control condition. If the experimental condition is found to lead to heightened risk of injury, rather than expressing the relative risk reduction as a negative number, the sign is changed to positive and this value is termed the *relative risk increase* (RRI). As with most epidemiologic statistics, the point estimate must be evaluated along with its 95% confidence interval. The key cutline for determining the efficacy of treatment for RRR is whether or not the confidence interval crosses the zero line (see Figure 14-5).

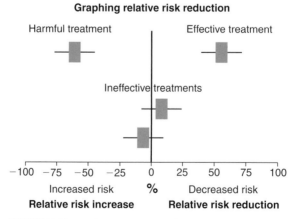

FIGURE 14-5   Interpretation of relative risk reduction point estimates and confidence intervals.

Another common statistic to compare the efficacy of a prevention intervention is the *absolute risk reduction* (ARR). The absolute risk reduction is the arithmetic difference between the injury rate (or risk) in the intervention group and the injury rate (or risk) in the control group. The control group incidence is always subtracted from the intervention group incidence. If converted to a percentage, the absolute risk reduction indicates the reduction in number of injuries per 100 people who received the intervention. If the experimental condition is found to lead to heightened risk of injury, rather than expressing the absolute risk reduction as a negative number, the sign is changed to positive and this value is termed the *absolute risk increase* (ARI).

Unlike the relative risk reduction, the absolute risk reduction is dependent on the magnitude of the injury incidence. With smaller injury incidence estimates (as seen with less common pathologies), the magnitude of the absolute risk reduction will remain small. For example, if condition A has an injury proportion of 20% in the control group and 10% in the intervention group, the relative risk reduction point estimate will be 50% and the absolute risk reduction will be 10%. However, if condition B has an injury proportion of 2% in the control group and 1% in the intervention group, the relative risk reduction will again be 50%, but the absolute risk reduction will only be 1%.

✔ CONCEPT CHECK

The absolute risk reduction is dependent on the magnitude of the injury incidence.

A statistic that builds on the absolute risk reduction is the *numbers needed to treat* (NNT). The NNT is calculated by simply taking the inverse of the absolute risk reduction (1/ARR) comparing two groups. The NNT represents the number of patients that need to be treated with the experimental treatment to prevent one injury in comparison with receiving the control condition. The ideal NNT is 1, meaning that for every patient treated with the experimental treatment, an injury is prevented. Conversely, the worst NNT is infinity (∞), meaning that an infinite number of patients would need to be treated to prevent one injury.

When NNT refers to a treatment that benefits patients, it is often termed the *numbers needed to treat to benefit* (NNTB), but when it refers to a treatment that is deleterious to patients (i.e., causing adverse events), it is referred to as the *numbers needed to harm* (NNTH). As with other epidemiologic statistics, the point estimate for NNT must be evaluated along with its 95% confidence interval. The key cutline for determining the efficacy of treatment for NNT is whether or not the confidence interval crosses the infinity line (see Figure 14-6).

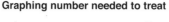

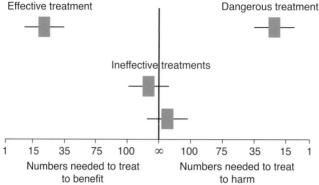

FIGURE 14-6   Interpretation of numbers needed to treat point estimates and confidence intervals. Note that the unique scale of this graph with 1 NNTB and 1 NNTH on the ends of the x-axis and infinity in the center.

✔ CONCEPT CHECK

The NNT represents the number of patients that need to be treated with the experimental treatment to prevent one injury in comparison with receiving the control condition.

The last statistic we will discuss in this chapter involves the *odds* of being injured. The odds of any given population becoming injured are calculated by dividing the injury risk by 1 minus the injury risk. Remember that odds must be in comparison to another number (i.e., the odds are 2:1 that a certain event will occur).

EXAMPLE

Odds of Being Injured

Using a fictitious example, if 15 out of 150 basketball players suffer an ankle sprain during the course of one basketball season, the odds of suffering an ankle sprain in this population are 0.11:1. When the first number in the expression of odds is less than one, interpretation can be quite difficult so we may want to take the inverse of this number (in this case, 1 divided by 0.11). In this case the odds of these

(continued)

basketball players not spraining their ankle are approximately 9:1. Assume that none of these basketball players used any type of prophylactic ankle supports such as bracing or taping. The following season, all of these athletes are taped for all practices and games and only 5 of 150 players suffer a sprain. The odds of suffering an ankle sprain with this intervention are 0.034:1. We could take the inverse of this and determine that the odds of these players not suffering an ankle sprain while being taped are approximately 29:1.

By themselves, the "raw" odds among the no intervention (control) group and the taping intervention group are difficult to interpret. However, by calculating an *odds ratio* between the two groups a more clear estimation of the treatment effect of the intervention becomes evident. By dividing the odds of athletes suffering an ankle sprain without tape (0.11:1) by the odds of athletes suffering a sprain while taped (0.034:1), we calculate an odds ratio of 3.2. This indicates that the odds of suffering an ankle sprain without tape compared to that with tape are 3.2:1 in this population of basketball players.

✔ CONCEPT CHECK

The odds of any given population becoming injured are calculated by dividing the injury risk by 1 minus the injury risk. Remember that odds must be in comparison to another number (i.e., the odds are 2:1 that a certain event will occur).

As with other epidemiologic statistics, the point estimate for odds ratios must be evaluated along with its 95% confidence interval. The key cutline for determining the efficacy of treatment (or increased risk) for odds ratio is whether or not the confidence interval crosses the 1.0 line on the log scale (see Figure 14-4).

Figure 14-7 provides an example of the calculation of incidence risk, incidence rate, odds ratio, relative risk reduction, and numbers needed to treat from an injury prevention study (McGuine & Keene, 2006).

CHAPTER SUMMARY

Studies of injury risk factors and injury prevention are extremely important to the advancement of the clinical practice of sports and occupational medicine. Injury surveillance lies at the heart of the identification of risk factors and the determination of the efficacy of injury prevention initiatives. When designing injury prevention studies, it is important that a "shotgun" approach to injury

McGuine & Keane, 2006

	Subjects	Exposures	Ankle Sprains	Incidence Risk	Incidence Rate (Per 1000 AE)
Control	392	20,828	39	(39/392) = 0.099	(39/20,828) * 1000 = 1.87
Experimental Treatment	373	20,250	23	(23/373) = 0.062	(23/20,250) * 1000 = 1.13

AE = Athlete Exposure

Statistic	Formula	Calculation	95% CI
Odds Ratio (Rates)	OR = CI Rate/EI Rate	1.87/1.13 = 1.65	(1.51 – 1.85)
Relative Risk	RR = EI Risk/CI Risk	0.062/0.099 = 0.63	(0.38 – 1.02)
Relative Risk Reduction	RRR = (1–RR)*100	(1–0.63)*100 = 37%	(2% RRI – 62% RRR)
Absolute Risk Reduction	ARR = CI Risk – EI Risk	0.099 – 0.062 = 0.037	(–0.001 ARI – 0.07 ARR)
Numbers Needed to Treat	NNT = 1/ARR	1/0.037 = 27	(13 NNTB to to 707 NNTH)

CI = Control Incidence   EI = Experimental Incidence

FIGURE 14-7   Example calculations from an injury prevention study. (McGuine TA, Keane JS. The effect of a balance training program on the risk of ankle sprains in high school athletes. *Am J Sports Med.* 2006;34(7):1103–1111.)

prevention not be used so that the factors that may lead to injury prevention may be clearly determined. The gold standard for the performance of studies of injury risk is the prospective cohort design. This type of study requires the baseline testing of a large number of participants and the following up of these individuals for injury occurrence over a defined period of time. An alternative is the case control design that compares measures between participants who have already suffered the injury of interest and matched controls who have not suffered the injury of interest. While easier to perform, there are inherent limitations to the case control study design that must be carefully weighed when developing a study of injury risk factors. These are important nuances in reporting and interpreting injury or illness risks and rates and the statistics utilized to assess these values.

KEY POINTS

- Determining an appropriate sample size is a critical step in designing a prospective study of injury risk factors.
- Due to the limitations of case control designs, results of case control studies must be put into their proper context.
- Care must be taken to avoid any bias when determining subject selection.
- The estimation of injury rates and risks is accomplished through injury surveillance systems.
- Prevalence may be presented as either a proportion or a percentage.
- The simplest comparison between two measures of injury incidence is to calculate the ratio of the injury incidence between two groups.
- Understanding the difference between injury *risk* and *rate* is a very important concept.
- Many case control studies rely on patient self-report for their injury history.
- In sports medicine and occupational medicine, the definition of "time loss" and "non–time loss" injuries must be considered.
- An athlete-exposure refers to one athlete participating in one practice or game.
- The ideal NNT is 1, meaning that for every patient treated with the experimental treatment an injury is prevented.
- The worst NNT is infinity (∞), meaning that an infinite number of patients would need to be treated to prevent one injury.

Critical Thinking Questions

1. List the steps in the Bahr et al. (2002) paradigm?
2. What is the preferred design of studies of injury risk factors?
3. What are the factors important to designing studies of injury risk factors?
4. List several nuances important to understanding the determination of the number of injuries or injured people within a given sample of interest.

Applying Concepts

1. Consider and discuss implications of the term "injury risk factor" when describing the results of a study that utilized a case control design.
2. Consider that retrospective design does have a serious limitation in comparison to the prospective design.

(continued)

3. Discuss issues associated with measures of "risk factors" being taken after the injury of interest has occurred.

   a. Consider the following:

   i. Why there is no way to know if these measures were present before the injury occurred (truly being a risk factor).

   ii. If the measures are a result of adaptation(s) to the injury that developed after the onset of injury.

REFERENCES

Agel J, Olson DE, Dick R, et al. Descriptive epidemiology of women's collegiate basketball injuries: National Collegiate Athletics Association Injury Surveillance System, 1988–1989 through 2003–2004. *J Athl Train.* 2007;42(2):202–210.

Bahr R, Kannus P, van Mechelen W. Epidemiology and sports injury prevention. In: Kjaer M, Krogsgaard M, Magnusson P, et al., eds. *Textbook of Sports Medicine: Basic Science and Clinical Aspects of Sports Injury and Physical Activity.* Malden, MA: Blackwell Science Ltd; 2003.

Basavarajaiah S, Wilson M, Whyte G, et al. Prevalence of hypertrophic cardiomyopathy in highly trained athletes: relevance to pre-participation screening. *J Am Coll Cardiol.* 2008;51:1033–1039.

Barratt A, Peter CW, Hatala R, et al. For the evidence-based medicine teaching tips working group. Tips for learners of evidence-based medicine: 1. Relative risk reduction, absolute risk reduction and number needed to treat. *CMAJ.* 2004;171(4). doi:10.1503/cmaj.1021197.

Knowles SB, Marshall SW, Guskiewicz KM. Issues in estimating risks and rates in sports injury research. *J Athl Train.* 2006;41:207–215.

McGuine TA, Keene JS. The effect of a balance training program on the risk of ankle sprains in high school athletes. *Am J Sports Med.* 2006;34(7):1103–1111.

TREATMENT OUTCOMES ACROSS THE DISABLEMENT SPECTRUM

If you do not expect the unexpected you will not find it, for it is not to be reached by search or trail.

—*Heraclitus from Heraclitus Quotes as quoted in BrainyQuote (www.brainyquote.com/quotes/authors/h/heraclitus.html)*

CHAPTER OBJECTIVES

After reading this chapter, you will:

- Understand why performing research on injured or ill patients is important to advancing the health sciences.
- Appreciate the challenges in conducting clinical research.
- Be able to explain the importance of selecting appropriate outcomes measures to assess in patients as their pathology progresses over time.
- Understand a conceptual framework for the measurement of treatment outcomes.
- Be able to delineate between disease-oriented and patient-oriented measures.
- Be able to describe global and region-specific measures.
- Understand how to choose the appropriate outcomes instruments.

KEY TERMS

conceptual framework
disease-oriented measures
global and region-specific measures

measurement
outcomes instruments
pathology

patient-oriented measures
treatment outcomes

INTRODUCTION

Performing research on injured or ill patients is of utmost importance to advancing the health sciences. One of the primary challenges in conducting clinical research is selecting the appropriate outcomes measures to assess in patients as their **pathology** progresses over time. The purpose of this chapter is to provide the **conceptual framework** for the **measurement** of **treatment outcomes**, delineate between **disease-oriented and patient-oriented measures**, describe **global and region-specific measures**, and provide guidance in choosing the appropriate **outcomes instruments**.

TYPES OF OUTCOMES MEASURES

Outcomes measures in the health sciences can be divided into two categories: those that provide *disease-oriented evidence* (DOE) and those that provide *patient-oriented evidence* (POE). DOE encompasses measures that provide insight into the physiology of illness or injury. Common examples include measures of blood pressure, electromyographic activity in a muscle during contraction, or the amount of circulating creatine kinase in a patient's blood. DOE measures provide information about a patient's pathology and are of utmost interest to health care providers, as opposed to being important to patients.

In contrast, POE consists of measures that are of direct interest to patients rather than clinicians. Examples include measures of the severity of symptoms, level of function, and quality of life. POE often involves information that is subjectively self-reported by patients as opposed to objective clinical or laboratory measures that are taken by health care providers or researchers. Epidemiologic measures that deal with the incidence or prevalence of a condition such as morbidity and mortality, and financial outcomes such as cost of health care services may also be considered as measures of POE. POE is sometimes referred to as *patient-oriented evidence* that *matters* (POEM).

The central difference between DOE and POE is that POE outcomes measures assess issues that are of the utmost interest to the patient, as opposed to information that is important to clinicians. This distinction is not intended to diminish the importance of DOE. In fact, DOE is critical to clinicians as they make decisions regarding the diagnosis and treatment of their patients' pathology. From a research perspective, DOE is critical to understanding the pathophysiology of specific conditions, and thus also the development of effective diagnostic and therapeutic interventions. POE outcomes measures, on the other hand, provide critical information regarding the impact that a person's health care status has on their ability to function in society and their quality of life. The remainder of this chapter focuses on POE.

> ✔ **CONCEPT CHECK**
>
> The central difference between DOE and POE is that POE outcomes measures assess issues that are of the utmost interest to the patient, as opposed to information that is important to clinicians.

DISABLEMENT MODELS

Any valid measurement system must be based on a sound theoretic rationale. The measurement of treatment outcomes in clinical research must be built upon disablement models. Several contemporary, but related, disablement models have been put forth by organizations such as the Institute of Medicine, World Health Organization, and National Center for Medical Rehabilitation Research. Each disablement model provides a framework using standard terminology for the description of health status. A common foundation for all of these models is the emphasis being placed on the psychosocial functioning of the individual patient (POE) as opposed to the physiologic or structural functioning of the patient (DOE). The concept of disability as a sociologic construct was initially championed by a sociologist, Saad Nagi, in the 1960s. The contemporary definition of *disability* is described as the inability or limitation in performing socially defined roles and tasks expected as an individual within a sociocultural and physical environment (Nagi, 1991). This is in contrast to the common perception of disability as a permanent physical or mental handicap.

> ✔ **CONCEPT CHECK**
>
> A common foundation for disablement models is the emphasis being placed on the psychosocial functioning of the individual patient (POE) as opposed to the physiologic or structural functioning of the patient (DOE).

Nagi's Model

Nagi's model (1991) is illustrated in Figure 15-1. In this model, the *active pathology* refers to the patient's injury or illness. *Impairment* refers to abnormality in physiologic function at the site of injury or illness. *Functional limitation* refers to limitations in actions due to the associated impairments. *Disability* is operationally defined in this model as an inability to perform normal socially expected activities due to functional limitations. *Quality of life* is defined as an individual's vitality and level of satisfaction with their current state of existence. Impairments, functional

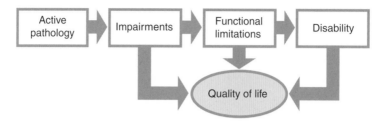

FIGURE 15-1   A visual representation of Nagi's disablement model showing the multiple impacts on quality of life.

limitations, and disability can all influence quality of life. In the context of health care outcomes, this concept is often referred to as *health-related quality of life* (HRQOL) to distinguish it from socioeconomic or interpersonal issues that may also influence an individual's overall quality of life.

Measures of impairments are typically considered DOE. Measures of functional limitations may represent DOE or POE depending on the context of the measures. Measures of both disability and quality of life are almost always considered POE. Examples of four patients using Nagi's disablement model are provided (see Table 15-1) to illustrate these distinctions.

Nagi's disablement model has been updated in the past decade in an effort to get beyond its linear approach to disability. Nagi's core concepts do, however, remain the foundation for the newer disablement models.

National Center for Medical Rehabilitation Research Disability Model

The National Center for Medical Rehabilitation Research (NCMRR) is a division of the United States National Institutes of Health. The NCMRR model is very similar to Nagi's model, however, it replaces "quality of life" with "societal limitations." *Societal limitations* refer to restrictions resulting from social policy or barriers, which limit fulfillment of roles or deny access to services and opportunities associated with full participation in society. This concept is hopefully less ambiguous than "quality of life" and clearly states the importance of societal role in health outcomes. The NCMRR is currently working to revise their disablement model (see Figure 15-2).

World Health Organization

The International Classification of Functioning, Disability and Health has been developed by the World Health Organization. This disablement model is pictured in Figure 15-3.

PATIENT DEMOGRAPHICS	20-YEAR-OLD FEMALE COLLEGIATE BASKETBALL PLAYER	35-YEAR-OLD MALE ROOFER	35-YEAR-OLD FEMALE LAWYER	70-YEAR-OLD-MALE RETIREE WHO VOLUN-TEERS REGULARLY AT A HOMELESS SHELTER
Active pathology	Knee ligament sprain	Knee ligament sprain	Irritable bowel syndrome	Early stage of Parkinson disease
Impairments	Knee pain Limited knee range of motion Quadriceps weakness	Knee pain Limited knee range of motion Quadriceps weakness	Frequent abdominal pain and bloating Chronic diarrhea Headaches	Minor tremors Slowed movements Diminished reflexes
Functional limitations	Unable to: • squat • kneel • climb stairs • jog • jump	Unable to: • squat • kneel • climb stairs • jog • jump	Unable to: • concentrate for extended periods of time • sit for long periods of time	Unable to: • perform upper extremity tasks without considerable shaking • walk as fast as he would like • maintain his balance as well as he previously did
Disability	Unable to: • play basketball • go to classes without using crutches	Unable to: • work as a roofer • play on the floor with his young children • maintain his home garden	Unable to: • work as productively as she would like as a lawyer • participate in social activities as she would like (no movies, no dinners out, etc.)	Unable to: • serve meals at the homeless shelter • maintain his home and yard as he would like
Quality of life	Increased anxiety because of loss of identity as an athlete Loss of social support from team members	Increased anxiety because of inability to work and provide financially for his family Depression because of inability to interact with his children as he would like to	Increased anxiety because of inability to work as much as she would like Extreme concern that she may not make partner at her law firm Loss of social role in her circle of friends	Increased anxiety about having to move out of his home because of his physical health Loss of social support from fellow volunteers at the homeless shelter

TABLE 15-1 Examples of four patients using Nagi's disablement model

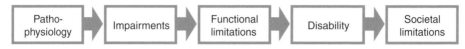

FIGURE 15-2   The NCMRR disablement model.

The WHO model has the same foundations as the Nagi model but also adds to it in unique ways. The WHO model uses a standardized documentation system that allows clinicians and health systems to classify and quantify specific descriptors of a patient's disability. At the top of the WHO disability model is a patient's *health condition*; this represents the patient's pathology that may be in the form of a disorder, disease, or injury. The cause of the health condition can typically be described in terms of abnormalities in *body functions and structures*. These represent altered physiologic functions and anatomic structures, respectively. At the center of the WHO Disablement Model is *activities* and these are operationally defined similar to functional limitations in the Nagi and NCMRR models. *Participation* involves the performance of activities in societal contexts.

The remaining portions of the WHO model are referred to as *contextual factors*. These include *personal factors* and *environmental factors* that influence a patient's ability to function. *Personal factors* include, but are not limited to, issues

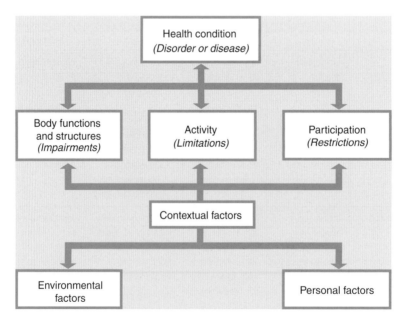

FIGURE 15-3   International Classification of Functioning, Disability and Health (ICF) model. (Reprinted with permission from World Health Organization (WHO).)

such as a patient's age, sex, socioeconomic status, and previous life experiences. *Environmental factors* refer to the physical, social, and attitudinal environments in which patients live and include support and relationships, attitudes, and services and policies; these can be considered at the level of the individual or society. The addition of these contextual factors allows for an individualization of the factors influencing a particular patient's disability. Without also considering personal and environmental factors of a patient, it is not possible to truly understand the barriers that exist to positively affect their disability.

Disability Model Summary

Arguments can be made for or against any of the three disablement models presented here, and there are sure to be new models proposed in the coming years. While these discussions are important, what is even more important is that the clinical outcomes measurement is done within the context of an accepted framework. The best existing outcomes assessment tools were created and validated using one of the accepted disability models described here. The biggest mistake an investigator can make is developing or adopting a new outcomes measurement tool that is not based on a sound disablement model and validated appropriately. The development of new measurement instruments should not be taken lightly.

✔ CONCEPT CHECK

The biggest mistake an investigator can make is developing or adopting a new outcomes measurement tool that is not based on a sound disablement model and validated appropriately.

CLINICIAN-DERIVED MEASURES

Most health care providers routinely take measures on their patients that could be considered clinical outcomes. These vary widely by specialty but could include measures such as core body temperature or body mass index. Almost always, these measures represent DOE. As state previously, measures of DOE are important but they also have limitations when they are used in clinical trials without accompanying POE.

Some clinical outcomes instruments exist that ask clinicians to rate the level of function or disability of their specific patient. Such items that involve a component of the physical exam (i.e., swelling, ecchymosis, etc.) that can be directly observed or perhaps even measured (these are examples of DOE), there is little concern over clinician bias in reporting. However, when clinicians are asked to subjectively assess their patient's outcome or level of disability, clinicians typically rate their patient's success substantially higher than the patients themselves do. Therefore, clinician subjective reports of patient outcomes should be considered DOE rather than POE.

 CONCEPT CHECK

When clinicians are asked to subjectively assess their patient's outcome or level of disability, clinicians typically rate their patient's success substantially higher than the patients themselves do.

PATIENT SELF-REPORT

The most common type of POE comes from those outcomes that patients self-report on their current health status. There are a huge number of patient self-report instruments that range from having patients rate a single question or item to having scores of specific questions and items. These instruments may be used to assess a subject's general or global health status or may be region- or condition-specific. It is essential that researchers and clinicians utilize outcomes instruments that are appropriate (i.e., valid) for the patients to whom they are being administered.

 CONCEPT CHECK

The most common type of POE comes for outcomes those patients subjectively self-report on their current health status.

GLOBAL HEALTH MEASURES

Survey instruments used to assess global health status typically focus on quality of life and disability. These often are multidimensional scales and include questions that specifically address both physical health and emotional well-being. Perhaps the best examples of global health measures are the SF-36 and the SF-12 (see http://www.sf-36.org/wantsf.aspx?id=1). These instruments have been widely studied and are frequently used to assess treatment outcomes in patients with chronic diseases. Instruments are often altered for specific age

> ## BOX 15.1 | Examples of common global health outcomes instruments.
>
> Short Form 36 Health Survey (SF-36)
> Short Form 12 Health Survey (SF-12)
> Sickness Impact Profile (SIP)
> Child Health Questionnaire (CHQ)
> Pediatric Outcomes Data Collection Instrument (PODCI)

groups (especially pediatrics) and also translated into other languages. In either case, it is essential that the revised instruments be validated before they are used extensively.

Challenges exist in assessing global health outcomes in patients who have pathologies (i.e., relatively minor musculoskeletal injuries) that are not chronic in nature and are associated with transient disability. In such cases, region-specific scales may be used, but it must be noted that efforts are underway to develop and validate outcomes instruments that focus on transient disability. Examples of common global health outcomes instruments are provided in Box 15.1.

CONDITION-, REGION-, OR DIMENSION-SPECIFIC MEASURES

A large number of outcomes instruments exist to assess patients with either distinct pathologies or groups of pathologies. These instruments are designed to address functional limitations and disabilities that are often associated with patients who have the specific injury or illness. For example, the Lower Extremity Functional Scale asks patients with lower extremity pathologies to answer questions about their ability to ambulate, squat, kneel, and perform other tasks that require lower extremity function (Binkley et al., 1999). Dimension-specific outcomes instruments are often designed to assess a specific physical or emotional phenomenon such as pain, anxiety, or depression (see Table 15-2). It is essential that clinicians and researchers utilize outcomes instruments that are appropriate (i.e., valid) for the specific patient population for which they are to be employed.

 CONCEPT CHECK

Dimension-specific outcomes instruments are often designed to assess a specific physical or emotional phenomenon such as pain, anxiety, or depression.

TABLE 15-2	Examples of condition-, region-, or dimension-specific outcomes instruments (not an exhaustive list)
INSTRUMENT	**PRIMARY PURPOSE**
Short Musculoskeletal Function Assessment (SMFA)	Musculoskeletal patients
Asthma Quality of Life Scale	Asthma patients
Lower Extremity Functional Scale (LEFS)	Lower extremity patients
Western Ontario MacMaster Osteoarthritis Index (WOMAC)	Knee and hip osteoarthritis patients
Anterior Knee Pain Scale (AKP)	Patellofemoral pain patients
Kujala Knee Score	Patellofemoral pain patients
International Knee Documentation Committee Scale (IKDC)	Knee surgery patients
Cincinnati Knee Scale	Knee surgery patients
Foot and Ankle Ability Measure (FAAM)	Foot and ankle patients
Sports Ankle Rating System (SARS)	Athletes with ankle injuries
Disability of the Arm, Shoulder, and Hand (DASH)	Upper extremity patients
Upper Extremity Function Scale (UEFS)	Upper extremity patients
Oswestry Disability Index	Low back pain patients
Roland Morris Low Back Pain Questionnaire	Low back pain patients
Fear Avoidance Beliefs Questionnaire	Musculoskeletal patients
Beck Depression Index	Depression
Pain Disability Index	Pain
McGill Pain Questionnaire	Pain

SINGLE ITEM OUTCOMES MEASURES

Having outcomes instruments with a limited number of questions is advantageous to patients, clinicians, and researchers. Eliminating redundancy in items is an important step in developing an outcomes instrument. Taken to the extreme, this has yielded the use of single item outcomes measures. When dealing with global health, these measures essentially ask patients to answer one question, "How are you?" Such measures are often referred to as Single

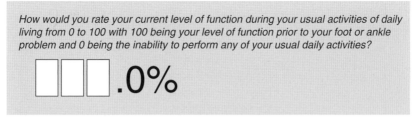

How would you rate your current level of function during your usual activities of daily living from 0 to 100 with 100 being your level of function prior to your foot or ankle problem and 0 being the inability to perform any of your usual daily activities?

.0%

FIGURE 15-4   Example of a Single Assessment Numeric Evaluation (SANE score) from the Foot and Ankle Ability Measure.

Assessment Numeric Evaluation, or SANE scores. Other single item tools might ask patients to judge only their level of pain or ask them if they have improved or gotten worse since their last assessment (see Figures 15-4, 15-5, and 15-6). The limitation of these single item scales is that they are unidimensional and do not assess health status across multiple aspects of the disablement scale. While seemingly convenient, single item outcomes measures should not be used in isolation, but instead should be used as part of a comprehensive outcomes assessment process.

CHOOSING THE APPROPRIATE OUTCOMES INSTRUMENTS

Clinicians and researchers have many choices when selecting outcomes instruments to employ in clinical practice or experimental studies. Two issues are critical when making these selections: (1) matching the purpose of measurement with the instrument's design and (2) ensuring that the instrument's clinimetric properties have been rigorously established.

Matching the purpose of using a specific outcomes instrument with the intended utility of the instrument is essential. For example, the WOMAC scale was specifically designed to assess clinical outcomes in patients with hip or knee osteoarthritis (Bellamy et al., 1998). To use the WOMAC scale on young adults

Mark an "X" on the spot on the line that represents the worst pain that you have been in over the past 24 hours. (Scored as a percentage of the length of the line.)

No pain   **Worst pain imaginable**

FIGURE 15-5   Example of a Visual Analog Scale for Pain.

"Since your last clinic visit, has there been any change in activity limitation, symptoms, emotions, and overall quality of life, related to your asthma?"	
−7	A very great deal worse
−6	A great deal worse
−5	A good deal worse
−4	Moderately worse
−3	Somewhat worse
−2	A little worse
−1	Almost the same, hardly any worse at all
0	No change
+1	Almost the same, hardly any better at all
+2	A little better
+3	Somewhat better
+4	Moderately better
+5	A good deal better
+6	A great deal better
+7	A very great deal better

FIGURE 15-6   Global rating of change example for asthma patients.

with knee meniscus injuries would be inappropriate because the instrument was not designed to be used in this population, nor have its clinimetric properties been validated in this population. Care must be taken not to overgeneralize the utility of an outcomes instrument to populations that it was not designed to measure.

In Chapter 10, the importance of establishing measurement properties of outcomes measures was discussed in detail. Survey instruments must be developed with the same rigor as laboratory or clinical measures employed in research. Clinimetric properties such as reliability, validity, sensitivity to change, and internal consistency must all be assessed during the development of an outcomes instrument. The process of creating a new outcomes scale is neither easy, nor brief, nor simple.

✔ CONCEPT CHECK

Clinimetric properties such as reliability, validity, sensitivity to change, and internal consistency must all be assessed during the development of an outcomes instrument.

CHAPTER SUMMARY

The importance of assessing patient-oriented evidence (POE) in addition to disease-oriented evidence (DOE) is critical to understanding the true effectiveness of clinical intervention. The most common measures of POE are instruments that require patients to self-report their health status. Outcomes instruments should be based on an accepted disablement framework. When selecting specific outcomes instruments, clinicians and practitioners must ensure that the instruments they select are appropriate for the population to be tested and that the instruments have had their clinimetric properties rigorously established.

KEY POINTS

- *Disease-oriented evidence* (DOE) is critical to understanding the pathophysiology of specific conditions.
- *Patient-oriented evidence* (POE) outcomes measures provide critical information regarding the impact that a person's health care status has on their ability to function in society and their quality of life.
- Each disablement model provides a framework using standard terminology for the description of health status.
- The WHO model uses a standardized documentation system that allows clinicians and health systems to classify and quantify specific descriptors of a patient's disability.
- Clinician subjective reports of patient outcomes should be considered DOE rather than POE.
- Eliminating redundancy in items is an important step in developing an outcomes instrument.
- Matching the purpose of using a specific outcomes instrument with the intended utility of the instrument is essential.
- Care must be taken not to overgeneralize the utility of an outcomes instrument to populations that it was not designed to measure.

 Critical Thinking Questions

1. Outcomes measures in the health sciences can be divided into two categories. What are those categories?
2. Following Nagi's (1991) model, consider how each of these measures would be considered:

   (a) measures of impairments;

(continued)

(b) measures of functional limitations; and

(c) measures of both disability and quality of life.

3. What is the key difference between the National Center for Medical Rehabilitation Research (NCMRR) model and Nagi's model?

 Applying Concepts

1. Consider the three disablement models presented in this chapter. Present arguments for or against any of the three disablement models presented here, then suggest and rationalize specific improvements that you expect to see in new models proposed in the coming years.

2. Discuss why it is imperative that clinical outcomes measurement is done within the context of an accepted framework.

REFERENCES

Bellamy N, Buchanan WW, Goldsmith CH, et al. Validation study of WOMAC: a health status instrument for measuring clinically important patient relevant outcomes to antirheumatic drug therapy in patients with osteoarthritis of the hip or knee. *J Rheumatol.* 1988;15:1833–1840.

Binkley JM, Stratford PW, Lott SA, et al. The Lower Extremity Functional Scale (LEFS): scale development, measurement properties, and clinical application. *Phys Ther.* 1999;79:371–383.

Denegar CR, Vela LI, Evans TA. Evidence-based sports medicine: outcomes instruments for active populations. *Clin Sports Med.* 2008;27(3):339–351.

Nagi S. Disability concepts revisited: implications for prevention. In: Pope A, Tarlov A, eds. *Disability in America: Toward a National Agenda for Prevention.* Washington, DC: National Academy Press; 1991:309–327.

Snyder AR, Parsons JT, Valovich McLeod TC, et al. Using disablement models and clinical outcomes assessment to enable evidence-based athletic training practice, part I: disablement models. *J Athl Train.* 2008;43(4):428–436.

Valovich McLeod TC, Snyder AR, Parsons JT, et al. Using disablement models and clinical outcomes assessment to enable evidence-based athletic training practice, part II: clinical outcomes assessment. *J Athl Train.* 2008;43(4):437–445.

CHAPTER 16

TREATMENT OUTCOMES: RESEARCH METHODS AND DATA ANALYSIS

… nothing ever goes away until it has taught us what we need to know.

—Pema Chodron (Source: When Things Fall Apart: Heart Advice for Difficult Times, p. 40)

CHAPTER OBJECTIVES

After reading this chapter, you will:

- Understand why assessment of the effectiveness of therapeutic interventions on patient outcomes is the centerpiece of clinical research.
- Be able to describe the tenets of evidence-based practice.
- Appreciate the value of evidence-based practice in making clinical decisions.
- Understand that the "best" research evidence ideally consists of patient-oriented evidence from well-conducted clinical trials.
- Appreciate the issues involving study design, statistical analysis, and interpretation of the results of clinical trials that assess treatment outcomes.

KEY TERMS

a priori	clinical trial	limitations
assessment	evidence	patient values
basic and translational research	infrastructure	translational research
clinician experience	levels of evidence	

INTRODUCTION

The **assessment** of the effectiveness of therapeutic interventions on patient outcomes is the centerpiece of clinical research. The tenets of evidence-based practice call for the use of the best research **evidence** in conjunction with **clinician experience** and **patient values** to make clinical decisions. The "best research evidence" ideally consists of patient-oriented evidence from well-conducted **clinical trials**. This chapter will focus on issues involving the study design, statistical analysis, and interpretation of the results of clinical trials that assess treatment outcomes.

BUILDING AN INFRASTRUCTURE TO MEASURE TREATMENT OUTCOMES

The performance of clinical trials to assess treatment outcomes must be done as part of a planned process with foresight. An **infrastructure** should be put in place that allows for the regular collection of treatment outcomes, including both disease-oriented and patient-oriented measures. Decisions among researchers, clinicians, and administrators need to be made **a priori** regarding which outcome measures will be systematically recorded and how often specific groups of patients will be assessed.

The means by which outcomes data will be collected and managed must also be determined. Historically, most patient self-report data were collected by having patients complete paper-based surveys. The patient responses then are entered manually into computer spreadsheets for data management and analysis. With large sample sizes, this can be very time consuming and also increases the chance that data are inaccurate due to data entry errors. Long-term follow-up surveys may also be administered by either phone or mail. More recently, systems have been implemented that allow patients to enter their data electronically on a handheld PDA or a laptop computer. This data are thus entered directly into both clinical and research databases. The former can be part of a patient's electronic health record. Long-term follow-ups can often be completed by patients with home computer access on either secure web sites or via e-mail. The use of direct electronic data entry by patients is recommended where feasible.

The performance of clinical trials often involves multiple clinical sites. This produces a challenge for researchers who must put in place mechanisms to capture outcomes data in different environments. The importance of building a strong research infrastructure for clinical outcomes research cannot be overemphasized.

> ✔ **CONCEPT CHECK**
>
> The performance of clinical trials to assess treatment outcomes must be done as part of a planned process with foresight. An infrastructure should be put in place that allows for the regular collection of treatment outcomes, including both disease-oriented and patient-oriented measures.

STUDY DESIGNS

The design of a clinical trial is the greatest factor that influences the "level of evidence" stemming from that study's results. The two most common schema for classifying **levels of evidence** are from the Centre for Evidence-Based Medicine (CEBM) and the Strength of Recommendation Taxonomy (SORT). For the purpose of this chapter we will utilize the CEBM classification.

The CEBM has five general categories of levels of evidence. Level 5 evidence is the lowest level and consists of expert opinion and disease-oriented evidence derived from the **basic and translational research**. Level 4 evidence is derived from case series. Level 3 evidence stems from case control studies, which are always retrospective in design. Level 2 evidence is derived from prospective cohort studies that lack randomization. The highest level of evidence is Level 1 evidence that comes from randomized controlled trials (RCTs), which are the gold standard for clinical trials methodology.

> ✔ **CONCEPT CHECK**
>
> Following the CEBM classification of levels of evidence, the highest level of evidence is Level 1 evidence that comes from randomized controlled trials (RCTs), which are the gold standard for clinical trials methodology.

Level 5 Evidence: Expert Opinion and Disease-Oriented Evidence

Expert opinion and disease-oriented evidence are considered the lowest level of evidence because these are not patient-oriented evidence. Expert opinion can be valuable in making healthcare decisions but the observations of experts have typically not been subjected to the scientific method. Disease-oriented evidence often comes from basic science research often consisting of experiments performed on cells, animals, or cadavers; or from surrogate outcomes that are more important to clinicians (i.e., physiological measures) than to their patients.

Level 4 Evidence: Case Series

A case series represents the reporting of the clinical outcomes of a number of patients with the same pathology who are treated with the same or similar intervention. The number of patients may vary from a handful to dozens depending on the prevalence of the pathology in the reporting clinician's clinical practice. A case series does not utilize an experimental design as there is no comparison group treated with a different intervention, thus limiting the internal validity of the study design.

Despite the lack of an experimental design, case series must still be performed in a structured and organized manner. Strict inclusion and exclusion criteria must be employed with a particular emphasis on comorbidities. Emphasis must also be placed on ensuring that the treatment intervention is standardized across all patients. Likewise, outcome measures must be taken at the same endpoints to be able to draw conclusions about the clinical outcomes of the patients. The results of case series may be used to justify the performance of a more rigorous scientific investigation of new treatment interventions, but they do not represent a high level of clinical evidence.

✔ CONCEPT CHECK

A case series does not utilize an experimental design, as there is no comparison group treated with a different intervention, thus limiting the internal validity of the study design. Despite the lack of an experimental design, case series must still be performed in a structured and organized manner.

Level 3 Evidence: Case Control Studies

Case control studies are by definition retrospective in nature. The clinical outcomes of two groups of patients are examined after interventions have already been administered. Patients treated with the experimental treatment are referred to as "cases," whereas patients treated with the standard treatment or no treatment are referred to as "controls." Patients in the two groups should match for relevant demographics such as age, sex, and severity of pathology. Case control studies have the advantage of being quicker to perform because potential study subjects already have the pathology of interest and have already received treatment. It is, however, that the follow-up times from intervention be standardized across subjects.

Patients are treated with the respective treatments based on clinician judgment, not because of experimental allocation. Numerous confounding factors may influence the decision to treat patients with respective interventions; the inherent weakness of this approach is that none of these confounding factors can be controlled for in the experimental design. Another limitation is that often there is no baseline data with which to compare the follow-up measures. While the results of case control studies must be interpreted in the context of the study design **limitations**, they may be used to justify the performance of a more rigorous prospective investigation of treatment interventions.

> ✔ **CONCEPT CHECK**
>
> In case control studies, patients are treated with the respective treatments based on clinician judgment and not because of experimental allocation. Numerous confounding factors may influence the decision to treat patients with respective interventions; the inherent weakness of this approach is that none of these confounding factors can be controlled for in the experimental design.

Level 2 Evidence: Prospective Cohort Studies

Prospective cohort studies involve baseline measurement before patients receive the prescribed treatment. The choice of treatment, however, is not randomly assigned but is instead left to the discretion of the treating clinician. As mentioned with the case control study design, numerous confounding factors may influence the decision to treat patients with the respective interventions. An advantage of this design is the ability to collect baseline data before administration of an intervention. When an RCT is not possible, a prospective cohort study is the next best alternative.

> ✔ **CONCEPT CHECK**
>
> Prospective cohort studies involve baseline measurement before patients receive the prescribed treatment.

Level 1 Evidence: Randomized Controlled Trials

The RCT is the gold standard for clinical investigation. Patients meeting the inclusion criteria are randomly assigned to intervention conditions and measures are taken at baseline and routine follow-up periods. By assigning interventions randomly, the potential of confounding biases between groups is limited. Several guidelines have been established to assure quality in the design and reporting of RCTs. These include the CONSORT statement (see Table 16-1) and the PEDro scale (see Table 16-2). While these instruments can be used to check the quality of published RCTs, they also serve a purpose in the design of RCTs.

TABLE 16-1 CONSORT checklist for RCTs			
SECTION AND TOPIC	**ITEM NO.**	**DESCRIPTION**	**REPORTED ON PAGE NO.**
Title and abstract	1	How participants were allocated to interventions (e.g., "random allocation," "randomized," or "randomly assigned").	
Introduction			
Background	2	Scientist background and explanation of rationale.	
Methods			
Participants	3	Eligibility criteria for participants and the settings and locations where the data were collected.	
Interventions	4	Precise details of the interventions intended for each group and how and when they were actually administered.	
Objectives	5	Specific objectives and hypotheses.	
Outcomes	6	Clearly defined primary and secondary outcome measures and, when applicable, any methods used to enhance the quality of measurements (e.g., multiple observations, training of assessors).	
Sample size	7	How sample size was determined and, when applicable, explanation of any interim analyses and stopping rules.	
Randomization			
Sequence generation	8	Method used to generate the random allocation sequence, including details of any restriction (e.g., blocking, stratification).	

Allocation conceal-ment	9	Method used to implement the random allocation sequence (e.g., numbered containers or central telephone), clarifying whether the sequence was concealed until interventions were assigned.	
Implementation	10	Who generated the allocation sequence, who enrolled participants, and who assigned participants to their groups.	
Blinding (masking)	11	Whether or not participants, those administering the interventions, and those assessing the outcomes were blinded to group assignment. If done, how the success of blinding was evaluated.	
Statistical methods	12	Statistical methods used to compare group for primary outcome(s); methods for additional analyses, such as subgroup analyses and adjusted analyses.	
Results			
Participant flow	13	Flow of participants through each stage (a diagram is strongly recommended). Specifically, for each group report the numbers of participants randomly assigned, receiving intended treatment, completing the study protocol, and analyzed for the primary outcome. Describe protocol deviations from study as planned, together with reasons.	
Recruitment	14	Dates defining the periods of recruitment and follow-up.	
Baseline data	15	Baseline demographic and clinical characteristics of each group.	

(continued)

TABLE 16-1   *(Continued)*

SECTION AND TOPIC	ITEM NO.	DESCRIPTION	REPORTED ON PAGE NO.
Numbers analyzed	16	Number of participants (denominator) in each group included in each analysis and whether the analysis was by "intention-to-treat." State the result in absolute numbers when feasible (e.g., 10/20, not 50%).	
Outcome and estimation	17	For each primary and secondary outcome, a summary of results for each group, and the estimated effect size and its precision (e.g., 96% confidence interval).	
Ancillary analyses	18	Address multiplicity by reporting any other analyses performed, including subgroup analyses and adjusted analyses. Indicating those prespecified and those exploratory.	
Adverse events	19	All important adverse events or side effects in each intervention group.	
Discussion			
Interpretation	20	Interpretation of the results, taking into account study hypotheses, sources or potential bias or imprecision, and the dangers associated with multiplicity of analyses and outcomes.	
Generalizability	21	Generalizability (external validity) of the trial findings.	
Overall evidence	22	General interpretation or the result in the context of current evidence.	

CONSORT Group, 2008. Accessed from http://www.consort-statement.org/consort-statement/flow-diagram/February 11, 2010.

TABLE 16-2 The PEDro Scale			
PEDRo SCALE			
Eligibility criteria were specified	No ❏	Yes ❏	Where:
Subjects were randomly allocated to groups (in a crossover study, subjects were randomly allocated an order in which treatments were received)	No ❏	Yes ❏	Where:
Allocation was concealed	No ❏	Yes ❏	Where:
The groups were similar at baseline regarding the most important prognostic indicators	No ❏	Yes ❏	Where:
There was blinding of all subjects	No ❏	Yes ❏	Where:
There was blinding of all therapists who administered the therapy	No ❏	Yes ❏	Where:
There was blinding of all assessors who measured at least one key outcome	No ❏	Yes ❏	Where:
Measures of at least one key outcome were obtained from more than 85% of the subjects initially allocated to groups	No ❏	Yes ❏	Where:
All subjects for whom outcome measures were available received the treatment or control condition as allocated or, where this was not the case, data for at least one key outcome was analyzed by "intention to treat"	No ❏	Yes ❏	Where:
The results of between-group statistical comparisons are reported for at least one key outcome	No ❏	Yes ❏	Where:
The study provides both point measures and measures of variability for at least one key outcome	No ❏	Yes ❏	Where:

✔ **CONCEPT CHECK**

By assigning interventions randomly, the potential of confounding biases between groups is limited.

A computerized randomization program typically does the randomization schedule for subjects. The individual responsible for coordinating the randomization should not be directly involved in deciding the inclusion criteria of potential subjects or the measurement of outcomes directly from patients.

Allocation of subjects to their respective intervention group should be done in a concealed manner. This is most often done by placing each subject's group assignment in a sealed opaque envelope that is not opened until the subject has been ruled to meet the study inclusion criteria and has provided informed consent to participate in the study. Off-site allocation is also sometimes used in which a clinician calls a clinical trials manager at another location to be informed of the particular subject's group allocation.

The maintenance of blinding of group allocations is important throughout clinical trials. This most often pertains to subjects and examiners taking measures being blinded to group assignment, but may also involve blinding of clinicians administering treatments such as drug therapies.

The issue of dropouts is an important consideration in RCTs. In clinical trials, some patients may choose to stop receiving the assigned intervention. In some cases, they may even end up receiving the intervention to which they were not allocated as part of their care after they have withdrawn from the study. It is important to compare the number of dropouts in each intervention condition to identify patient dissatisfaction with a given treatment. When dropouts occur, rather than discarding the data from subjects who drop out, the data should be analyzed using *intention to treat analysis*. In this case, subjects are analyzed in the group to which they were allocated regardless of whether or not they actually received the full course of the assigned intervention. This analysis is seen as a conservative method to dealing with dropouts.

Another issue that may arise in RCTs (and other types of clinical trials) is missing data points. Rather than discarding subjects who drop out completely, *imputation* of their data should be performed. In clinical trials, this most often involves carrying the subjects' most recent scores forward by using these scores for all future time points as well. This conservative approach assumes that had subjects continued in the trial, they would not have gotten any better with further intervention. Other methods also exist for imputation of missing data, but these statistical techniques are beyond the scope of this text.

A CONSORT flow chart is recommended in the reporting of RCTs to illustrate issues of subject retention throughout the entire course of the trial (see Figure 16-1).

DATA ANALYSIS: STATISTICAL SIGNIFICANCE VERSUS CLINICAL MEANINGFULNESS

Traditional statistical analysis in the health sciences has focused on hypothesis testing. Using this approach, the null hypothesis (there are no differences between comparisons) is either confirmed or refuted. This approach assesses the statistical

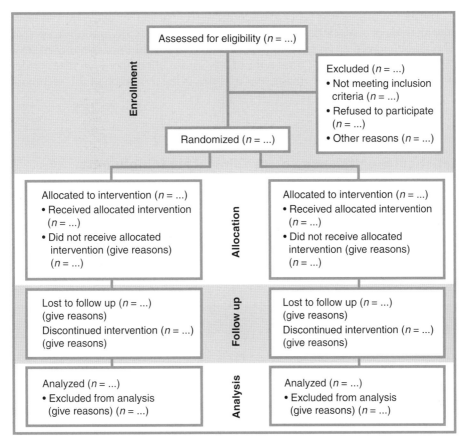

FIGURE 16-1 CONSORT flow chart. (CONSORT Group, 2008. Accessed from http://www.consort-statement.org/consort-statement/flow-diagram/ February 11, 2010.)

significance of the involved comparisons, but does not necessarily assess the clinical meaningfulness of the results. Is it possible to have statistically significant results that are not clinically meaningful? Is it possible for results to not be statistically significant but to have clinical meaningfulness? The answer to both questions is an emphatic, yes.

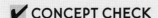 **CONCEPT CHECK**

Traditional statistical analysis assesses the statistical significance of the involved comparisons, but does not necessarily assess the clinical meaningfulness of the results.

The aim of this section is not to discount the role of statistical hypothesis testing in the analysis of clinical trials data. There is clearly a role for hypothesis testing and it should be viewed as an integral part of data analysis, but not the only means of analysis. Hypothesis testing does not provide information about the magnitude of mean differences between comparisons and this is the limitation of this technique.

EXAMPLE

Statistical Significance versus Clinical Meaningfulness

A certain flexibility exercise may lead to small increases in joint range of motion in all subjects. A controlled study of this intervention may find that it results in a significant ($P<0.05$) increase in joint range of motion compared to a control intervention. However, if the mean difference between groups is only 2 degrees of motion, astute clinicians will question whether or not an increase of that small magnitude is of any clinical importance.

✔ CONCEPT CHECK

There is clearly a role for hypothesis testing and it should be viewed as an integral part of data analysis, but not the only means of analysis. Hypothesis testing does not provide information about the magnitude of mean differences between comparisons and this is the limitation of this technique.

In the above example, the unit of measurement (degrees) is quite easy for clinicians to interpret and thus the meaningfulness of the results can be easily ascertained.

When measures are not so easily understood on face value, other analysis concepts such as confidence intervals, effect sizes, and minimal clinically important differences may be employed.

Confidence Intervals

Confidence intervals are an estimate of dispersion, or variability, around a point estimate. In the case of treatment outcomes data, the point estimate is typically a mean, or average, value for a given sample. (It is important to recognize that confidence intervals can be calculated around almost any statistical measure that gives a point estimate.) If a different sample were measured out of the entire relevant population, the point estimate would likely vary somewhat from the original point estimate. If different samples were taken continually and the means graphed, we would eventually be likely to have a normal distribution of point estimates (see Figure 16-2).

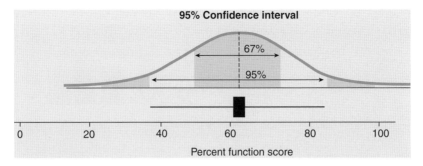

FIGURE 16-2   Point estimate (represented by the black rectangle) and 95% confidence interval (represented by the horizontal black lines extending from the rectangle). We are 95% confident that the true population mean lies within the confidence interval.

✔ **CONCEPT CHECK**

Confidence intervals are an estimate of dispersion, or variability, around a point estimate.

The confidence intervals between two comparisons can be evaluated visually by assessing whether the confidence intervals overlap or not. If confidence intervals do overlap, there is uncertainty as to whether a meaningful difference exists between the two conditions (see Figure 16-3).

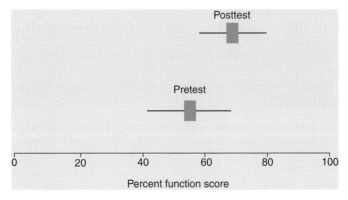

FIGURE 16-3   The two confidence intervals overlap so there is considerable uncertainty that a difference exists between the two conditions.

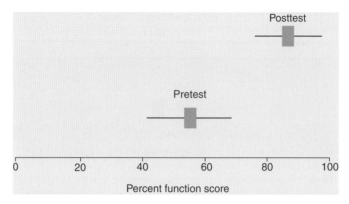

FIGURE 16-4   The two confidence intervals do not overlap so there is certainty that a difference exists between the two conditions.

In contrast, if there is no overlap between the confidence intervals of two comparisons, we are at least 95% certain that there is a clear difference between the two conditions (see Figure 16-4).

Confidence intervals are determined as $M \pm w$, where M represents the point estimate and w represents the width of the confidence interval. To calculate the width, $w = T_c(SE)$, where T_c represent an established critical value to be used as a multiplier (95% CI: 1.96, 99% CI: 5.2), and SE represents standard error. SE is calculated as $SD/\sqrt{n}$, where SD is the standard deviation associated with the point estimate and n is the sample size. The width of the confidence interval is thus influenced by two factors, the variance in the data (indicated by the SD) and the sample size. Wider confidence intervals are associated with larger SD, low sample size, or both. Narrower, more precise, confidence intervals occur with smaller SD, higher sample size, or both.

The assessment of confidence intervals provides an estimate of the certainty that differences actually exist or do not exist in the entire population, as opposed to the sample used for the particular study.

✔ CONCEPT CHECK

The width of the confidence interval is influenced by two factors: the variance in the data (indicated by the SD) and the sample size.

Effect Sizes

Another way to interpret data is the use of effect sizes. Effect sizes provide an estimate of the strength of a treatment effect and, thus, an indication of the meaningfulness of results. Where confidence intervals involved the unit of measurement, effect sizes are on a standardized, unitless scale. There are several ways to compute effect sizes, but the most straightforward method is Cohen's d. Quite simply, d = (Mean 2 − Mean 1)/SD 1, where Mean 2 represents the experimental condition, and Mean 1 and SD 1 represent the control condition. Essentially, this effect size estimate treats the mean difference between conditions as a proportion of the standard deviation.

✔ CONCEPT CHECK

Effect sizes provide an estimate of the strength of a treatment effect and, thus, an indication of the meaningfulness of results.

In cases where there is not a clear control condition, effect size can be calculated as d = (Mean 2 − Mean 1)/pooled SD. In this case the denominator represents the pooled standard deviation of both conditions.

The most common interpretation of effect size estimates is derived from the social sciences (Cohen, 1988). Effect sizes greater than 0.8 are considered "strong," those between 0.5 and 0.8 "moderate," between 0.2 and 0.5 "small," and less than 0.2 "weak." There is some debate about whether this same scale can be simply applied to health outcomes measures, but at this time these values are widely accepted (Rhea, 2004).

Whether an effect size estimate is positive or negative simply reflects which condition is placed first in the numerator of the effect size equation. In general, effect sizes are reported as positive values unless there is a specific reason to report them as negative values. It must be noted that confidence intervals can also be created around effect size point estimates as a method of providing an assessment of the precision, or certainty, of the treatment effect. The interpretation of these confidence intervals is very similar to those previously described in this chapter.

✔ CONCEPT CHECK

In general, effect sizes are reported as positive values unless there is a specific reason to report them as negative values.

Minimal Clinically Important Difference

The topic of receiver operator characteristic (ROC) curves is introduced in Chapter 13. That chapter is devoted to issues of diagnostic accuracy. ROC curves can also be applied to analyses of data related to treatment outcomes and prognosis. Specifically, ROC analysis provides one a means of identifying the change in a health status measure that is associated with improvements that are meaningful to patients. This value is referred to as the *minimally clinically important difference* (MCID) or *minimally important difference* (MID). ROC analysis has also been applied in the development of clinical prediction rules, discussed in detail in Chapter 17, to identify findings from patient history, observation, and physical examination that predict success when a specific intervention is applied.

✔ CONCEPT CHECK

ROC analysis provides one a means of identifying the change in a health status measure that is associated with improvements that are meaningful to patients. This value is referred to as the *minimally clinically important difference* (MCID) or *minimally important difference* (MID).

The structure of the ROC for these applications is very similar to that previously described in Chapter 13. Recall that the use of an ROC analysis in diagnostic studies is needed when the measure in question is continuous rather than dichotomous. The point on that continuous measure that best differentiates those with and without the condition or disease of interest based on a dichotomous "gold" standard is identified on the ROC. In the case of estimating an MCID, the continuous measure is the change reported on a patient self-report measure or a clinician-derived measure such as range of motion while the dichotomous measure may be a report of being at least "much improved" on a Global Rating of Change (GROC) scale or the ability to return to work or sport. As with ROC analyses applied in diagnostic studies a point (remember northwest corner) can be identified on the continuous measure that best differentiates those that are improved or return to an activity from those patients that do not.

In the case of clinical prediction rules the continuous measure is the number of factors present following patient evaluation that are related to the outcome of treatment. Along this scale there will be a point representing the number of factors present that best differentiates patients who responded well (e.g., much improved based on GROC or >50% reduction in pain) from those who did not (e.g., no change in condition reported on GROC or <50% reduction in pain). Examining examples from the clinical literature best reveals the value of these analyses in estimating MCID and deriving clinical prediction rules.

✔ CONCEPT CHECK

In the case of clinical prediction rules the continuous measure is the number of factors present following patient evaluation that are related to the outcome of treatment.

There are multiple approaches to estimating an MCID including ROC analysis, use of standard error measurement values, and effect size estimates. Each approach has advantages and disadvantages and this discussion is not intended to suggest that the use of an ROC analysis is always preferable. The impact of these different approaches is not trivial and each is discussed in detail by Copay et al. (2008).

Stucki et al. (1995) investigated the use of Physical Function Scale, Symptom Severity Scale, Roland–Morris scale, and Sickness Impact Profile to differentiate between levels of satisfaction 6 months following surgery in patients with spinal stenosis (see Figure 16-5). Examining the Roland scale result the ROC analysis revealed that a difference of 1.25 units change differentiated patients who were unsatisfied with their outcome from those that were somewhat satisfied or better. Interestingly, if the mean differences in Roland scale scores were used, the difference between unsatisfied and somewhat satisfied patients was 1.4 units. Either estimate of MCID might be considered appropriate but it is important, as noted by Copay et al. (2008), that the means of calculating the MDIC be made clear to the reader. Figure 16-5 and the paper by Stucki et al. (1995) illustrate another application of ROC analyses. Note that the area under the curve is greatest for the Physical Function Scale. This finding suggests that the Physical Function Scale better discriminates between unsatisfied patients and the others. The construction of 95% confidence intervals would reveal whether these differences are statistically significant. An illustration of this application is found in McBrier et al. (2009).

CLINICAL PREDICTION RULES

Flynn et al. (2002) derived a clinical prediction rule to guide the treatment of patients with low back pain with spinal manipulation. Ultimately, five factors were selected that best discriminate between patients who have a favorable response to spinal manipulation defined as a greater than 50% improvement on the Modified Oswestry Disability Questionnaire and those that did not. The identified factors were a duration of symptoms <16 days, having at least one hip with >35° of internal rotation, hypomobility with lumbar spring testing, Fear Avoidance Beliefs Questionnaire (FABQ) work subscale score <19, and no symptoms distal to the knee. Three of these measures (duration of symptoms, hip range of motion, and FABQ scores) are continuous measures. The authors assessed the ability of each of these and other continuous measures to differentiate between patients who had favorable responses from those that did not. The result of this research was that patients with four or more predictors of success were 24.38 times (+LR = 24.38, 95% CI 4.63 − 139.41) more likely to respond favorably to manipulation than patients with 3 or fewer predictors of success. For those with three or more predictors the associated +LR = 2.61 (95% CI 1.78 − 4.15), demonstrating a substantial decrease in the likelihood of achieving >50% improvement on the Modified Oswestry Disability Questionnaire following manipulation.

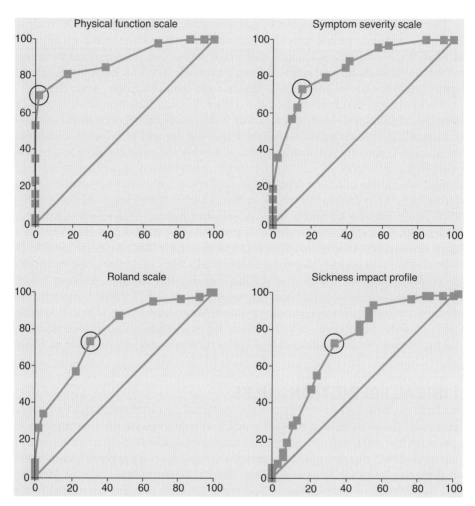

FIGURE 16-5   ROC curves of different self-reported measures in spinal stenosis patients. The y-axis represents sensitivity and the x-axis represents 1-specificity. The red circles represent the most "northwest" point on the ROC curve, indicating the best combination of sensitivity and specificity. The unit measures for the most "northwest" points were 0.45 for the Symptom Severity Scale, 0.40 for the Physical Function Scale, 1.25 for the Roland Scale, and 4.0 for the Sickness Impact Scale. (Reprinted with permission from Stucki G, Liang MH, Fossel AH, et al. Relative responsiveness of condition-specific health status measures in degenerative lumbar spinal stenosis. *J Clin Epidemiol.* 1995;48:1369–1378.)

The papers by Stucki et al. (1995) and Flynn et al. (2002) are examples of the utility of ROCs across varying research purposes. The analyses essentially identify cut-offs or points along continuous data that best correspond to dichotomous sub-groups of a sample drawn from a population. Although the concept of ROCs may appear foreign and perhaps intimidating, once an understanding of sensitivity and specificity (see Chapter 9 for a detailed explanation) is gained the use of ROC analysis in research and interpretation of these analyses in the clinical literature we read become much more user-friendly.

COMPREHENSIVE DATA ANALYSIS

The purpose of this section is to identify multiple ways to interpret data from clinical outcomes studies. Traditional hypothesis testing is the most common way to analyze data statistically, but its limitations in assessing clinical meaningfulness must be acknowledged. We are not advocating the replacement of hypothesis testing with alternative techniques such as confidence intervals, effect sizes, and MCIDs, but instead are suggesting that these be used as adjuncts to hypothesis testing as part of a comprehensive data analysis plan.

✔ CONCEPT CHECK

Traditional hypothesis testing is the most common way to analyze data statistically, but its limitations in assessing clinical meaningfulness must be acknowledged.

CHAPTER SUMMARY

Clinical outcomes studies form the basis of much of evidence-based practice. Performing successful clinical trials requires a solid infrastructure for data collection and management, the use of a sound study design, and a comprehensive data analysis plan. Careful planning is essential for successful execution of clinical outcomes research.

KEY POINTS

- The importance of building a strong research infrastructure for clinical outcomes research cannot be overemphasized.
- The design of a clinical trial is the greatest factor that influences the "level of evidence" stemming from that study's results.

- Evidence derived from expert opinion and disease-oriented evidence resulting from basic and translational research is the lowest level of evidence in the evidence hierarchy set by the Centre for Evidence-Based Medicine (CEBM).
- A case series represents the reporting of the clinical outcomes of a number of patients with the same pathology who are treated with the same or similar intervention.
- Case control studies are by definition retrospective in nature.
- The randomized controlled trial (RCT) is the gold standard for clinical investigation.
- The individual responsible for coordinating the randomization should not be directly involved in deciding the inclusion criteria of potential subjects or the measurement of outcomes directly from patients.
- Hypothesis testing does not provide information about the magnitude of mean differences between comparisons and this is the limitation of this technique.

Critical Thinking Questions

1. What are the two most common schemas for classifying levels of evidence?
2. What are the five general categories of levels of evidence utilized by the CEBM?
3. Why are case control study designs *not* randomized?

Applying Concepts

1. Consider and discuss what is meant by the phrase "best research evidence." Provide historical and current examples from clinical and health-related research.
2. Discuss and debate the advantages and disadvantages of prospective cohort studies. Keep in mind that the choice of treatment is *not* randomly assigned but is instead left to the discretion of the treating clinician. What are some of the confounding factors that may influence the decision to treat patients with the respective interventions? Provide specific examples and details to support your position.
3. Is it possible to have statistically significant results that are not clinically meaningful? Is it possible for results to not be statistically significant but to have clinical meaningfulness? The answer to both questions is an emphatic, yes. Discuss and explain why the answer to both of these questions is "yes."

REFERENCES

Chodron P. *When Things Fall Apart: Heartfelt Advice for Difficult Times*. Boston, MA: Shambala Publication, Inc.; 1997.

Cohen J. *Statistical Power Analysis for the Behavioral Sciences*. 2nd ed. Hillsdale, NJ: Lawrence Erlbaum Associates; 1988.

Copay AG, Glassman SD, Subach BR, et al. The minimum clinically important difference in lumbar spine surgery: a choice of methods using the Oswestry Disability Index, Medical Outcomes Study Questionnaire Short Form 36, and pain scales. *Spine J*. 2008;8:968–974.

Flynn T, Fritz J, Whitman J, et al. A clinical prediction rule for classifying patients who demonstrate short-term improvement with spinal manipulation. *Spine*. 2002;27: 2835–2843.

McBrier NM, Neuberger T, Denegar CR, et al. MR imaging of acute injury in rats and effects of Buprenex® on limb volume. *J Am Assn Lab Animal Sci*. 2009;48:1–5.

Rhea MR. Determining the magnitude of treatment effects in strength training research through the use of the effect size. *J Strength Cond Res*. 2004;18:918–920.

Stucki G, Liang MH, Fossel AH, et al. Relative responsiveness of condition-specific health status measures in degenerative lumbar spinal stenosis. *J Clin Epidemiol*. 1995;48: 1369–1378.

SUGGESTED READING

Hopkins WG, Marshall SW, Batterham AM, et al. Progressive statistics for studies in sports medicine and exercise science. *Med Sci Sports Exerc*. 2009;41(1):3–13.

CHAPTER 17

CLINICAL PRACTICE GUIDELINES AND CLINICAL PREDICTION RULES

*The men of experiment are like the ant, they only collect
and use; the reasoners resemble spiders, who make cobwebs
out of their own substance.*

—Francis Bacon, from Aphorism 95 from Bacon's 1620 work
The New Organon, or True Directions Concerning the
Interpretation of Nature, as quoted on goodreads
(http://www.goodreads.com/quotes/)

CHAPTER OBJECTIVES

After reading this chapter, you will:

- Understand the difference between clinical prediction guides (also known as clinical prediction rules) and clinical practice guidelines.
- Understand the grading system for clinical practice guidelines.
- Understand the concept and application of clinical prediction guides.
- Be able to explain and describe why and how the Ottawa Ankle Rules are used as prediction guides.
- Be able to discuss how practice guides are connected to diagnostic studies.
- Discuss how patient care is improved through the use of clinical practice guidelines and clinical prediction guides.
- Explain and describe the concept of "strength of evidence" in clinical research.
- Identify outside influences when implementing a strategy to take care of a patient.

KEY TERMS

clinical practice guidelines
clinical prediction guides
clinical prediction rules
intervention

likelihood ratios
population values
position statements
predictor variables

receiver operator characteristic curve
regression analysis
strength of the evidence

INTRODUCTION

This section of the book has been devoted to research methods and data analyses across a spectrum of clinical research. We have addressed diagnostic procedures, screening and treatment outcomes, and explored systematic review and meta-analysis. Before closing out this section two additional topics warrant attention: **clinical prediction guides** (also known as clinical prediction rules) and **clinical practice guidelines**. These topics could be addressed in separate short chapters. However, while quite different in scope and developmental process each helps answer the question of how to proceed with specific patients based on presentation and examination findings. Thus, we have chosen to include these topics in a single chapter.

CLINICAL PREDICTION GUIDES

Clinical Prediction Guides as Evaluative Procedures

Clinical prediction guides (also known as clinical prediction rules) are developed from a cluster of exam findings or characteristics and may assist in the evaluative or treatment phase of patient care. We prefer the term clinical practice guide, as opposed to rule, since the true purpose of these reports is to guide, rather than dictate, clinical decisions.

EXAMPLE

Ottawa Ankle Rules

In Chapter 13 we introduced the Ottawa Ankle Rules. The Ottawa Ankle Rules are an example of a clinical prediction guide that has evolved into a clinical practice guideline in some centers. The Ottawa Ankle Rules are based on the observation of weight-bearing status and areas of tenderness upon palpation. Patients presenting following lateral sprains that are able to bear weight for four steps and are not tender over posterior 6 cm of the medial or lateral malleoli, the base of the fifth metatarsal or navicular, are very unlikely to have sustained a fracture and thus radiographic evaluation is not indicated. If the patient is unable to bear weight for 4 steps or has pain with palpation at distal 6 cm of the medial or lateral malleolus, the base of the fifth metatarsal or the navicular radiographic evaluation is needed to determine whether a fracture has occurred. This clinical prediction guide has been studied in a number of settings using a variety of assessors (e.g., orthopaedic surgeons [Springer et al., 2000], family physicians [McBride, 1997], physical therapists [Springer et al., 2000], nurse practitioners [Mann et al., 1998], and nurses [Derksen et al., 2005; Fiesseler et al., 2004; Karpas et al. 2002]) and settings (e.g., emergency department [Broomhead & Stuart, 2003; Karpas et al., 2002; Papacostas et al., 2001; Yazdani et al., 2006] and clinics [Papacostas et al., 2001; Wynn-Thomas et al., 2002]) has performed well. As noted previously, this level of development has resulted in the Ottawa Ankle Rules emerging as practice guidelines, addressed at the end of this chapter, in some settings.

✔ CONCEPT CHECK

The Ottawa Ankle Rules are an example of a clinical prediction guide based on the observation of weight-bearing status and areas of tenderness upon palpation.

Clinical prediction guides for the use of radiographic examination have also been developed for patients presenting with knee pain and a history of cervical spine injury. The Ottawa Health Research Institute web site (http://www.ohri.ca/emerg/cdr.html) provides descriptions of each of these examination procedures. Clinical prediction guides have also been developed to assist in the identification of conditions where single examination procedures provide unacceptable results and "gold standard" assessment is difficult. Laslett et al. (2005) identified a cluster of tests which when collectively positive are strongly predictive of low back pain of sacroiliac joint origins. Specifically, the tests employed by these investigators were distraction, right-sided thigh thrust, right-sided Gaenslen test, compression, and sacral thrust. When three or more of these tests provoked pain the patients were 4.29 (+LR = 4.29) times more likely to experience pain resolution following sacroiliac joint injection with an anesthetic than patients with two or fewer positive tests.

✔ CONCEPT CHECK

Clinical prediction guides are developed from a cluster of exam findings or characteristics and may assist in the evaluative or treatment phase of patient care.

Clinical Prediction Guides as Treatment Procedures

As noted, clinical prediction guides are not isolated to evaluative procedures. Flynn et al. (2002) identified a cluster of characteristics of patients with low back pain likely to benefit from spinal manipulation. These investigators reported that patients with low back pain that met at least four of five criteria (duration of current episode less than 16 days, no symptoms distal to the knee, Fear-Avoidance Beliefs Questionnaire work subscale less than 19, evidence of lumbar spine segmental hypomobility, and the presence of at least 1 hip with at least 35 degrees of internal rotation range of motion) had a more favorable outcome to manipulation than those meeting few or none of these criteria. In a subsequent study Childs et al. (2004) reported a 92% chance of successful outcome when patients meeting the same criteria were treated with spinal manipulation. Moreover, patients positive on the guide that were treated with exercise experienced substantially and statistically significantly less improvement on all **outcomes measures**. Similar investigations have identified clusters of signs and symptoms that predict optimal outcomes with stabilization (Hicks et al., 2005) and spinal extension–based exercises (Browder et al., 2007).

DATA ANALYSIS

Data analysis in studies conducted to develop and validate clinical predication guides may compare outcomes measures between groups as described in Chapters 15 and 16 devoted to outcomes measures. Childs et al. (2004) compared patients receiving or not receiving care based on the clinical predication guide developed by Flynn et al. (2002). As noted above, those that were treated with spinal manipulation based on the criteria proposed by Flynn et al. (2002) had superior outcomes at 6 months in comparison to patients identified as candidates for manipulation but assigned to treatment with exercise alone. The analyses conducted by Flynn et al. (2002) used data from a single cohort to generate **likelihood ratios** that translated into the probability of a successful outcome based on a dichotomous measure when a patient presents with a set of predictive characteristics. This process is further illustrated in the following example.

EXAMPLE

Estimating the Likelihood of a Successful Treatment Outcome from Medical History and Physical Examination Findings

Cleland et al. (2007) provide an excellent example of this approach. The purpose of the investigation was to identify patients with neck pain likely to benefit from thoracic spine manipulation. Seventy-eight patients with neck pain were treated with thoracic spine manipulation of whom 42 were deemed to have benefited from one treatment of thoracic spine manipulation based on a global rating of change score of 5 or more corresponding to at least being "quite a bit better." Through **regression analysis** six variables were retained as being predictive of outcomes: symptom duration of <30 days, no symptoms distal to the shoulder, subject reports that looking up does not aggravate symptoms, Fear-Avoidance Beliefs Questionnaire Physical Activity subscale score of <12, diminished upper thoracic spine kyphosis (T3–T5), and cervical extension of <30 degrees. Treatment outcomes were dichotomized as successful or unsuccessful based on the global rating of change score (see Table 17-1) permitting the generation of a **receiver operator characteristic curve** (introduced in Chapter 13).

Table 17-1	The six variables forming the clinical prediction rule and the number of subjects in each group at each level[a]

- Symptoms <30 days
- No symptoms distal to the shoulder
- Looking up does not aggravate symptoms
- FABQPA score <12
- Diminished upper thoracic spine kyphosis
- Cervical extension ROM <30 degrees

NO. OF PREDICTOR VARIABLES PRESENT	SUCCESSFUL OUTCOME GROUP	NONSUCCESSFUL OUTCOME GROUP
6	2	0
5	3	0
4	9	1
3	18	4
2	7	11
1	3	14
0	0	6

[a]FABQPA, Fear-Avoidance Beliefs Questionnaire Physical Activity subscale; ROM, range of motion. (Reprinted with permission from Cleland JA, Childs JD, Fritz JM, et al. Development of a clinical prediction rule for guiding treatment of a subgroup of patients with neck pain: use of thoracic spine manipulation, exercise, and patient education. *Phys Ther.* 2007;87:9-23.)

These investigators reported an $+LR = 5.9$ (95% CI = 2.72 to 12.0) when three or more predictors were present meaning that these patients were, on average, 5.9 times more likely to benefit from thoracic spine manipulation than those with fewer **predictor variables**. The $+LR$ increased to 12 (95% CI = 2.28 to 72.8) when four or more predictor variables were present. The presence of three or more predictor variables raised the probability of a successful outcome from 54% (42 of 78 patients) to 86% (32 of 37 patients).

Clinical prediction guides, like other clinical trials, are single research endeavors that provide estimates of **population values**. Repetition of studies is warranted. When similar results are reported in subsequent studies the prediction guide is strengthened and point estimates can be refined through meta-analysis.

CLINICAL PRACTICE GUIDELINES

Clinical Practice Guidelines versus Clinical Prediction Guides

Clinical practice guideline sounds similar to clinical prediction guides; however, a clinical practice guideline is quite different. While practice guidelines and prediction guides assist in the diagnosis and treatment of patients, clinical practice guidelines are broader in scope and development. Clinical practice guidelines are "systematically developed statements to assist practitioner and patient decisions about appropriate health care for specific clinical circumstances" (Institute of Medicine, 1990). The primary distinctions between practice guidelines and prediction guides are that guidelines are developed by a team of clinician–scholars after systematic review of the literature rather than from a single investigation and are generally more comprehensive.

The task of authors of clinical practice guidelines, also sometimes labeled as **position statements**, is to synthesize the best available evidence and provide concise recommendations for patient care. The strength of the research evidence can vary between and even within a clinical practice guideline depending on the quality and quantity of research available. In some cases recommendations are well founded in the research literature. Sometimes, however, recommendations are based on expert consensus because sufficient research data is not available. Therefore those that generate clinical practice guidelines, often subgroups of professional organizations, should periodically update practice guidelines to reflect the current best evidence.

A Word of Caution About Implementing Clinical Practice Guidelines

Clinical practice guidelines can be very useful to the busy clinician. Clinical practice guidelines can provide a quick reference for a course of action in the evaluation and treatment of a particular patient. Unlike systematic reviews that may conclude insufficient evidence exists to recommend or not recommend a particular test or **intervention**, clinical practice guidelines are likely to offer direction. Despite a common desire to "cut to the chase" and implement a plan, the clinician should review clinical practice guidelines as carefully as any other type of research addressed in this text. Sackett et al. (2000) provided an excellent summary of clinical practice guidelines to help the reader appraise the guideline and consider whether it is appropriate to apply the guideline in the management of a particular patient. As noted above, the evidence at the foundation of a clinical practice guideline may range from the review of one or more high-quality systematic reviews to reliance primarily on expert consensus. The **strength of the evidence** supporting a clinical practice guideline should be provided to the consumer by the authors of clinical practice guideline. Sackett et al. (2000) presented a system of grading recommendations with letters A, B, C, and D based on the strength of the research evidence available for diagnostic, intervention (treatment and prevention), prognostic, and economic analysis clinical practice guidelines. Table 17-2 provides a summary of grading of recommendations related to diagnosis and intervention. This summary can assist in the critical appraisal of clinical practice guidelines. The highest levels of evidence generate grade A recommendations. Highest levels of evidence are not, however, always available. B grade recommendations derived from studies of patient cohorts might, for example, be the best available evidence under some circumstances (e.g., management of rare conditions). The clinician–consumer of the medical literature must ultimately decide to abide by a clinical practice guideline or deviate from a guideline in the management of a particular patient. To best weigh and ponder the options the clinician should be informed as to the level of evidence considered in developing a clinical practice guideline.

✔ CONCEPT CHECK

Sackett et al. (2000, pp. 173, 177) presented a system of grading recommendations with letters A, B, C, and D based on the strength of the research evidence available for diagnostic, intervention (treatment and prevention), prognostic, and economic analysis clinical practice guidelines. Table 17-2 is adapted from Sackett et al. to summarize grades and levels of evidence from intervention (prevention and treatment) and diagnostic studies.

Table 17-2 Grades and levels of evidence in intervention (treatment and prevention) and diagnostic studies

GRADE	LEVEL	INTERVENTION	DIAGNOSIS
A	1a	Systematic reviews with homogeneity of data derived from randomized controlled clinical trials	Systematic reviews with homogeneity of data derived from level 1 diagnostic studies or clinical practice guides validated in independent testing
	1b	Single randomized controlled clinical trial with narrow confidence interval	High-quality study of a diagnostic test including independent blind comparison of appropriately selected consecutive patients undergoing both the diagnostic test and reference standard test
	1c	All or none—either all patients achieve desired outcome when only some had or some patients achieve a desired outcome when previously none had[a]	Absolute Spin of Snout[b]
B	2a	Systematic reviews with homogeneity of data derived from cohort studies	Systematic reviews with homogeneity of data derived from level 2 diagnostic studies
	2b	Single cohort study or lower-quality randomized controlled clinical trial	Independent blind comparison of diagnostic test and reference clinical trial standard in nonconsecutive patients or a narrow spectrum of patients or nonvalidated clinical prediction guide
C	3a	Systematic reviews with homogeneity of data derived from case control studies	None
	3b	Single case control study	Independent blind comparison of diagnostic test and reference standard without reference standard testing for all patients
	4	Case series and low-quality case control studies	Diagnostic studies where reference standard was not applied to blind clinicians conducting the diagnostic test
D	5	Expert opinion without explicit critical appraisal (systematic review) or expert opinion based on nonclinical research	Expert opinion without explicit critical appraisal (systematic review) or expert opinion based on nonclinical research

[a]All or none is generally associated with death and survival but might be applied to functional recovery (e.g., before the development of a surgical technique no athletes returned to professional level sports and now some do).

[b]See page 226 for discussion of SpPIn and SnNOut. (Adapted with permission from Sackett DL, Straus SE, Richardson WS, et al. *Evidence-based medicine: how to practice and teach EBM.* Edinburgh: Churchill Livingston; 2000.)

LEVELS OF EVIDENCE

Level of Evidence and Grade of Recommendation

Grade A recommendations are the result of the availability of level 1 evidence which in the case of interventions consists of systematic reviews of randomized controlled trials with homogeneous results (1a) (a "-" is added to identify recommendations where there is concern resulting from heterogeneity of findings or wide confidence intervals), individual randomized controlled trials with narrow confidence intervals (1b), or all or none results (1c) where either all patients died prior to the intervention in question and some now survive or where some patients died prior to the intervention and now some survive. Grade B recommendations stem from systematic reviews based on level 2 evidence consisting of systematic reviews of cohort studies with homogeneous results (2a), individual cohort studies or RTC with less than 80% follow-up (2b), outcomes research (2c), systematic reviews of case control studies with homogeneous results (3a), or individual case control studies (3b). Grade C recommendations are based on case series or lower-quality case control or cohort studies (evidence level 4) while grade D recommendations stem from expert opinions, logical applications of physiologic principles, or bench science (evidence level 5).

DIAGNOSTIC PRACTICE GUIDELINES AND GRADE OF RECOMMENDATION

In the case of diagnostic practice guidelines, grade A recommendations also result from systematic reviews of high-quality diagnostic studies (see Chapter 18) with homogeneous results (1a), from well-conducted studies meeting the standard for level 1 systematic review (1b), or in situations with absolute sensitivity or specificity (1c). Grade B recommendations result from systematic reviews of diagnostic studies where one or more sources of bias were introduced (e.g., not all patients received the "gold standard" assessment, assessors were not blinded, etc.) (2a) or single clinical trials in which not all patients received the "gold standard" assessment. Grade C recommendations stem from single clinical trials without assessor blinding (evidence level 4), while grade D recommendations are the results of expert opinions, logical applications of physiologic principles, or bench science (evidence level 5). As with the grading of evidence related to intervention a "-" is used to signify that there is concern resulting from heterogeneity of findings or wide confidence intervals.

ADDITIONAL CONSIDERATIONS

Once the consumer has ascertained that the clinical practice guidelines have resulted from a comprehensive (all languages, all journals) review and is up to date and considered the strength of the recommendations, there are additional considerations before proceeding with the recommended patient care. In the case of prevention efforts one must decide if the event rate and/or seriousness of the problem warrant the expenditure and effort required to implement the intervention. In all cases where a patient or the patient's guardians are able to provide input one must also consider whether a proposed plan for diagnosis or treatment is in conflict with their beliefs and values. Lastly, one must consider whether there are barriers to implementation. For example, while the work of Childs et al. (2004) cited previously might result in a clinical practice guideline calling for thoracic spine manipulation in a 40-year-old patient presenting with thoracic kyphosis, limited cervical extension, and an absence of radicular symptoms, the treatment may not fall within the practice domain based on the state in which a clinician is credentialed to practice. Organizational rules, entrenched local traditions, and resource availability may also pose barriers that the clinician cannot overcome in an effort to implement a clinical practice guideline.

✔ CONCEPT CHECK

In all cases where a patient or the patient's guardians are able to provide input one must also consider whether a proposed plan for diagnosis or treatment is in conflict with their beliefs and values.

CHAPTER SUMMARY

In summary, while attractive and frequently very helpful, the clinician must be prepared to critically review clinical practice guidelines as with other forms of clinical literature. The development of clinical prediction guides and clinical practice guidelines, combined with the evolution of the Internet however, greatly expands access to information likely to improve patient care. For example, Fritz et al. (2007) investigated the impact of following guidelines recommending active intervention in the treatment of patients with low back pain. Those treatments that adhered to the clinical prediction guide experienced greater pain relief, greater functional recovery, and were 77% more likely to be deemed to have a successful outcome in physical therapy despite requiring less care rendered at a lower cost. Thus, when appropriately assessed and implemented, prediction guides and practice guidelines enhance care and may lower health care costs.

KEY POINTS

- Clinical prediction guides are formed from a cluster of exam findings and may help with forming a diagnosis or the treatment of a patient.
- Position statements are often clinical practice guidelines developed to improve health care practice.
- Implementation of clinical practice guidelines can be hindered by factors including organizational rules, availability of proper resources, and tradition.
- The goal of clinical practice guidelines is to combine the best evidence and provide the most useful recommendations for the patient care.
- Clinical practice guidelines should be regularly updated in order to reflect the best evidence to date.
- Clinical prediction guides can help with identifying a problem when a single examination does not provide results.
- Clinical prediction guides can be used to help determine the need for referral for radiographic examination and other diagnostic work-up.
- Clinical practice guidelines are professional edicts developed by a team of clinician–scholars.
- While clinical practice guidelines are valuable resources, the practice of evidence-based care calls for the integration of patient's values and clinician experience into clinical decision-making. Thus, a patient's values and preferences must be taken into consideration when deciding the appropriate course of action.

Critical Thinking Questions

1. What outside influences have to be considered when deciding the appropriate course of action for a patient?
2. If a new treatment exists, what must be done to determine its effectiveness?

Applying Concepts

1. Use Sackett's grading recommendations with letters (A, B, C, and D) to base the strength of the research evidence available for diagnostic, intervention (treatment and prevention), prognostic, and economic analysis clinical practice guidelines for a current clinical study of your choice.
2. Discuss how you would use the Ottawa Ankle Rules as prediction guidelines to help determine the need for radiographic evaluation to judge the chances of an ankle fracture following a lateral sprain.

REFERENCES

Broomhead A, Stuart P. Validation of the Ottawa Ankle Rules in Australia. *Emerg Med (Fremantle)*. 2003;15:126–132.

Browder DA, Childs JD, Cleland JA, et al. Effectiveness of an extension-oriented treatment approach in a subgroup of subjects with low back pain: a randomized clinical trial. *Phys Ther*. 2007;87:1608–1618.

Childs JD, Fritz JM, Flynn TW, et al. A clinical prediction rule to identify patients with low back pain most likely to benefit from spinal manipulation: a validation study. *Ann Intern Med*. 2004;141:920–928.

Cleland JA, Childs JD, Fritz JM, et al. Development of a clinical prediction rule for guiding treatment of a subgroup of patients with neck pain: use of thoracic spine manipulation, exercise, and patient education. *Phys Ther*. 2007;87:9–23.

Derksen RJ, Bakker FC, Geervliet PC, et al. Diagnostic accuracy and reproducibility in the interpretation of Ottawa ankle and foot rules by specialized emergency nurses. *Am J Emerg Med*. 2005;23:725–729.

Fiesseler F, Szucs P, Kec R, et al. Can nurses appropriately interpret the Ottawa ankle rule? *Am J Emerg Med*. 2004;22:145–148.

Flynn T, Fritz J, Whitman J, et al. A clinical prediction rule for classifying patients with low back pain who demonstrate short-term improvement with spinal manipulation. *Spine*. 2002;27:2835–2843.

Fritz JM, Cleland JA, Brennan GP. Does adherence to the guideline recommendation for active treatments improve the quality of care for patients with acute low back pain delivered by physical therapists? *Med Care*. 2007;45:973–980.

Hicks GE, Fritz JM, Delitto A, et al. Preliminary development of a clinical prediction rule for determining which patients with low back pain will respond to a stabilization exercise program. *Arch Phys Med Rehabil*. 2005;86:1753–1762. Available at http://www.ohri.ca/emerg/cdr.html, accessed January 5, 2010.

Institute of Medicine. *Clinical Practice Guidelines*: *Directions for a New Program*. Washington, DC: National Academy Press; 1990.

Karpas A, Hennes H, Walsh-Kelly CM. Utilization of the Ottawa ankle rules by nurses in a pediatric emergency department. *Acad Emerg Med*. 2002;9:130–133.

Laslett M, Aprill CN, McDonald B, et al. Diagnosis of sacroiliac joint pain validity of individual provocation tests and composites of tests. *Man Ther*. 2005;10:207–218.

Mann CJ, Grant I, Guly H, et al. Use of the Ottawa ankle rules by nurse practitioners. *J Accid Emerg Med*. 1998;15:315–316.

McBride KL. Validation of the Ottawa ankle rules. Experience at a community hospital. *Can Fam Physician*. 1997;43:459–465.

Papacostas E, Malliaropoulos N, Papadopoulos A, et al. Validation of Ottawa ankle rules protocol in Greek athletes: study in the emergency departments of a district general hospital and a sports injuries clinic. *Br J Sports Med*. 2001;35:445–447.

Sackett DL, Straus SE, Richardson WS, et al. *Evidence-based Medicine: How to Practice and Teach EBM*. Edinburgh: Churchill Livingston; 2000.

Springer BA, Arciero RA, Tenuta JJ, et al. A prospective study of modified Ottawa ankle rules in a military population. *Am J Sports Med*. 2000;28:864–868.

Wynn-Thomas S, Love T, McLeod D, et al. The Ottawa ankle rules for the use of diagnostic X-ray in after hours medical centres in New Zealand. *NZ Med J*. 2002;115(1162):U184.

Yazdani S, Jahandideh H, Ghofrani H. Validation of the Ottawa ankle rules in Iran: a prospective survey. *BMC Emerg Med*. 2006;6:3.

CHAPTER 18

SYSTEMATIC REVIEW AND META-ANALYSIS

Computers are useless. They can only give you answers.

—Pablo Picasso from Pablo Picasso Quotes as quoted
in BrainyQuote (www.brainyquote.com/quotes/
quotes/p/pablopicas102018.html)

CHAPTER OBJECTIVES

After reading this chapter, you will:

- Learn how to complete a systematic review.
- Understand the hierarchy of evidence.
- Be able to identify the domains and elements of a systematic review.
- Understand the difference between narrative and systematic reviews.
- Identify obstacles clinicians must overcome to practice evidence-based medicine.
- Be able to describe and explain the differences between systematic review and meta-analysis.
- Understand how to conduct a meta-analysis.
- Be able to discuss the concept of validity in systematic review.
- Explain the role of the Cochrane Collaboration in evidence-based health care.
- Understand the concept and implications of publication bias in systematic review.

KEY TERMS

case reports
clinical research
Cochrane Collaboration
evidence-based medicine (EBM)

interpretation
intervention
intervention outcomes
patient-important outcomes

randomized treatment
order trials
strength of evidence
systematic review

INTRODUCTION

Throughout the preceding chapters attention has been directed toward the design of studies and analysis of data related to the prevention, diagnosis, and treatment of illness and injury. In these chapters attention has been directed to the fact that data derived from samples drawn from populations provide only estimates of true population values. For instance, the positive likelihood ratio (+LR) = 3.9 and negative likelihood ratio (−LR) = 0.28 generated from our mock data set (see pages 228–230) provide only an estimate of the diagnostic usefulness of the diagnostic test. The calculation of confidence intervals provides a range (+LR 1.4 to 11.0 and −LR 0.12 to 0.64 in this case) within which we can be 95% confident that a true population value lies. The larger a sample, the more likely the values derived are reflective of the true population values and thus "truth." For example, if one maintains the same proportions of true positives, true negatives, and false findings as described in Table 13-3 with a 10-fold increase in sample size (see Table 18-1) the +LR and −LR values are unchanged but the confidence intervals narrow substantially +LR = 3.9 (95% CI = 2.8 to 5.4), −LR = 0.27 (95% CI = 0.21 to 0.35). Thus, it would seem that what is needed to answer the multitude of clinical questions facing health care providers are large, well-designed studies that generate narrow confidence intervals and thus confidence that the findings reflect the usefulness of diagnostic tests in a population or responses to **interventions**.

This simple solution crumbles when we are faced with the realities of the time, effort, and costs associated with **clinical research**, challenges of recruiting patients into studies, losing patients to drop-out and balancing research with clinical prac-

TABLE 18-1 Gold standard result			
	POSITIVE (CONDITION PRESENT)	**NEGATIVE (CONDITION ABSENT)**	**TOTAL**
Positive examination Using test under study	*Cell A* True positive $n = 180$	*Cell B* False positive $n = 30$	210
Negative examination Using test under study	*Cell C* False negative $n = 50$	*Cell D* True negative $n = 120$	140
Total	230	150	350

Sensitivity = 18/23 = 0.78; Specificity = 12/15 = 0.80; +LR = 3.9 (95% CI = 2.8−5.4); −LR = 0.27 (95% CI = 0.21−0.35).

tice, teaching, and daily responsibilities. Moreover, while communication across the research and clinical communities has increased through the advances in information technology, multiple groups may have and may continue to investigate similar problems simultaneously in various areas of the world.

The clinician seeking to practice **evidence-based medicine** faces two significant obstacles. First, even in the most specialized environments the problems patients bring to us differ. A clinician practicing in an outpatient sports medicine environment may focus on the care of patients following reconstructive knee surgery and total knee arthroplasty. Through training, continuing education, and repetition, patterns of treatment evolve that reflect current best evidence. But we all encounter less common conditions even in specialized practice. How should one treat a patient with pigmented villonodular synovitis? A quick literature search (May 6, 2010) on Pubmed identifies 1018 titles. Perhaps the clinician has sufficient interest and time to read several promising titles and apply the evidence to the care of this patient. But then another unique case presents and it becomes increasingly difficult to catch up.

Moreover, the clinician searching for an answer to a problem will likely find not only multiple papers but also differing and sometimes conflicting results. Wouldn't it be nice if the data from multiple studies could be synthesized and analyzed to guide clinical decisions without individual clinicians having to sort through multiple papers? **Systematic review** provides the clinician the results compiled from multiple clinical trials in a single document, sometimes with the effect of defining current best practice. Such reviews are not always available, frustrating for the clinician but perhaps creating an opportunity for the would-be investigator. In the case of pigmented villonodular synovitis none were found, but several databases (see Table 18-2) contain collections of systematic reviews or ref-

TABLE 18-2	Examples of databases that contain collections of systematic reviews or references to systematic reviews	
DATABASE	**URL**
The Cochrane Collaboration includes Cochrane Database of Systematic Reviews (CDSR), Database of Abstracts of Reviews of Effects (DARE), and Cochrane Central Register of Controlled Trials. The Cochrane Collection includes Cochrane Database of Systematic Reviews (CDSR), Database of Abstracts of Reviews of Effects (DARE), and Cochrane Central Register of Controlled Trials.	http://www.cochrane.org/index.htm
The Physiotherapy Evidence Database	http://www.pedro.fhs.usyd.edu.au/index.html
Center for Review and Dissemination	http://www.crd.york.ac.uk/crdweb/

erences to systematic reviews. The purpose of this chapter is to describe how to complete a systematic review.

 CONCEPT CHECK

The clinician seeking to practice evidence-based medicine faces two significant obstacles.

SYSTEMATIC REVIEW

What For? And, How To?

Before we move forward with the "how to" of systematic review one additional point needs to be made regarding the "what for." Systematic reviews are clinician-friendly and summarize the evidence into a single paper. But how are systematic reviews viewed in comparison to other forms of "evidence"? Several authors have described hierarchies of the strength of the evidence provided in various forms of clinical research (see Boxes 7.1, 18.1, and Figure 18-1)

In each of the hierarchies described in Box 18.1 and Figure 18-1, systematic review takes a rightful place as the most compelling evidence in most circumstances. Note that within patient, **randomized treatment order trials,** while excellent, require that each patient enrolled in a study receives all interventions for prescribed periods of time in randomized order. While possible in studying interventions in

---

BOX 18.1	**A hierarchy of strength of evidence for treatment decisions.**

Within patient, randomized treatment order trial

Systematic review of clinical trials with random assignment to treatment

Clinical trial with random assignment to treatment

Systematic review of non-random assignment of treatment trials

Single trial with non-random assignment of treatment

Laboratory studies related to physiological and biomechanical mechanisms underlying disease, injury or treatment

Opinion developed through informal clinical observations

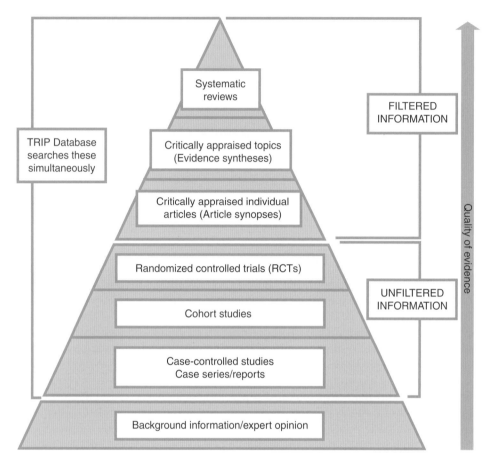

FIGURE 18-1   Evidence-based medicine pyramid. (Reprinted with permission from Harvey Cushing/John Hay Whitney Medical Library, Yale University School of Medicine, available at http://www.ebmpyramid.org/samples/complicated.html.)

chronic or recurrent conditions, there is a very limited spectrum of conditions for which studies of this design are feasible.

What is a Systematic Review?

Now to the questions of "What is a systematic review?" and "How is a systematic review conducted?" Systematic review is a research process where the investigators identify previous studies that address a particular question, summarize findings, and when possible collapse data for meta-analysis, a process where statistical analysis is performed on data combined from multiple studies. Perhaps the best way to better understand systematic review is to contrast the process with a traditional literature review (see Table 18-3).

TABLE 18-3	Key distinctions between narrative and systematic reviews, by core features of such reviews	
CORE FEATURE	NARRATIVE REVIEW	SYSTEMATIC REVIEW
Study question	Often broad in scope.	Often a focused clinical question.
Data sources and search strategy	Which databases were searched and search strategy are not typically provided.	Comprehensive search of many databases as well as the so-called gray literature. Explicit search strategy is provided.
Selection of articles for study	Not usually specified, potentially biased.	Criterion-based selection, uniformly applied.
Article review or appraisal	Variable, depending on who is conducting the review.	Rigorous critical appraisal, typically using a data extraction form.
Study quality	If assessed, may not use formal quality assessment.	Some assessment of quality is almost always included as part of the data extraction process.
Synthesis	Often a qualitative summary.	Quantitative summary (meta-analysis) if the data can be appropriately pooled; qualitative otherwise.
Inferences	Sometimes evidence-based.	Usually evidence-based.

Available at http://www.ncbi.nlm.nih.gov/books/bv.fcgi?rid=hstat1.table.71502. (Adapted with permission from Cook DJ, Mulrow CD, Haynes RB. Systematic reviews: synthesis of best evidence for clinical decisions. *Ann Intern Med.* 1997;126:376–380.

TRADITIONAL LITERATURE REVIEW VERSUS SYSTEMATIC REVIEW

Literature reviews that populated the medical journals in the past provide a discussion around multiple references related to an issue but often limit the included literature to that which supports a position taken by the author or authors a priori. A reader searching the literature might identify additional reports, some containing conflicting conclusions. In a systematic review the investigators begin with an answerable question and work through a planned process.

The Agency for Healthcare Quality and Research outlined the essential elements of systematic review (see Table 18-4). As noted previously, systematic review like other research begins with a question. As with other types of clinical

TABLE 18-4	Domains and elements for systematic reviews
DOMAIN	**ELEMENTS**[a]
Study question	• **Question clearly specified and appropriate**
Search strategy	• *Sufficiently comprehensive and rigorous with attention to possible publication biases* • *Search restrictions justified (e.g., language or country of origin)* • Documentation of search terms and databases used • Sufficiently detailed to reproduce study
Inclusion and exclusion criteria	• **Selection methods specified and appropriate, with a *priori* criteria specified if possible**
Interventions	• **Intervention(s) clearly detailed for all study groups**
Outcomes	• **All potentially important harms and benefits considered**
Data extraction[b]	• Rigor and consistency of process • Number and types of reviewers • Blinding of reviewers • Measure of agreement or reproducibility • Extraction of clearly defined interventions/exposures and outcomes for all relevant subjects and subgroups
Study quality and validity	• *Assessment method specified and appropriate* • Method of incorporation specified and appropriate
Data synthesis and analysis	• *Appropriate use of qualitative and/or quantitative synthesis, with consideration of the robustness of results and heterogeneity issues* • Presentation of key primary study elements sufficient for critical appraisal and replication
Results	• **Narrative summary and/or quantitative summary statistic and measure of precision, as appropriate**
Discussion	• **Conclusions supported by results with possible biases and limitations taken into consideration**
Funding or sponsorship	• *Type and sources of support for study*

[a]Elements appearing in italics are those with an empirical basis. Elements appearing in bold are those considered essential to give a system a Yes rating for the domain.

[b]Domain for which a Yes rating required that a majority of elements be considered. (Reprinted from West S, King V, Carey TS, et al. Systems to Rate the Strength of Scientific Evidence. Evidence Report/Technology Assessment No. 47 [Prepared by the Research Triangle Institute-University of North Carolina Evidence-based Practice Center under Contract No. 290-97-0011]. AHRQ Publication No. 02-E016. Rockville, MD: Agency for Healthcare Research and Quality. April 2002. Accessed from http://www.ncbi.nlm.nih.gov/bookshelf/br.fcgi?book=hserta&part=A73054 February 18, 2010.)

research the subsequent description of the research methods should appear appropriate to address the question. In the case of systemic review the description of the research methods begins with a clear description as to how the investigators conducted their search. Most will begin by describing the search terms entered and the databases searched.

✔ CONCEPT CHECK

Systematic review is a research process where the investigators identify previous studies that address a particular question, summarize findings, and when possible collapse data for meta-analysis, a process where statistical analysis is performed on data combined from multiple studies.

SYSTEMATIC REVIEW AS A RESEARCH PROCESS

It is important to note that because systematic review is a research process, the research methods impact upon the validity of the data and thus the conclusions drawn. Much like understanding research methods of clinical trials improves one's ability to critically review clinical reports the consumer can assess the methodologic quality of a systematic review by applying the standards found in Table 18-4. As noted by Jewell (2008, p. 370), clinicians "should evaluate systematic reviews carefully before accepting them at face value because of their high rankings on evidence hierarchies."

A well-prepared systematic review offers a comprehensive analysis of the clinical literature available at the time it is prepared. In some cases strong conclusions can be drawn and in others insufficient data are available from which to make recommendations. In the first instance the systematic review may lead to firm practice recommendations and clinical practice guidelines. When conclusions cannot be drawn from the existing data new avenues for research are identified. Moreover, we may question how certain we are that our practice habits provide accurate assessments and optimize **intervention outcomes**.

Once an overview of a problem has been presented and the purpose of the research stated, a description of the research methods should follow. The literature search strategy in a systematic review must be described in a manner that is fully reproducible. This means that the reader following the described methods would identify the same papers published at the time the research was conducted. Thus, a detailed description of the criteria and methods employed to include papers for final analysis or exclude papers from further consideration. Investigators may, for example, limit the systematic review to randomized, controlled clinical trials and thus eliminate cohort studies, **case reports**, and literature reviews from further consideration. Papers may be limited by language such as including only those published in English. Regardless of the criteria, a reader reproducing this process should obtain the same results. Flow diagrams (see Figure 18-2) can help the reader follow the process from search to a final pool of papers included in the review.

Once a description of the search process that identified papers for consideration is provided a description of how final papers were included for data analysis should be provided. The incorporation of multiple reviewers using criteria determined a priori and blinded to the assessment of other investigators reduces the potential for bias.

Similarly, methods by which data are extracted from individual papers for analysis should be described, including a description of investigators blinded to the assessment of others. Additional concerns may include the grading of methodologic quality of included papers. There are multiple grading scales of methodologic quality of diagnostic and intervention studies, since studies of differing methodologic quality can lead to differences in the results of individual trials. Thus the assessment of methodologic quality can become an important element in the **interpretation** of data analysis.

✔ CONCEPT CHECK

Literature reviews provide a discussion around multiple references related to an issue but often limit the included literature to that which supports a position taken by the author or authors a priori. By comparison, a systematic review begins with an answerable question and works through a planned process of investigation.

DATA SYNTHESIS

Data synthesis is the process through which data from multiple studies are combined. Data from studies using similar research methods and measurements can be combined through meta-analysis. This process can substantially increase the size of the sample contributing data for analysis thus increasing statistical power and narrowing confidence intervals. Several factors, however, warrant consideration before combining data for meta-analysis. One must consider whether the patients included in individual studies are sufficiently similar to warrant combining data. For example, Verhagen et al. (2007) did not pool data in their systematic review of the treatment of whiplash pain. One consideration in this decision was the fact that, while all of the patients in the trials included for review-fulfilled criteria for having suffered whiplash mechanism injuries, the timing of interventions varied from acute to chronic symptoms. It is certainly reasonable to suspect patients with chronic symptoms may respond differently to treatment than those entering a clinical trial more acutely.

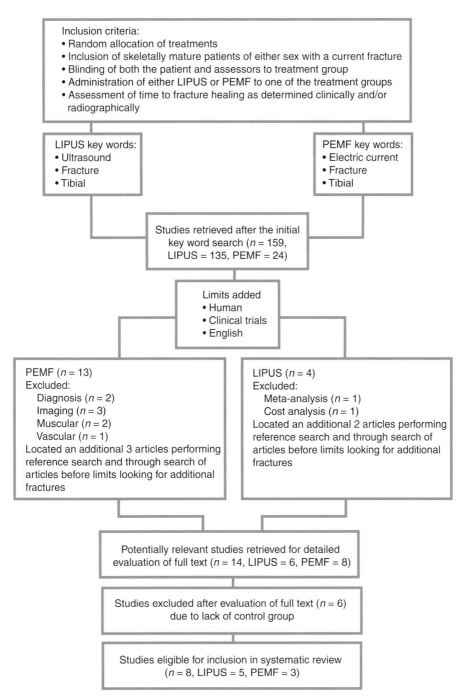

FIGURE 18-2 Flow diagram depicting the process from establishment of criteria for inclusion through search process to a final pool of papers included for review of low-intensity pulsed ultrasound and pulsed electromagnetic field treatments of tibial fractures. (Reprinted with permission from Walker NA, Denegar CR, Preische J. Low-intensity pulsed ultrasound and pulsed electromagnetic field in the treatment of tibial fractures: a systematic review. *J Athl Train.* 2007;42:530-535.)

The similarity between treatments is also of concern. For example, Bjordal et al. (2001) reported that the response to LASER therapy in the treatment of lateral epicondylalgia is dependent on the parameters of the stimulus. By analyzing data from clinical trials that delivered LASER at a dose between 0.5 and 3.5 J/cm^2 these authors concluded that LASER benefits patients with this condition. This is in contrast to a report by Stasinopoulos and Johnson (2005) who included treatments with LASER were ineffective based on trials where LASER was applied across a broader dose spectrum. Additional investigation into the dose response to LASER is warranted but it is possible that incorporating data from trials where heterogeneous treatments parameters were applied would lead to conclusions that do not reflect responses to specific treatment parameters.

The variables being measured and the units of measurement may also preclude meta-analysis. For example, Walker et al. (2007) attempted to compare the efficacy of low-intensity pulsed ultrasound (LIPUS) to pulsed electromagnetic fields (PEMF) in the treatment of tibial fractures. These efforts were thwarted because the identified studies of LIPUS reported days to fracture healing while those investigating PEMF reported the proportion of fractures healed at predetermined times.

In each of these situations the independent opinions of multiple investigators using the same criteria strengthen the decisions made regarding the pooling of data for meta-analysis. When meta-analysis is not possible qualitative analysis can yield important information. Despite being unable to perform meta-analysis, Morgan (2005, p. 361) was able to draw conclusions favoring exercise incentives "in certain populations, namely individuals who are not sedentary but already slightly active, older adults and those who are overweight (but not obese)." He noted further that "increases in the level of physical activity may not be sustained over time."

Once decisions regarding pooling of data are made qualitative data analysis or quantitative meta-analysis is performed. More discussion of meta-analysis is forthcoming but let's turn to issues of harm and the presentation of results first. The issue of harm related to diagnostic procedures and interventions is an important and sometimes overlooked issue. However, many diagnostic procedures and treatments have potential side effects. Those that are minor and commonly known may not require special comment but others may weigh into decisions regarding recommendations related to testing or treatment.

Kerkhoffs et al. (2007), for example, completed a meta-analysis on outcomes data to compare surgical and nonsurgical management of acute lateral ankle injuries in adults. The authors concluded that "there is insufficient evidence available from randomised controlled trials to determine the relative effectiveness of surgical and conservative treatment for acute injuries of the lateral ligament complex of the ankle." Moreover, they reported that "there was some limited evidence for longer recovery times, and higher incidences of ankle stiffness, impaired ankle mobility and complications in the surgical treatment group" (Kerkhoffs et al., 2007, p. 1). Thus, while surgical management may have benefits, they must be weighed against the frequency and severity of side effects in the clinical decision process.

It is incumbent on researchers directing clinical trials and systematic reviews to report adverse events and the researcher consumer to consider the incidence and morbidity associated with the events. When possible independent reviewers should catalog side effects and adverse events using a strategy agreed to a priori. However, all investigators must be encouraged to identify reports of unusual events so that such occurrences are reviewed and included within the systematic review.

META-ANALYSIS

Raw data or mean difference data from multiple studies can be pooled for meta-analysis. The reader of meta-analyses will find reference in the methods section of these papers to fixed or random effects models. Katz (2001, p. 162) summarized the differences by describing fixed effects models as asking the question, "is there evidence here (within the data available) of an outcome effect" while random effects models address whether "the available data indicate that the larger population of data from which they were drawn provides evidence of an outcome effect." Thus, random effects analysis projects greater generalizability of the results of an investigation.

When mean difference values are pooled the values should be weighted based on the sample size of the study. Mean values calculated in studies with larger samples are more likely to reflect population values than mean scores reported in smaller studies. The details of these calculations are beyond the scope of this text. However, there are several software packages (e.g., RevMan, see http://www.cc-ims.net/RevMan/) available to assist in the completion of meta-analysis. Furthermore, weighing can be used to account for other factors that may affect the results of an analysis such as controlling for publication bias by placing more weight on studies failing to show a treatment effect or funding bias by giving more weight to studies not funded through industry sources. The reader is referred to the writings of Petitti (2000) for more detailed discussions of these issues.

CONSIDERATIONS FOR APPLYING THE RESULTS FROM SYSTEMATIC REVIEW TO THE CARE OF THE INDIVIDUAL PATIENT

Considerations in the execution and consumption of a systematic review were addressed previously in this chapter. This discussion addressed the control of potential threats to the validity of data that subsequently affects the conclusions of the study. In clinical practice the provider must go beyond these considerations when deciding how to proceed with the care of individual patients. The Systematic Review (of therapy) Worksheet (Figure 18-3) from the University of Toronto's University Health Network illustrates a process through which clinicians can

SYSTEMATIC REVIEW (OF THERAPY) WORKSHEET

Citation:

Are the results of this systematic review valid?

Is this a systematic review of randomised trials?
Does it include a methods section that describes: a) finding and including all relevant trials? b) assessing their individual validity?
Were the results consistent from study to study?
Were the individual patient data used in the analysis (or aggregate data)?

Are the valid results of this systematic review important?

Translating odds ratios to NNTs:

The numbers in the body of the tables are the NNTs for the corresponding odds ratio at that particular patient's expected event rate (PEER).

1. When the odds ratio (OR) < 1
   This table applies when a bad outcome is prevented by therapy.

		OR < 1				
		0.9	0.8	0.7	0.6	0.5
Patient's expected event rate (PEER)	0.05	2.09[a]	104	69	52	41[b]
	0.10	110	54	36	27	21
	0.20	61	30	20	14	11
	0.30	46	22	14	10	8
	0.40	40	19	12	9	7
	0.50	38	18	11	8	6
	0.70	44	20	13	9	6
	0.90	101[c]	46	27	18	12[d]

[a] The relative risk reduction (RRR) here is 10%
[b] The RRR here is 49%
[c] For any OR, NNT is lowest when PEER = 0.50
[d] The RRR here is 9%

(continued)

2. When the odds ratio (OR) > 1

This table applies both when a good outcome is increased by therapy and when a side-effect is caused by therapy.

		OR > 1				
		1.1	1.2	1.3	1.4	1.5
Patient's expected event rate (PEER)	0.05	212	106	71	54	43
	0.10	112	57	38	29	23
	0.20	64	33	22	17	14
	0.30	49	25	17	13	11
	0.40	43	23	16	12	10
	0.50	42	22	15	12	10
	0.70	51	27	19	15	13
	0.90	121	66	47	38	32

Can you apply this valid, important evidence from a systematic review in caring for your patient?

Do these results apply to our patient?	
Is your patient so different from those in the study that its results cannot apply?	
Is the treatment feasible in your setting?	
What are your patient's potential benefits and harms from the therapy?	
Method I: **In the OR tables above, find the intersection of the closest odds ratio from the systematic review and your patient's expected event rate (PEER)**	
Method II: **To calculate the NNT from any OR and PEER:** $$NNT = \frac{1 - \{PEER \times (1 - OR)\}}{(1 - PEER) \times PEER \times (1 - OR)}$$	

(continued)

Are your patient's values and preferences satisfied by the regimen and its consequences?	
Do you and your patient have a clear assessment of their values and preferences?	
Are they met by this regimen and its consequences?	

Should you believe apparent qualitative differences in the efficacy of therapy in some subgroups of patients?—Only if you can say "yes" to all of the following:

Do they really make biologic and clinical sense?	
Is the qualitative difference both clinically (beneficial for some but useless or harmful for others) and statistically significant?	
Was this difference hypothesised before the study began (rather than the product of dredging the data), and has it been confirmed in other, independent studies?	
Was this one of just a few subgroup analyses carried out in this study?	

FIGURE 18-3   The Systematic Review (of therapy) Worksheet from the University of Toronto's University Health Network. (Reprinted with permission from University of Toronto's University Health Network, available at http://www.cebm.utoronto.ca/teach/materials/sr.htm.)

make decisions about the extent to which the results of a systematic review should influence a plan of care.

The components of the "Are the results of this systematic review valid?" section provide a check sheet regarding issues of validity. The worksheet then leads the clinician to patient-specific concerns that must be considered before allowing the evidence to direct recommendations for care. The first question raised under *"Can you apply this valid, important evidence from a systematic review in caring for your patient?"* is *"Is your patient so different from those in the study that its results cannot apply?"* This is a rather rhetorical question in that it suggests the need for an absolute yes or no response. First, each patient is an individual who possesses a unique history and physical state. Second, the clinician treating a patient that is very different from those included in a systematic review will rarely find evidence from the study of a group representative of the patient to guide their decisions. This question, however, forces a weighing of the evidence from which a rationale for treatment recommendation can be developed and presented to the patient.

The next question *"Is the treatment feasible in your setting?"* leads to further deliberation. Obviously, if a treatment has been shown to be highly effective in similar patients and can be administered, the clinician will likely proceed in recommending the treatment. However, if the treatment is not feasible in the current setting, the clinician must decide whether treatment in that setting is likely to be of similar benefit and poses a similar risk or whether referral for the therapy in question is warranted. Referral is sometimes an easy process but in some cases the patient's circumstances and preferences weigh heavily in the decision.

Once these questions are answered and the clinician is prepared to apply the results from a systematic review in recommending a course of treatment it is time to consider the likelihood that the patient will benefit from the intervention and the potential for adverse responses to treatment. There are a number of ways to convey the response to an intervention, either preventative or therapeutic. These measures have been introduced in previous chapters but are summarized here. The response to an intervention can be conveyed as the magnitude of change on one or more measures or as a probability of a favorable or adverse outcome. For example, Medina et al. (2006) completed a systematic review of the response to hyaluronic acid injections on pain, stiffness, and function in patients with osteoarthritis of the knee. The paper identified modest benefits based on analysis of confidence intervals derived from the data. While useful, these data do not help the clinician or the patient in knowing the probability of an intervention resulting in improvement or harm in an individual case. Some patients, in fact, report feeling much better after a series of hyaluronic injections. The potential for such outcomes is estimated with odds ratios, risk reduction measures, and numbers-needed-to-treat (NNT) measures. Since NNT is the inverse of absolute risk reduction (ARR) the same information is provided in differing units. It is also possible to calculate NNT from odds ratio data if the patient's expected event rate (PEER) is known. The tables found in Figure 18-3 assist in this conversion and will be applied shortly.

Consider the works of Grindstaff et al. (2006) and Myklebust et al. (2003). The first is a meta-analysis developed from studies where specific exercise programs were designed and implemented in an effort to prevent anterior cruciate ligament injuries. These authors completed an NNT analysis estimating that 89 athletes need to be enrolled in an intervention program to prevent one ACL injury per season. Mykleburst et al. (2003) completed an investigation of the effects of an ACL injury prevention program in team handball players. These authors reported a reduction in ACL injuries, especially in elite level players. Although the injury reduction was not statistically significant, the point odds ratio estimate for ACL injury in elite players completing the exercise program was 0.51 in the first year and 0.37 during the second year. During the year prior to initiating the prevention program 29 ACL injuries were recorded in 924 players (PEER = 0.031). If we round up to a PEER = 0.05, an odds ratio of 0.50 yields an NNT = 41. Thus, a clinician could be fairly confident that enrolling female team handball players in a prevention program will reduce ACL injuries at least as effectively as has been reported in studies of a wider array of athletes.

NNT is a measure familiar to clinicians but a concept that can be difficult to convey to patients. ARR may be less confusing since it is a percentage. ARR is simply the event rate in a control group minus an event rate in a treatment group. In the Mykleburst et al. (2003) paper the event rate of ACL injuries in female athletes was reduced to 0.02. Thus the risk of injury was reduced from 3 in 100 athletes per season to 2 in 100 athletes per season. A 1% reduction in injury doesn't sound like much. Relative risk reduction (RRR) calculated by (event rate in a control group − event rate in treatment group)/(event rate in control group) may yield a different perspective. Using the values above, RRR = (0.031 − 0.02)/0.031 or 0.35. Thus the RRR reflects a 35% reduction in the risk of ACL injury with participation in an exercise regimen that sounds a lot different from a reduction of 1 injury per 100 athletes per season.

Why are these values so different and which is most useful? The differences in ARR and RRR lie in the incidence rate of the problem. In this example, the incidence rate is low and thus the ARR is small. When the incidence rate is low, however, small differences in incidence rate can yield a large RRR. While this explains the differences in ARR and RRR, it does not answer the latter question of which value is most useful. Unfortunately, all of the measures can provide helpful information and thus no single measure is most useful.

In this case we are concerned with a serious musculoskeletal injury that is costly in terms of lost productivity, diminished quality of life, and health care expenditure. The injury may preclude future high-level sport participation and will lead to early degenerative changes in the affected knee. While neither of the studies noted above addressed adverse events during the exercise intervention, it would be reasonable to assume that such events (serious injury occurring during the exercise training) are very rare. The intervention can also be offered at relatively low cost. Stop and consider these last statements. Notice that the ARR, RRR, and NNT are being discussed in a new context rather than as isolated values. Many clinicians would interpret these data as a reason to recommend an ACL injury prevention program. Interventions that pose a greater risk, require more time or money, or conflict with a patient's values or willingness to participate might yield recommendations that differ markedly despite being associated with identical NNT, ARR, and RRR measures.

The worksheet (Figure 18-3) leads the clinician to two final considerations, patient preferences and decisions regarding patient subgroups. The role patient preferences and choices play in the clinical decision-making process was discussed by Haynes et al. (2002). Figure 18-4A depicts a model where patient preference, research evidence, and clinical expertise impact upon clinical decisions. Figure 18-4B presents a more contemporary model that leaves the clinician at the center of the decision-making process and introduces the clinical state of the patient and the surrounding circumstances into the process. This model returns the

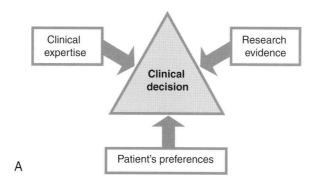

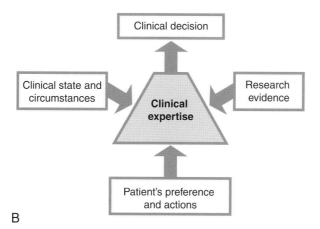

FIGURE 18-4   Schematic representations of clinical decision-making. **A:** Early model. **B:** Contemporary model with the clinician as the actor making and being responsible for clinical decisions. (Adapted with permission from Haynes RB, Devereux PJ, Guyatt GH. Clinical expertise in the era or evidence-based medicine and patient choice. *Evid Based Med.* 2002;7(2):36–38.)

clinician to that active role of decision-making in a broader context of practice. Clearly, clinicians must consider the circumstances (e.g., access to exercise equipment, time constraints) surrounding a case as well the patient's preferences in developing and implementing plans of care. The issues that influence how patients are cared for could be discussed at length but are beyond the scope of this chapter. This limited discussion is intended to serve as a reminder that we should not get carried away interpreting the numbers and forget that each patient is a unique story and that the individual, not the research, is the focus of our attention. The last section of the worksheet addresses situations where there is evidence to suggest that a subset of patients may respond differently from a larger sample. In the desire to help the patient clinicians may consider an intervention despite a lack of evidence suggesting benefit because their individual patient differs in some respect to the "average" patient studied. This may be quite reasonable in some cases but by completing the worksheet the clinician is once again forced into a critical analysis of the evidence supporting the effectiveness of the intervention being considered. Once again the values of the patient and the clinician expertise will influence the ultimate plan of care but the best available evidence will have been critically assessed.

CHAPTER SUMMARY

Systematic review with or without meta-analysis is a research strategy that often provides clinicians with the best current evidence to integrate into patient management. Systematic review can also identify where further investigation is needed to guide effective, cost-efficient health care. As with all clinical research the methods employed in an investigation can threaten data validity. The investigator should strive to control threats validity by employing sound research methods and convey the conduct of the research to the consumer. The consumer must appraise systematic reviews critically before applying the results of an investigation in their practice.

This chapter was written from the perspective of the research consumer. In identifying the components of the systematic review, however, the investigator is also provided a sound foundation from which to pursue an investigation. The busy clinician will continue to seek well-conducted systematic reviews to provide summaries of the clinical literature on selected topics in a time-efficient manner. Since larger samples are more likely to represent true population values a systematic review also is at the top of the evidence value hierarchy. The clinician will continue to be challenged by conflicting results and a dearth of research in some areas. Systematic reviews however have become common features across much of the health care research literature and often a click away on the computer.

KEY POINTS

- Systematic review provides the clinician with results compiled from multiple clinical trials in a single document, sometimes with the effect of defining the best current practice.
- A literature review is often limited because it supports a position taken by the author, whereas a systematic review begins with an answerable question and works through a planned process.

- Because systematic review is a research process, the research methods impact the validity of the data and the conclusions drawn.
- Data from studies using similar research methods and measurements can be combined through meta-analysis.
- Systematic reviews are used to provide clinicians with the most well-supported evidence of solutions to clinical problems.
- Hierarchies were put into place to rank reviews based on the strength of the argument made and the evidence given.
- Sample size affects the weight of a meta-analysis.
- In a systematic review, once a description of the search process that identified papers for consideration is provided a description of how final papers were included for data analysis should be provided.
- Since larger samples are more likely to represent true population values a systematic review is at the top of the evidence value hierarchy.
- Consideration of patient values serves as a reminder that clinicians should not get carried away interpreting numbers and forget that the patient is the focus of attention.

Critical Thinking Questions

1. What advice does Jewell (2008) offer clinicians interested in using systematic reviews?
2. What is a systematic review?
3. How can time affect the credibility of a systematic review?
4. Why might specialized medical professionals need to rely on evidence-based medicine?
5. Why do larger sample sizes provide a more accurate view of a true population tendency?

Applying Concepts

1. Discuss the use of systematic review with or without meta-analysis in a research strategy and consider how/if it provides clinicians with the best current evidence to integrate into patient management.
2. Following the notion of EBP, consider and discuss the extent to which that patient values serve as a reminder that we should not get carried away interpreting the numbers and forget that the patient is the focus of our attention. Provide examples from historical and current research.

REFERENCES

Bjordal JM, Couppe C, Ljunggren AE. Low level laser therapy for tendinopathy. Evidence for a dose-response pattern. *Phys Ther Rev*. 2001;6:91–99.

Grindstaff TL, Hammill RR, Tuzson AE, et al. Neuromuscular control training programs and noncontact anterior cruciate ligament injury rates in female athletes: a numbers-needed-to-treat analysis. *J Athl Train*. 2006;41:450–456.

Haynes RB, Devereaux PJ, Guyatt GH. Clinical expertise in the era of evidence-based medicine and patient choice. *Evid Based Med*. 2002;7:36–38. Available at http://www.cc-ims.net/RevMan; accessed March 12, 2008.

Jewell D. *Guide to Evidence-Based Physical Therapy Practice*. Boston, MA: Jones & Bartlett Publishers; 2008:370.

Katz DL. *Clinical Epidemiology and Evidence-Based Medicine*. Thousand Oaks, CA: Sage Publications; 2001:162.

Kerkhoffs GM, Handoll HH, de Bie R, et al. Surgical versus conservative treatment for acute injuries of the lateral ligament complex of the ankle in adults. *Cochrane Database Syst Rev*. 2007;2:CD000380.

Medina JM, Thomas A, Denegar CR. Effects of hyaluronic acid on pain, stiffness and disability: a meta analysis. *J Fam Pract*. 2006;55:669–675.

Morgan O. Approaches to increase physical activity: reviewing the evidence for exercise-referral schemes. *Public Health*. 2005;119:361–370.

Myklebust G, Engebretsen L, Braekken IH, et al. Prevention of anterior cruciate ligament injuries in female team handball players: a prospective intervention study over three seasons. *Clin J Sport Med*. 2003;13:71–78.

Petitti DB. *Meta-analysis, Decision Analysis and Cost Effectiveness Analysis. Methods for Quantitative Synthesis in Medicine*. 2nd ed. New York: Oxford University Press; 2000.

Stasinopoulos DI, Johnson MI. Effectiveness of low-level laser therapy for lateral elbow tendinopathy. *Photomed Laser Surg*. 2005;23:425–430.

Verhagen AP, Scholten-Peeters GGGM, van Wijngaarden S, et al. Conservative treatments for whiplash. *Cochrane Database Syst Rev*. 2007; 2. Art. No.: CD003338. DOI: 10.1002/14651858.CD003338.pub3.

Walker NA, Denegar CR, Preische J. Low-intensity pulsed ultrasound and pulsed electromagnetic field in the treatment of tibial fractures: a systematic review. *J Athl Train*. 2007;42:530–535.

PART IV

DISSEMINATION OF RESEARCH

CHAPTER 19

PRESENTATION OF FINDINGS

A scholar's ink lasts longer than a martyr's blood.

—*Irish saying, from Irish Proverb Quotes as quoted in World of Quotes.com Historic Quotes and Proverbs Archive (www.worldofquotes.com/author/Irish-Proverb/1/index.html)*

CHAPTER OBJECTIVES

After reading this chapter, you will:

- Develop an appreciation for the dissemination of research findings as a part of the research process.
- Understand the differences between presentation and publication of findings.
- See the point of poster and platform presentations at professional meetings.
- Recognize the advantages and unique features of each presentation forum.
- Understand why publication of peer-reviewed papers is held in higher regard than presentations at professional meetings.
- Appreciate the advantages of publishing research findings.
- Recognize the workings of a well-prepared presentation.
- Understand the components of a well-written research paper.

KEY TERMS

call for abstracts	peer reviewed	relevant literature
CINAHL	publication guidelines	scientific paper
limitations	PubMed	validity

INTRODUCTION

The preceding 18 chapters are intended to provide a foundation for conducting research that generates data that guide clinical decision-making and to prepare practitioners in evidence-based clinical care and students in professional preparation allied health care programs to use research data in their daily practice. The advancement of evidence-based practice requires investigators and clinicians to work together in collecting data and disseminating the results of their research. This chapter is devoted to the dissemination of findings and therefore targeted more to the investigator than the research consumer. We believe, however, that the more insight consumers have into the research process the better prepared they will be to critically appraise what they read. The dissemination of research findings is as much a part of the process as is the development of research methods and for some a more daunting task. This chapter provides an overview of research presentation and manuscript preparation with an emphasis on the latter subject.

TYPES OF PRESENTATIONS

The dissemination of research findings occurs almost exclusively through presentations at professional meetings and publication of manuscripts. It is common that research findings are first made public at professional meetings with subsequent publication in a **peer-reviewed** scholarly journal. Each forum has advantages and unique features. For the consumer the opportunity to see data presented for the first time at a professional meeting, pose questions, and discuss the research as well as the application of results is often enjoyable and professionally rewarding. From the perspective of the investigator/presenter professional meetings provide an opportunity to showcase their work and receive feedback that often refines and directs future projects.

The publication of peer-reviewed papers is held in higher regard than presentations at professional meetings. This forum also offers some distinct advantages. The reasons that publication is viewed as being a greater accomplishment than presentation include the fact that manuscripts receive the most thorough and critical review from peers since journals receive far more submissions than they have the capacity to print. The great advantages of publishing, especially in this electronic age, are the opportunity to reach a worldwide audience with work that is permanently available.

Professional Meetings: Posters and Platform Presentation

The invitation to present one's research findings at a meeting is exciting and a professional honor. Just how does an investigator get invited to present? In order to present research findings at a professional meeting the investigators must respond to a **call for abstracts** from the organization sponsoring the meeting and submit an abstract for review. Each organization provides guidelines regarding the length and style of the abstract and publishes submission deadlines. As with all **publication guidelines** it is important that the submitted materials conform to the guidelines of the organization. Abstracts are typically limited in length with a 400 to 600-word limit being common. Writing a good abstract is challenging since the author has relatively few words to convey the findings from an extensive research effort. We suggest following the example format guidelines and tips for abstract preparation given in Box 19.1.

Once an abstract is submitted, a panel of professionals within the organization usually reviews the work with those submissions meeting the standards for acceptance being included in the meeting program. The accepted abstracts are then presented either in poster or platform (oral) presentations. These formats of presentation, which are usually assigned rather than selected by the presenter, require different presentation skills. Posters that describe an entire research project must convey the most important points in an orderly format within a limited space. Consumers attending a meeting often have large blocks of time to browse through and read groupings of posters. Authors are typically assigned to be present to discuss their work at prespecified times during the meeting. The opportunity to discuss

BOX 19.1	Tips, example format, and guidelines for abstract preparation.

TITLE OF RESEARCH PROJECT AND AUTHORS
Introduction: (1 to 2 sentences). Identify the problem or question of study. Identify the need for the research being reported. *Purpose:* (1 to 2 sentences). Clearly state the point of the research. Briefly put in plain words why the study or experiment was done. Hint—research rationale is typically to determine or investigate or test or explore the connection between or among variables of interest. *Methods and Procedures:* (3 to 4 sentences). Briefly describe what was being measured in the study and how it was tested. What was the general idea behind the nitty-gritty "nuts and bolts" of the study? Identify independent variables (IV) and dependent variables (DV) of interest. State how variables of interest were measured. Provide brief objective detail to highlight key points and summarize what was done and how it was done to collect and/or test the variables of interest. *Results:* (2 to 3 sentences). Note what was found out from the study or experiment. How did one variable influence or change another? Describe the statistical relationship between IV(s) and DV(s) in the population sampled. Report significant results, only. Report numbers and/or precise statistical results such as means, percentages, chi square, level of significance, etc. *Conclusions:* (1 to 2 sentences). Must be based on results reported. What did you interpret or infer from the results? Explain the "take-home message" of this research. Hint—remember that the conclusion must connect to the purpose. Directly address the main question or questions posed in the statement of purpose.

research one-on-one with an author can lead to dynamic discussions and professional collaborations. The challenge of preparing a really good poster requires skills in layout and design. Posters that appear poorly organized, cluttered, or generally unattractive tend to attract few readers regardless of the quality of the research. We suggest the tips for producing effective posters in Table 19-1. See also

TABLE 19-1	Tips for producing effective posters
POSTER CHECKLIST	
✓	Follow required format, size limits, and presentation specifications
✓	Expand abstract and stick to the key points and "big picture" concepts
✓	Information should be concise, yet provide logical, organized, easy-to-follow flow of relevant details
✓	Balance use of text and graphics
✓	Effective use of graphics, tables, and figures to communicate information
✓	Eye-catching, professional use of color
✓	Avoid combinations of color vision deficiencies (red-green deficiency, blue-yellow deficiency, monochromacy)
✓	Overall layout should have balanced organization and appear aesthetically pleasing
✓	Avoid over-information, cluttered, or messy display
✓	When viewing the poster from a distance of approximately 3 feet, your eye should be drawn to the most important graphic, table, or figure
✓	Title should be readable from a distance of approximately 3 feet
✓	Identify your university or place of employment
✓	Provide author contact information
✓	Make sure there is a clear, easily identifiable, and understandable 'take-home' message
✓	Poster must present professional quality appearance (i.e., use of materials, fonts, color(s), graphics, etc.)
✓	Proof read
✓	Check spelling, grammar, and typos
✓	Bring extra push-pins or Velcro buttons
✓	Bring copies of abstract

http://www.posterpresentations.com, which provides free PowerPoint poster presentation templates for research presentations.

Platform presentations require a different set of skills. First and foremost for many is the challenge of public speaking in front of an audience of one's peers. Most novices and many experienced presenters will experience some degree of anxiety before their presentation. At the extreme we have witnessed presenters faint in the midst of their talk! Besides overcoming stage fright good platform presentations require the development of effective graphics. Once the domain of the slide projector, computer-generated graphic presentations now allow for animation, video, and greater creativity. The latitude in developing a presentation has resulted in many a message being lost in the production. The graphics used must support the presentation, not become the presentation. Consumers should be able to glean the salient information from graphics rather than being overwhelmed by the extent of information presented. The final but not trivial challenge in rendering an effective platform presentation is the effective use of time. Platform presentations are timed events with each speaker being strictly limited most often to 15 minutes (including 3 to 5 minutes for questions!). Meeting sessions must stay on schedule in order for attendees to attend the presentations they most want to hear. Thus, it is typical that once a presenter has used his or her allotted time the presentation is ended without regard to the state of completion. Platform presentations require planning, practice, and to the extent possible anticipation of the questions liable to be posed during a brief question and answer session. We suggest the following as tips for preparing effective platform presentations (Table 19-2).

✔ CONCEPT CHECK

The latitude in developing a presentation has resulted in many a message being lost in the production. The graphics used must support the presentation, not become the presentation.

As noted in the introduction, research findings first reported at professional meetings are often subsequently published in the peer-reviewed professional literature, although it is not necessary to present in a public forum before submitting a manuscript for consideration. The ultimate goal, however, is to publish reports from research in journals that are widely read and indexed in commonly used databases such as **PubMed** and **CINAHL**. Scientific information is more rapidly and widely disseminated than at any time in history speeding the professional development of clinicians and the delivery of advanced care to patients.

TABLE 19-2	**Tips for preparing effective platform presentations**

PLATFORM PRESENTATION CHECKLIST

✓	**General planning** • Know your audience • Know your time limit • Know your material • Know your technology • Practice, practice, and practice your presentation

✓	**Effective PowerPoint slides**
	• Design tactfully yet skillfully
	• Follow basic presentation structure in slideshow
	   ◦ Title slide
	   ◦ Overview slide
	   ◦ Content slides (cover no more than 1–2 slides per minute)
	   ◦ Summary slide
	   ◦ Reference slide
	• Use consistent appearance (layout, background, font style)
	• Include copyright and citation documentation
	• Do not use clip art
	• Check for mistakes (i.e., spelling, grammar, citations, etc.)

✓	**Effective PowerPoint slide appearance** • Use light font on dark backgrounds • Avoid combinations of color vision deficiencies (red-green deficiency, blue-yellow deficiency, monochromacy) • Slides should appear balanced and proportional • Use font size between 24 and 48 points • Bullet key points; avoid full, long sentences ◦ Limit bulleted points to 3–5 per slide • Avoid hard-to-read font styles (i.e., italics, all capitals) • Limit or avoid transition and animation/sound effects • Follow consistent use of capitalization and punctuation
✓	**Effective presentation delivery** • Dress professionally and appropriately • Speak clearly, project your voice, and pace your rate of speech • Smile appropriately • Make eye contact with your audience • Talk off the slides; don't read the slides to the audience; avoid use of notes • Never turn your back toward the audience • Say thank you! • Invite and allow time for questions

Scientific Writing

Conveying and discussing the results of an investigation in a manuscript is an essential final step in the research process. Reading the research literature can foster new research ideas and identify strategies to improve patient care. A well-written research paper leads the reader through the purpose of the work, carefully describes the research methods, presents the results, and concludes with a discussion of the meaning and application of the findings in a logical and easily understood manner. The relative ease of reading a well-prepared paper belies the work required in the writing process. A few scholars simply write well in a manner that seems effortless. The extensive editing and revision of most published papers, however, reveals the reality that for most writing is hard work. Nearly all papers published in scientific journals are considerably improved from the submitted and earlier draft versions through the input of reviewers and editors. Since manuscripts receive such scrutiny authors must develop "thick skin" so as to see the merits in constructive criticism rather than taking such criticism personally.

While writing well requires effort and practice, there are some recommendations that can be applied that can make it easier to get your first and subsequent papers published.

Author Guidelines

As noted previously, following the published guidelines is essential for professional success and acceptance of submitted work. Professional journals publish Authors' Guides, which explain the format and style requirements for papers published in that journal. The more closely the guidelines are adhered to, the better the chances of success. In some cases a failure to comply with an Authors' Guide may lead to the rejection of a paper without peer review. The guidelines relate to all aspects of the manuscript including the title, abstract, body of the paper, and standards for the format of tables, figures, and references. In some cases limits are placed on the length of an abstract, or the entire manuscript and the number of tables, figures, and references permitted.

Title and Abstract

The title of a paper is the first thing readers see and often the last consideration of the author. Titles are applied to projects in the development of research and often carried forward throughout the research process. Titles, however, should be given careful consideration once the manuscript has been fully developed. The title should concisely describe the paper in a manner that will attract the interested reader to it. Some journals limit the length of a title to, for example, 150 characters (Physical Therapy) or 16 words (Journal of Athletic Training). While length may be limited, titles that are too short may not adequately convey the purpose of the research. Thus, the best titles are usually highly descriptive without being exceedingly long.

An abstract precedes the full text of a paper and "should be viewed as a miniversion of the paper" (Day, 1988, p. 28). The format and length of the abstract are typically specified in an authors' guide with the format dependent on nature of the paper. For example, the abstract of a laboratory research report will differ from that of a systematic review or a case study. Regardless of the type of manuscript being prepared the challenge of summarizing an entire paper in 250 or 300 words requires a careful consideration regarding the most salient aspects of each section of the paper as well as word choice. The advent of electronic databases such as PubMed where abstracts are readily available has raised the importance of a well-written abstract. Abstracts are invaluable in assisting readers locate the information they seek. Titles are often insufficient in detail to decide whether time should be spent reviewing an entire paper when a reader is faced with dozens or hundreds of "hits" from a search based on key terms. Abstracts can be rapidly scanned to glean a more specific sense of the paper before committing the time required to retrieve and read the entire manuscript. While it is necessary to review an entire paper to appropriately assess its relevance and importance to one's work, it is simply not possible to read everything related to most specific topics. Thus, authors need to attend to the details of preparing an abstract that best represents their work while consumers must be able to scan abstracts to identify the research that is priority reading.

✔ CONCEPT CHECK

Authors need to attend to the details of preparing an abstract that best represents their work while consumers must be able to scan abstracts to identify the research that is priority reading.

The Body of a Manuscript

The body of a **scientific paper** is divided into sections, which provide order and enhance the transitions through the course of the manuscript. Although there may be some small variations the structure of a research paper published in a health science journal consists of Introduction, Methods, Results, and Discussion sections.

The Introduction.   Over time, scientific writing has evolved resulting in changes to instructions to authors and generally accepted writing style. The greatest change to the body of a research paper has occurred in the Introduction section. From an editor's perspective the problem with many an introductory section is length. A well-written Introduction identifies a problem or a question in need of study, provides a relatively brief review of the most important **relevant literature**, and concludes with a clear statement of purpose for the research. In most cases three or perhaps four paragraphs are sufficient to introduce the reader to the research and capture their interest. There appear to be a few problems common to Introduction sections that miss the mark for quality. The first is the tendency to cite more of the literature than required to orient the reader and substantiate the need for the research being reported. Perhaps this common problem, which most often is found in the writing of younger scholars, is attributable to experiences in the writing of theses and dissertations. While there is more latitude in the format of these documents today a lengthy and detailed Introduction demonstrating the student's mastery of the subject remains a common expectation. The reader of a scientific manuscript is not interested in judging the cumulative scholarly accomplishments of the author(s). Moreover, a lengthy Introduction poses the risk of losing the interested reader when the text drifts from the central purpose of the research. In summary, save the detail related to previously published literature for the Discussion section of the paper and "cut to the chase" in the Introduction.

Perhaps the second greatest problem encountered as editors and reviewers of scientific papers is the failure to concisely define the purpose of the investigation and "weave the thread" through the entire paper to a concluding statement. When the research methods, reported results, and/or discussion of the Results do not reflect the stated purpose something is amiss. Hopefully, such a paper does not survive the review process and get published without revision; however, when one does, readers beware for greater than usual effort will be required to sort how the value of the information in one's research and practice.

The last concern with Introduction sections that bears mentioning here is the effort on the part of authors to identify the need for the research being reported. On the one hand, implying that the work isn't of importance but of merely of some interest will be a death blow to the attention to all but the most dedicated readers. More commonly, however, the importance of the work is overstated. Big problems are usually solved over time through multiple research efforts while smaller problems, often of limited importance to most and greater importance to a few, are just that, smaller problems. Moreover, how often do the **limitations** imposed on the research and the inability to study a very large sample lead to statements such as "we conclude that ..., however further investigation is needed to ...." The point is that a balance is needed to capture the reader's attention without overstating (or overselling) the importance of one's work.

✔ CONCEPT CHECK

A well-written Introduction identifies a problem or a question in need of study, provides a relatively brief review of the most important relevant literature, and concludes with a clear statement of purpose for the research.

Methods.   If the challenge of writing a really good Introduction is conveying important information concisely, then the challenge of preparing a really good Methods section is attention to detail. In short, the Methods section of a paper should permit the reader to replicate the study completely. In addition, the Methods section should also provide the reader with detailed information on the subjects (mean and standard deviation for age, height, and mass as well as other relevant baseline variables, gender, race/ethnicity, and details related to other important nominal data) and the measurement process (reliability and measurement precision estimates, **validity**, study results, etc.). The Methods section should convey exactly how, when, and where data were acquired and provide sufficient detail to replicate the data analysis. The manufacturer or producer of instruments and software used in data collection and analysis as well as model numbers and software versions should also be reported.

Although there is great latitude given in the length of a Methods section, the reader (seeking information promised in the Introduction) is hoping to be led to the Results in an efficient manner. To that end, the use of subheadings in a Methods section is encouraged and often required as per many Authors' Guidelines.

EXAMPLE

Structure of Methods Section

Physical Therapy Information for Authors (http://www.ptjournal.org/misc/ifora.dtl) calls for the Methods section of a clinical trial to be structured as follows:
- Design Overview
- Setting and Participants
- Randomization and Interventions
- Outcomes and Follow-up
- Statistical Analysis
- Role of the Funding Source

Reports of laboratory investigations often include Subjects, Instruments, Procedures, and Statistical Analyses as subheadings of the Methods section. Additional subheadings such as Data Analysis when data are processed prior to statistical analysis or Participant Screening and Assignment may also be appropriate. It is easier to reduce the number of subheadings when it is apparent that sections provide overlapping information or that text will flow best in a single section than it is to insert subheadings when sections become too lengthy and cumbersome.

✔ CONCEPT CHECK

The Method section of a paper should permit the reader to replicate the study completely.

The methods used to analyze data should be explained in sufficient detail to permit replication of the study in the Methods section of a paper. This is typically the last subheading in a Methods section and serves not only to fully describe the methods used but as a transition into the reporting of results.

Results.   In sports, one may hear the phrase "results are what is important." For the consumer, learning the results of an investigation is the reason for investing the time to read a paper. Much like sports, one gains far more appreciation for the results when one understands the method. Many of us enjoy learning more about the coaching that leads to success or on occasion the cheating that compromises the validity of success. Thus, as a reader of research it is important to carefully consider the methods used to acquire and analyze data so one can make some judgment regarding the validity of the data reported. No short cuts to the Results section.

In writing the Results section of a report it is important for the author to appreciate and provide what the reader is seeking: answers to the question or questions posed in the Introduction. Those answers should be provided directly with sufficient references to statistics, tables, and figures that complete and enhance the presentation. Two of the more common problems we encounter as editors and reviewers are the presentation of statistical method in the Results section of a paper and the tendency to report statistics over answers to the key question or questions. The first of these issues has been addressed in the previous section of the chapter but the latter warrants some further attention.

First and foremost, authors should report the most important results first. It is common to collect data and report results on multiple variables during a study. If information related to one or two variables is considered paramount then the results related to these variables should be reported first. If the importance of the variables is relatively equal, statistically significant findings should be reported first. In reporting statistically significant differences authors should report the results and reference the statistic rather than report the statistical outcome.

EXAMPLE

Statements of Results

Consider the following two statements of hypothetic results from a study of a 6-week home exercise program involving stationary cycling versus normal daily activity in patients with arthritis of the knees that included a 20-point self-report of daily pain (0 = no pain, 20 = completely disabling pain).

First statement:

ANOVA revealed a significant reduction ($P < 0.05$) in pain after the completion of the 6-week cycling program compared to continuing of normal daily activities.

Second statement:

We found that at the completion of a 6-week cycling program participants reported a reduction in daily knee pain (−7.2 points [95% CI = 4.1 to 10.3]) compared to the participants who continued with normal daily activity (+0.2 points [95% CI = −1.4 to 2.8] [$P < 0.05$]).

In the first statement, the statistical procedure (ANOVA) is noted before the result of interest, which is distracting to the reader. If the Method section was properly developed, the fact that the analysis of variance (ANOVA) was performed should already be known to the reader. Furthermore, the inclusion of confidence intervals (CI) in the latter provides estimates of the magnitude of change in each group in addition to addressing the issue of differences due to chance.

In addition to reporting the results of those participants having completed a study, a Results section should account for participants that drop out and to the greatest extent possible the reasons for discontinuing participation.

EXAMPLE

Discontinuation of Participation

An author might report:

Five participants (three cycling and two normal daily activity) dropped out of the study. Two of the cycling participants reported increases in knee pain and

(continued)

swelling after 5 and 8 days of participation and one moved to another country. Of the normal activity group one was injured in an accident and the other failed to respond to reminders about follow-up.

As noted previously, clinical investigations may measure multiple variables sometimes at multiple points in time resulting in large data sets. Tables and figures should be used to provide the reader with as much information as needed to understand the results of the study and apply the findings to their practice or research. At a minimum, mean values with confidence intervals, variance estimates, or both should be provided for all groups across time. The use of tables and figures allows for the presentation of far more information than could be captured in a readable narrative. In some cases a Results section may consist of a single paragraph supported by several tables and/or figures. It is important that the reader be directed to the appropriate tables and figures with statements such as "mean +/− standard deviation pain values at baseline, 6-weeks and 12-week follow-up are found in Table X." Moreover, information presented in tables and figures should not be repeated in the text of a Results section. Despite the fact that it is the focus of the reader's interest the Results section of many well-written papers is elegantly concise and to the point.

✔ CONCEPT CHECK

As a reader of research, it is important to carefully consider the methods used to acquire and analyze data so that one can make some judgment regarding the validity of the data reported.

Tables and Figures.   The subject of tables and figures also warrants discussion at this point. Tables are set off from the main text and used to present numerical as well as textual information. Each table should have a unique title and be arranged with clearly labeled column headers and row identifiers or headings. The units of measure should be clearly identified when appropriate. Footnotes that add clarity to the table are encouraged. A well-developed table will convey extensive information to the reader yet occupy relatively little space in the paper. The format of tables is prescribed in the authors' guide of journals.

Figures include an array of materials that convey information to the reader, often far more effectively than can be accomplished with words alone. Figures may include photographs, computer-generated images, algorithms, and graphic displays of data. Bar graphs and line graphs can convey information regarding trends and uncover the meaning of interactions between variables in the most effective manner. Regardless of the structure of a figure each figure should be accompanied by a legend that adds clarity to the figure and be in a format consistent with a journal's authors' guide. The information within a figure should not repeat information from the text or a table. When the data represented in a figure is interval or ratio, error bars to convey the precision of estimated mean values should be included. Estimated error cannot be conveyed in all graphical presentations (e.g., pie charts) and is but one consideration in choosing the format of a figure. When developing figures and choosing a format, it is important that the needs of the reader and limitation of production in black, white, and gray scale be kept in mind. Figures that include a lot of lines or multiple subtle contrasts in tone are difficult to read and interpret. In some cases it might be possible to develop two figures to convey results while in others it may be best to confine data to one or more tables rather than generate a busy, and therefore difficult to interpret single figure.

Discussion and Conclusion.   The last section of a scientific paper is devoted to a discussion of the results and a conclusion. The Discussion section may include the authors' conclusions or may be followed by a brief Conclusion paragraph. The Discussion section likely has a greater impact as to how favorably a paper is judged once published than any other portion of the work and plays a significant role in seeing a paper accepted for publication. Certainly, a flawed research design that poses a significant threat to the validity of data is good reason for rejecting a paper from consideration for publication. Barring "fatal" design flaws, however, the Discussion permits the author(s) the opportunity to suggest applications for their results, compare their results to works previously published, probe theoretical foundations, and identify topics for future research. A well-written Discussion brings data to life and leaves the reader filled with new insights and ideas. Poorly prepared Discussion sections first suffer from the plague of the poor Introduction; they are simply too long. A lengthy Discussion often drifts from the central focus of the research and puts the reader at risk of losing the key points. Aside from being too lengthy, the most common problem we have encountered in editing and reviewing papers is the excessive speculation that some authors are prone to. While the Discussion should not simply repeat the Results, the results should be kept in perspective. The generalization of results beyond the bounds of the study setting and population must be addressed with caution and the limitations of the study fully disclosed. In reviewing papers we frequently refer back to the purpose of the research stated in the Introduction. When the Discussion extends beyond the purpose it is likely too long and perhaps excessively speculative. Regardless of whether the conclusion is imbedded in the Discussion or placed under a unique heading labeled Conclusion, the final words should directly address the main question or questions posed in the statement of purpose. It is always concerning when the end does not appear directly tied to the beginnings of a scientific paper. In those cases where the conclusions do not appear directly related to the purpose one is likely to find more confusion than clarity in between.

> ✔ **CONCEPT CHECK**
>
> It is always concerning when the end does not appear directly tied to the beginnings of a scientific paper. In those cases where the conclusions do not appear directly related to the purpose one is likely to find more confusion than clarity in between.

Final Suggestions

Scientific writing is hard, time-consuming work. It is, in our experiences, not difficult to get lost in the forest that is a scientific paper and lose track of the path from Introduction through to Conclusion. While there is not a single solution we suggest, we do offer some final suggestions to keep in mind throughout your writing process:

1. Writing mud
2. Seek review
3. Be patient

The concept of writing mud comes from recollections of the late Dr. George Sheehan, the philosopher of the exercise boom in the 1960s and 1970s. His books and columns are still most enjoyable reading and over the course of his writing career which overlapped with his career as a cardiologist he wrote a lot. He confessed in some of his writings and lectures to struggling at times to get ideas onto paper (in the age of the manual typewriter!) and talked of writing what came to mind or what he referred to as mud. It is advice we still share particularly with students and young scholars. He made the point that it is not possible to revise and edit until something is in writing. Certainly, some of this book began as mud and some of the mud was discarded. However, you have to begin somewhere and we concur with Dr. Sheehan, if all of the thoughts are not coming together begin with mud.

Once the mud has taken form seek constructive criticism. Does the paper make sense to those knowledgeable of the subject and can the interested reader not an expert in the subject follow the logic and identify the most important findings? Once the feedback has been incorporated into the paper the last step is to let the paper sit for a few days.

Be patient rather than rushing to submit the work for review by an editorial board in consideration of publication. After a few days where other activities distract from near full focus on the paper, read from a fresh perspective. If all is in order the paper is ready to submit, but we have found this is the prime time to revise wording, shorten and generally fine-tune the writing.

CHAPTER SUMMARY

This chapter is devoted to the dissemination of research results through presentation and publication. Public speaking and scientific writing are skills that require practice to hone. Unfortunately, it is not possible to write an instructional chapter that will decrease the work of writing or assure immediate proficiency. However, the advice shared in this chapter is, to a large extent, passed down from our mentors and certainly helped us in our personal development as presenters and writers. Hopefully, it will help some who read this book through the challenges of presenting their work to the health care community.

KEY POINTS

- Titles should be highly descriptive without being exceedingly long.
- Abstracts are typically limited in length with a 400 to 600-word limit being common.
- The body of a scientific paper is divided into sections, which provide order and enhance the transitions through the course of the manuscript.
- The use of subheadings in a Method section is encouraged and often required as per many authors' guidelines.
- The Methods section should convey exactly how, when, and where data were acquired and provide sufficient detail to replicate the data analysis.
- The Results section should provide answers to the question or questions posed in the Introduction.
- Authors should report the most important results first.
- Information presented in tables and figures should not be repeated in the text of a Results section.
- A well-written Discussion brings data to life and leaves the reader filled with new insights and ideas.

Critical Thinking Questions

1. Why is the publication of peer-reviewed papers held in higher regard than presentations at professional meetings?
2. What is a common problem when writing the Introduction section of a scientific paper?
3. What is the risk of a lengthy Introduction section?
4. Why is it important that the discussion of results does not extend beyond the purpose of a study?

(continued)

Applying Concepts

1. Consider the potential problems encountered as editors and reviewers of scientific papers if the author of the paper fails to concisely define the purpose of the investigation and "weave the thread" through the entire paper to a concluding statement. Discuss the likely implications if the research methods, reported results, and/or discussion of the results do not reflect the stated purpose of the study/paper.

2. Locate a "Call for Papers" or "Call for Abstracts" for an upcoming or recent professional meeting. Bring it to class with you for review and comparison of authors' guidelines.

3. Choose three abstracts on a topic of interest to you in three different scholarly journals. Bring them to class with you for review and comparison of style format.

REFERENCES

Day RA. *How to Write and Publish a Scientific Paper*. 3rd ed. Phoenix, AZ: Oryx Press; 1988:28.

Physical Therapy Information for Authors. Available at http://www.ptjournal.org/misc/ifora.dtl, accessed January 5, 2009.

CHAPTER 20

WRITING THE FUNDING PROPOSAL

The individual has always had to struggle to keep from being overwhelmed by the tribe. If you try it, you will be lonely often, and sometimes frightened. But no price is too high to pay for the privilege of owning yourself.

—Friedrich Nietzsche (1844–1900), as found in Classic Quotes Quotation #5087 quoted in The Quotations Page (www.quotationspage.com)

CHAPTER OBJECTIVES

After reading this chapter you will:

- Understand the "culture of grants."
- Understand how to search for funding sources.
- Understand how to write a competitive grant proposal.

KEY TERMS

grants	internal culture	procurement principles

INTRODUCTION

The preceding chapters provide detailed steps for conducting research with a focus on problem solving using the research process. In particular, Chapter 1 outlines nine steps to frame a method of problem solving, including: (1) identifying a topic;

(2) searching and reviewing the literature; (3) defining a topic; (4) stating a general question or a problem; (5) phrasing an operationally defined hypothesis; (6) planning the methods to test the hypothesis; (7) data collection; (8) data analysis and interpretation of results; (9) writing about the findings. Generally, these steps mirror the sequence used to develop a well-conceived and convincing grant proposal.

Although the grant proposal process is anxiety provoking in many people, such anxiety is unnecessary. With careful preparation and critical review of successful proposals, the grant writing neophyte becomes fully capable of submitting a competitive grant proposal designed to improve evidence-based practice. This chapter provides a brief overview of the culture of **grants**, identifies resources helpful in locating funding opportunities, and draws upon the nine steps of research problem solving to compose and create a competitive grant application.

HISTORY AND CULTURE OF GRANTS

The successful entry into a new discipline or field of endeavor requires recognition of its **internal culture**. All professional disciplines, including proposal writing and research administration, adopt practices that must be followed or adhered to. The underlying concepts of grant "giving" and "getting" are long established within a profession that expects conformity to its policies, practices, and protocols. This history of conformity provides an important context and rationale for the existence of certain procedures and policies within the submission process. Understanding the historical evolution of grant funding can provide valuable insight for orienting the grant process and can significantly increase the competitiveness of the grant application.

The founding principles of grant proposal and award have historical basis as early as 1215 as contained within the Magna Carta. This English charter is considered a landmark legal document in the history and evolution of democracy and whose premise is based on improving the general human condition (Pallister, 1971). This commitment to improving the conditions of society helped shape much of the US Constitution, the Bill of Rights, and current English-based common law practice. This embodiment of democratic principles is echoed within the United States' principles of equal taxation, free trade, and equal access to tax dollars. The access to tax dollars is a key principle in early US procurement law that has eventually translated into equal access for all citizens. This guarantees all US citizens the right to compete for federal funds that would allow them to perform research benefiting society.

For over 200 years, the US Constitution has helped guide **procurement principles**. The protection of due process, equal access to opportunities, and the receipt of funding for research to benefit society are codified in statutes governing the procurement process. Examples of some of the federal statutes are: The Truth in Negotiations Act (TIN), The Competition in Contracting Act (CICA), The Federal Procurement Reform Act (FPRA), The Federal Property and Administration

Services Act (FPASA), The Armed Services Property Act (ARPA), The Contracts Disputes Act (CDA), and several additional statutes that govern ethics, labor laws, environmental laws, and small business development. These acts establish the principles governing the competition for federal funds and the process by which the awards are issued. Using the acts (also called laws or statutes), Congress creates regulations through legislation applicable to all federal agencies. Although oversimplified, these regulations provide the framework for open access to funding information via public announcements of all funding opportunities for grant and contract activity supported by US tax dollars.

Today, the federal Office of Management and Budget (OMB) is the central agency responsible for overseeing procurement regulations for federal grants and contract activity. The OMB uses well-established management systems and tools to assist federal agencies with their compliance with Congressional provisions. All federal agencies announcing calls for proposals require OMB clearance for the use of certain proposal forms to assure compliance with federal statutes. For example, OMB approval numbers appear at the top and/or bottom of proposal face pages and budget and certification forms of federal grant applications. The numbers indicate that agency procurement procedures meet federal mandates and regulations for fair and unbiased competition.

Additionally, the OMB manages the federal budget and communicates research and development allocations to the broader community. The OMB communicates through announcements using the *Federal Register* and the *Commerce Business Daily*, and also posts information alerts on their website and the central government announcement portal for federal funding opportunities, Grants.gov (http://www.grants.gov). Lastly, the OMB staff regularly present workshops and seminars describing federal research priorities and budgetary allocations at national conferences targeted at research investigators and administrators.

✔ CONCEPT CHECK

Understanding the historical evolution of grant funding can provide valuable insights for orienting the grant process and can significantly increase the competitiveness of the grant application.

GRANT VERSUS CONTRACT

The federal government defines research as a systematic investigation, including research development, testing, and evaluation, designed to develop or contribute to generalizable knowledge. The definition is found within Section 45 of the Code of Federal Regulations, Part 46.102(f) and, by its very nature, research is considered a process that benefits society. "Generalizable knowledge" is most often interpreted as an investigator having the *intent* to conduct research with the purpose of presenting or publishing findings in the public domain intended for the common good.

There are two primary mechanisms used to fund research activities; the first is termed "assistance" that is synonymous with "grant." The second is called "acquisition" that is the equivalent of "contract."[1] In addition, there exists a plethora of combinations or amalgamations of grants and contracts that are often described as "cooperative agreements."

The distinctions between a grant, contract, and cooperative agreement are important. Grants, by virtue of their definition, are an allocation of resources intended to improve the human condition. In contrast, contracts are issued when the purpose of the funding is to benefit the sponsor. Grants are governed by the OMB Circulars. Acquisitions are governed by procurement law, otherwise known as contract law, by the Federal Acquisition Regulations (FARs). The regulations control the award terms and conditions that further mandate the prior approvals required for researchers and define the conditions upon which funds can be disbursed. For example, when a grant is awarded, the recipient must use reasonable efforts to complete the project as originally proposed and approved. When a contract is issued, the recipient must comply with the deliverables outlined in the application or penalties (typically financial withholdings or termination) may be assessed. An applicant should fully understand and delineate whether their research seeks to make improvements to society (grant) or whether the research is undertaken to help solve a problem for the sponsor (contract). Cooperative agreements generally include a combination of grant and contract terms and conditions and typically involve collaborative relationships and shared oversight of the project with the sponsor. Almost every large company, college, or university hires specialists within their research offices whose responsibilities require expertise in procurement law and negotiations to ensure acceptable terms and conditions for researchers to carry out grant or contract activity. These persons keep constant surveillance to remain current regarding any changes described in the OMB Circulars and more than 4000 laws that currently affect government contracting.

All institutions receiving federal research funding are required to establish procedures and policies that adhere to the governing statutes and regulations administered by OMB and the federal agencies. The federal agencies are responsible for ensuring that each and every award adheres to OMB or FAR regulations. The awardee, in turn, must ensure adherence from all other entities that may contract or subcontract on the proposed project. The regulations specific to federal agencies are available on the OMB website in the form of circulars (http://www.whitehouse.gov/omb/). The Federal Acquisition Regulations, Section 48 CRR 1 through 53,

---

[1]There are also several other types of procurement applications such as memorandum of agreements, fixed priced agreements, material transfer agreements, subcontracts, consulting agreements, and intellectual property agreements. These agreements inclusively fall under the header of "contract."

are the core regulations that apply to all government agencies issuing contracts for research and development activity. The FAR is also available on the World Wide Web at http://www.acqnet.gov/FAR/.

SOURCES OF FUNDING

Currently, over $400 billion dollars is awarded for research annually, through 22 different federal agencies. These monies represent approximately 17% of the federal budget and 11% of the US Gross National Product. All federal funding opportunities are announced in the *Federal Register*, *Commerce Business Daily*, and on the government's central information and grants application portal, www.grants.gov. In addition to the central World Wide Web portal, funding announcements are listed on each individual federal agency's website. The announcements are easily accessed by entering the term "grants" or "program announcements" or "funding" in the website's main search field. For those investigators seeking funding from a specific federal agency, automated e-mail alerts announcing funding opportunities are generally available via an agency-specific listserv.

The management of funding opportunities has itself developed into a challenging and respected profession, where talented and experienced individuals are highly sought after by both academia and industry. Inevitably, any institution of higher education that performs research of some sort will have an individual or an entire department dedicated to the search and pursuit of funding opportunities. For example, in 2005, the number of grant-making foundations totaled 71,095 (The Foundation Center, 2007). Given the number of US foundation and corporate giving programs it is impractical to attempt to search individual foundation websites one at a time. Instead, a new industry has been created to provide database mining software specifically designed to assist academic institutions with the search for funding opportunities.

The three leading search engines that colleges and universities use today to conduct funding opportunity searches are the Sponsored Programs Information Network (SPIN), the Illinois Research Information System (IRIS), and the Community of Science (COS). Each of these database systems allows an investigator to input key words to attempt to match their research interest(s) to key words contained within the description of funding opportunities. Once an investigator enters key words, the software searches all applicable funding opportunities and announcements and generates a report of funding announcements with key word matches. The announcements provide a brief synopsis describing the funding opportunity, including the name of the sponsor, their location, amount and average size of awards, deadline, and geographic limitations. The investigator can conduct advanced searches using Boolean logic (using quotes around "and" or "or" to narrow a search) or take advantage of links within a search that cast a wider net to other opportunities. For example, at the end of a SPIN search, the investigator is provided with a list of key words synonymous to those originally supplied. The synonymous or related key words provide links to new searches, effectively expanding the yield of funding opportunities.

State funding opportunity announcements vary depending on state congressional sponsorship, state priorities or procedures, and budgetary constraints. The state funding opportunity announcements usually lag behind the electronic notifications of other sponsors. To locate state sources, the investigator is advised to search the website of a specific state agency(s) and contact an agency representative to discuss pending opportunities proposed for funding in the state legislature. Investigators should also request enrollment on the agency's e-mail distribution list or mailing list. Some states, such as New York, fund regional libraries. A regional library receives congressional funding to maintain a collection of periodicals, funding directories and searchable databases for funding opportunities for the region it serves. A reference librarian can assist users unfamiliar with the indexes and databases.

For those investigators interested in funds dispersed from the more than 71,095 (2005) US foundations or corporate giving programs, the leading searchable databases are the Foundation Directory and Metasoft Systems' BigDatabase and Foundationsearch program. These are just two of many commercially available products used to navigate and yield targeted searches for specific research and other funded projects. Universities, regional libraries, and even some economic development agencies like business bureaus and chambers of commerce may provide access to users depending on community needs and any licensing arrangements with database vendors.

Locating the optimum funding source requires advanced planning, practice, and patience. The challenge presented is not the lack of funding opportunities, rather locating the *right* funding opportunity. The proper funding opportunity is one that is targeted to an investigator's interest and expertise. The opportunity must be closely aligned with the investigator's research program and the sponsor should provide sufficient funding to complete the research plan. If the announcement matches the mission of the sponsor and the interest and intent of the investigator, two additional criteria must be met: (1) the sponsor awards funds in the investigator's geographic location; and (2) the investigator's host institution or employer meets the eligibility criteria.

Every announcement or request for proposal (RFP) includes a description of eligibility criteria to permit interested applicants to determine an announcement's suitability. The previously described databases also include fields that allow Boolean searches to factor in geographic limitations and eligibility criteria.

Once the investigator has found the right source of funding, further work ensues. Take, for example, attempting to procure funding from the National Institutes of Health (NIH) for research. According to survey data collected from colleges and universities in 2006, "the Department of Health and Human Services (HHS), including the NIH, continues to provide the majority of the federal government's funding to universities and colleges. In FY 2006 HHS contributed 57% of the total federal funding ($17.1 billion), primarily in support of the medical and biological sciences" (Britt, 2007). Every year the NIH budget contains the largest amount of competitive funding in the United States for research in health care and disease prevention (Britt, 2007). According to *Federal Grants and Contracts Weekly* (2007), the total funds administered by the NIH for research, health care, injury prevention, and treatment for all sectors of the economy including universities and colleges comprise approximately $30 billion annually with about 10,000 new research projects receiving awards in the same period.

There are hundreds of NIH program announcements made available each year. In order to identify the announcements most relevant to an investigator's particular research interests, the search for opportunities may need to be culled by targeting a specific Institute within the overall NIH. Although the NIH is one sponsor, the NIH is actually comprised of 26 different Institutes, with multiple programs available in each Institute and many funding opportunities cross listed among different Institutes for joint funding. It is up to the investigator to browse the Institutes to match their expertise to the individual Institute's mission. Once the investigator chooses a specific Institute, then the individual Web pages of the Institute(s) should be examined in depth to assure that the correct program announcement has been chosen.

As with other federal agencies, within the NIH there exist many programs tailored to the higher education research community. For example, the NIH offers program opportunities that are specifically designed for new investigators, primarily undergraduate institutions, small business innovation research programs, training programs, international programs, and so forth. Finding the *right* funding source takes advanced planning, communication with the sponsor and with any collaborators, and with the investigators' organization to ensure that the investigator has identified a viable opportunity for which he/she can realistically compete.

Investigators are strongly advised to contact their institutional research officer(s), if available, to help match their expertise and interests with the best-fit funding opportunities and programs. Institutional research officers receive thousands of funding opportunities from hundreds of sponsors each year. These advisors have valuable experience and knowledge concerning which programs best match their institutions' eligibility, geographic restrictions, and investigators' strengths. In addition, they are also familiar with the particular nuances and intricacies of the agency divisions and programs within their state, the federal government, and any particular requirements of specific foundations.

✔ CONCEPT CHECK

All federal funding opportunities are announced in the *Federal Register, Commerce Business Daily,* and on the government's central information and grants application portal. In addition to the central World Wide Web portal, funding announcements are listed on each individual federal agency's website.

GRANT WRITING FOR THE TWENTY-FIRST CENTURY: A RECIPE FOR SUCCESS

Advanced Planning

Despite the annual availability of billions of dollars for research, there remains stiff competition for grant funds. The National Science Foundation (NSF), the second largest contributor to federal research expenditures, reported receipt of over 43,000 grant applications in 2006–2007.[2] The NSF average funding success rates have steadily declined over the past 7 years from 36% in 2000 to 24% in 2005 to most recently 22% in 2006. The NSF attributes the decline to a reduction in federal funding allocations, coupled with an exponential increase in the number of proposals. In 2005, the success rate for first-time applicants was 13% compared to a 24% success rate for investigators with prior NSF awards. The NIH funding rates follow similar patterns.

One answer to the challenges of effectively competing in the federal market place is that "the top 100 research performers accounted for 80% of all R&D (research and development) dollars in FY 2006. These proportions have varied little during the past two decades" (Britt, 2007). Because of the low funding rated for new investigators, far more new proposals are rejected than funded. There are many reasons that applications are rejected, but one important and often overlooked reason is that applicants underestimate the importance of advanced planning in cultivating relationships with the sponsors or administrators of an agency or foundation. Advanced planning also allows a neophyte investigator the opportunity to acquire the necessary experience developing a well-conceived proposal that adheres to the expectations of the grant's "culture."

As part of the grants and contracts award process, a panel of reviewers meet to discuss, rank, and recommend funding for the top proposals. In order to receive funding, investigators need to convincingly present both sound science and convincing arguments. An effective proposal writer engages a reviewer in wanting to read more and will hopefully create in the reviewer some positive emotion, action, or thought. The ability to move a reviewer is truly an art form. The genre of effective proposal writing is mostly defined by persuasive writing.

Persuasive proposals are written using can-do, action verbs and motivate the reviewer toward wanting to help solve the problem being presented. Proposals *move* reviewers to action through piquing curiosity and leaving the reviewer with the desire to fund the proposal to determine exactly how the investigator will solve the questions or problems raised. A good proposal writer presents information clearly and is committed to the argument they are presenting. A strong

---

[2]As reported by Jean Feldman, Director of NSF Policy Division, at the National Council of University Research Administrator's Conference, Annual Meeting, Washington, DC, November, 2007.

commitment to the subject makes the proposal believable and literally makes the words come alive through the passion and drive of the author. Those authors not fully committed to a particular philosophy, hypothesis, or strategy quickly lose the attention of the reviewer. A proposal should tell a compelling story: a story that the investigator believes in and sees clearly the tasks at hand.

Cultivating a Sponsor Relationship

An essential strategy to assist writers *move* readers to action and *engage* reviewers in wanting to help solve a particular problem begins with contacting the appointed program officer of the agency to which the proposal will be directed. Contact should occur well before the established deadline. Early contact helps establish the credibility of the investigator by reflecting a character of a preplanner, one serious about wanting to compete for the funding opportunity, and one keenly interested in feedback to be successful. Adopting a collaborative approach with a program officer helps engage the officer in dialogue to shape the emphasis of the proposal text based on what feedback is offered during the discussion process.

In addition to communicating with potential applicants, the program officer's role includes responsibility for administering the "request for proposals," or overseeing the release of the public announcement of the funding opportunity and assuring the eligibility of applicants encouraged to submit to the competition. The program officer also oversees and coordinates the assignment of the proposal's review by peers and, based on reviewer's comments, typically has significant input as to who receives an award. During the review process, the program officer gives the peer reviewers a specific protocol and timeline to rank each proposal. For federal proposals, ranking occurs by using established criteria or scoring rubrics. Whether federally funded or not, almost every set of proposal guidelines provide applicants with a list of the established criteria that will help guide the reviewers in their decisions. Sometimes the criteria are labeled "review criteria" while other times the format and header sections listed in the application guidelines, although not specifically identified as review criteria, are used for ranking. Most often reviewers assign percentage points to each review criterion.

According to grants guru David G. Bauer,[3] a highly sought-after national consultant on grant seeking, before writing a proposal the investigator should inquire from the program officer what percentage points are assigned to each section of the narrative. Knowing the ranking percentages allows the investigator to write the narrative while focusing on the most highly weighted areas. By communicating with the program officer, the investigator can more easily determine the scoring rubric, how the percentages are assigned, what key points are of most

---

[3]David G. Bauer is author to 15 books on grant writing and getting and is nationally renowned for his work with training university faculty in increasing the odds of their proposals being funded.

importance to the agency, and the background, experience, and training of the reviewers scoring the application. The reviewers' background information is essential for attempting to target the proposal to a receptive audience. For example, a frequent mistake made by new investigators is assuming that the reviewers of the proposal are as knowledgeable as they are in their specific discipline. Often that is not the case. Proposers need to be cognizant of composing in an easily understandable style so that all readers can comprehend what is being proposed. Consider an investigator writing a proposal suggesting the creation of a significant new manufacturing procedure, followed by a detailed methodological design, using acronyms and discipline-specific jargon. Although the proposal might "wow" the reviewer with a similar technical background, another reviewer may have little knowledge of the acronyms and significance of the new method because the language is written in such a way as to exclude some readers while including others. It is the responsibility of every investigator to write in such a manner that invites the fundamental understanding of the topic, its significance, and application to specific disciplines.

However, a certain balance of lyric, prose, and technical description is required. The composition cannot be so general as to dilute or minimize the content. Rather, difficult concepts should be clearly articulated and presented in a manner that educates the reviewer without being condescending. This process is often termed "scaffolding." The basic concept of scaffolding is to introduce a general concept and build upon the concept's foundation with increasing complexity so that the reviewer expands their understanding as they progress through the text.

Having acquired information about scoring priorities and the background and types of reviewers scoring the proposal, the prepared investigator now has a distinct advantage over other applicants who did not contact the program officer. According to David G. Bauer, almost all successful applicants have had some prior contact with an appointed program officer. In his book titled *The "How To" Grants Manual*, Bauer shares that "in a study of 10,000 federal proposals, the only variable that was statistically significant in separating the funded and rejected proposals was pre-proposal contact with the funding source. Chances for success increased an estimated threefold when contact with the funding source takes place before the proposal is written" (Bauer, 1984, p. 106).

Early and frequent contact with the program officer may help the investigator discover other useful elements. Program officers often offer advice in interpreting guidelines and may share information that is not included in the written RFP. As an example, perhaps a current award cycle or "request for proposals" seeks specific proficiencies in the use of technology to improve scientific methodology. Those applicants unaware of the technology proficiency criteria would be at a disadvantage in composing their proposal. Through constructive dialogue with the program officer, the applicant may discover hints, nuances, and subtle interpretations of the evaluation guidelines. These nuances and interpretations help target the content and better align the writing style and level of detail provided based on the intended audience.

Given the responsibility of reviewing hundreds of research proposals each year, program officers become particularly proficient at recognizing cutting edge research, and having a general awareness of the current state-of-the-art. Via dialog and open communication with this valuable resource, the investigator can gain perspective about similar projects that have received funding, and which specific topics are most interesting to the sponsor. The information obtained in this exchange will place the investigator in an excellent position for effectively proposing the research topic, assuring alignment within the larger context of the sponsor's interests.

✔ CONCEPT CHECK

An effective proposal writer engages a reviewer in wanting to read more and will hopefully create in the reviewer some positive emotion, action, or thought.

Literature Review

Before beginning the composition of a grant application, investigators need to conduct a thorough literature search to understand the history, evolution, and current and potential future trends in the research topic being considered. An appropriate start to a literature review begins in a library or in the library's electronic holdings via remote access using discipline-specific databases, online catalogs, and periodicals. The sponsor's website is also an excellent resource. Most sponsors provide a list of prior awardees and some provide a brief synopsis, abstract, or project summary of previously funded grants.

By using both library resources and sponsor databases and archives, the applicant can comprehensively search past and current literature on their subject. Investigators should also learn to scrutinize publications' acknowledgment sections. Almost all sponsors require an acknowledgment statement indicating that the published research was supported in full, or in part, by the sponsor and that the ideas presented are not necessarily endorsed by the sponsor. The investigator can glean important clues about funding sources in the acknowledgment section and follow up with that source to determine if any current or pending funding opportunities would be applicable to their area of interest.

Distilling Broad Concepts into Fundable Ideas

In addition to persuasive writing, the most successful proposal writers build and support their study on prior research obtained through their literature review. Via this process the investigator is able to expand their vision in a new direction or re-configure procedures, interventions, or treatments in comparison to previous study designs. Establishing and validating a sound methodological procedure is the foundation for which a grant proposal is conceived and reviewed for funding. However, the crucial first step to grant writing is having a good idea. Ideas need to be novel. Novel in this context means having an interesting and potentially useful idea.

Many proposals are effectively written and convincing, but the concept itself appears insignificant or inconsequential. The letters received by the authors of nonfunded proposals typically state "We are sorry that your project was not funded. The topic did not match the XYZ's highest priority this round." In other words, sponsors do not want to fund projects that do not appear important, useful, or are of low priority.

Basing an idea on the significance of prior work as demonstrated through a literature search develops the idea's credibility and usefulness. An effective way to hone an idea is to select a broad concept that you want to explore, conduct an exhaustive literature search, and then identify gaps in knowledge or inconsistencies in published results that merit further exploration. Writers must demonstrate to sponsors that they are familiar with previously published research, and that the proposed research study builds upon past practices to make improvements to the future. Once the idea is demonstratively sound, then the writer can begin partitioning the concept(s) into methodological steps. It is these "gaps" in knowledge that sponsors are funding and that are considered novel and important to science.

GRANT WRITING VERSUS PUBLICATION AUTHORSHIP

Once the preplanning strategies have been addressed, the program officer(s) contacted, and the thorough literature review completed, the investigator is now ready to begin composing the proposal. By this time, the applicant should have a clear understanding of what constitutes a fundable concept, who has done what in the field, and what interesting, significant, and potentially fundable new work needs to be performed. Additionally, the applicant should have acquired a working knowledge of what methodologies have been previously used in funded studies, what information has been disseminated, and in which journals that information has been published.

Begin by using a proactive writing style. Grant writing differs from publication authorship in that the text is active, rather than reflective. Grant writing purposefully builds an argument that the proposed research or project is important and that the time is of the essence. The presented ideas need to be developed in a succinct, clear, and persuasive writing style. A passionate commitment to an idea helps create belief in the mind of the reviewer that the proposal is important, exciting, and deliverable. The composition style engages the reviewer and convinces the reviewer to support the proposal.

Understanding the psychology of grant writing greatly helps the writer in choosing their examples, selecting evidence, and articulating a "plan of action." A good reviewer wants to be involved in selecting projects that are worthy and takes his/her role seriously in selecting the best proposals that will simultaneously advance the mission of the sponsor or match the program announcement's objectives. Therefore, writing to the readers, understanding and using the terms identified in the program announcement, familiarity with the sponsor's history, prior grants, and priorities, and combining those with your own knowledge and interest in the project being proposed is the best recipe for successfully engaging reviewers and being awarded funding.

Elements of a Proposal

Most proposals include the following sections:

1. A title page that identifies the institution and investigator
2. An abstract that provides a quick summary of the project
3. Project narrative, which includes:
   a. An introduction of the organization submitting the proposal and the idea being presented
   b. A description of the significance of or need for the research
   c. An overview of the background of the problem, what previous work has been performed to address the problem, and how the applicant will either fill a gap in the existing science or build upon prior work
   d. A description of the specific methods to be used to investigate the problem
   e. A description of the qualifications of the key personnel leading the proposed research
   f. A timeline to chronicle the order and sequence of events and activities
   g. A description of how the methods will be evaluated to quantify and validate the progress
   h. The plans for disseminating results so that others can learn from the work
   i. A reference section to identify the sources used, quoted, or referred to throughout the proposal.

Each of these sections is discussed below. There are variations in the number or content of the sections, but in general the information presented is fairly standardized. In every case, the investigator should read and reread proposal guidelines to assure that the directions are carefully followed. Proposals that do not adhere to formatting instructions (margins, paginations, fonts, page or character limitations, order, appendices, etc.) will not be reviewed. If there are any questions about the instructions, investigators should contact the sponsor for guidance. Additionally, investigators should familiarize themselves with the review criteria and any specialized requirements such as supplemental instructions or electronic proposal submission details. Unfortunately, many of the electronic proposal processing systems are in their infancy and require more time and effort than anticipated. As with the case of new programs, multiple data entry fields occur and some of the bridges/crosswalks between computer systems are not understood or even retrievable. Therefore, plan well in advance and test the sponsor's proposal processing system to avoid unnecessary stress in order to successfully meet the proposal deadline.

Title Page

A title page provides useful contact information and a basic description of the proposal. Generally, a title page includes a descriptive, yet succinct title for the project. The title of the project will establish an immediate image in the reviewer's mind of what is expected in the narrative. Put some effort into choosing a good title. The title page also includes the name(s) of the principal investigator, any co-investigators, office address, phone number and e-mail information, and the name of the investigators' home institution. Additionally, the title page typically contains project start and end dates, and the total funding requested. Note that state and federal title pages require the name and position of the authorizing official who assumes legal responsibility for assuring the contents of the proposal adhere to state and federal statutes governing grants and contracts. The title page is either hand or electronically signed by the authorizing official prior to submission to the sponsor. Authorizing officials generally reside in the research or grants office, but on occasion may be the chief executive officers of the institution or agency.

Abstract

The abstract, or proposal summary, is in some ways the most important text of the entire proposal. It is often the only section of the proposal that all reviewers read. The abstract serves as a summation of the project. It includes a description of what problems the researcher is trying to address, why the project is significant, and what impact the project will have if funded. Abstracts should be no longer than one page, succinctly written and composed as the last task of the writing phase in order to capture a full summation of the entire project. Abstracts should include the research questions and procedures used to address the questions, and should be written in terms understandable to anyone. If the proposal is funded, the abstract can be published verbatim and many sponsors release the abstract for public announcements about the project.

EXAMPLE

Abstract

Below is an example of an abstract.

The purpose of this study is to investigate therapeutic exercises to reduce the common ailments and foot pain in females diagnosed with plantar fasciitis, an inflammation caused by excessive stretching of the fibrous tissue that runs along the bottom surface of the foot and, when excessively stretched, can lead to plantar fasciitis that results in heel pain, arch pain, or heel spurs. The study will explore therapeutic exercises for improvements in gait to increase participants exercise length and strength. Although several studies conducted by leading podiatrists (list authors names in parenthesis) show multiple strategies of stretching, the use of orthotics, low-dose pain medication, and weight control as effective "treatment" for managing plantar fasciitis, significant numbers of patients continue to complain of pain and therefore reduced exercise duration and selection. This study will evaluate the efficacy of diet, massage therapy, and yoga on pain reduction and increased length and strength for women golfers who regularly walk 18 holes of golf and who have been diagnosed with plantar fasciitis. At least 50 female participants will be enrolled in the study, each at least 15 lbs overweight, between 45 and 50 years old, active in the sport, and interested in a lifestyle change of dieting, foot massage therapy, and yoga. The study will take place in upstate New York and provide valuable information for women's health, sport and fitness practitioners, and alternative treatments to enhance the quality of life of women golfers who suffer from plantar fasciitis.

Table of Contents

Currently, most proposals require electronic submission via the World Wide Web with many sponsors relying on the use of software programs that automatically enter the applicant's information in the table of contents page. The advantage of using automated forms is that the investigator receives an effective management tool for following page limitations and staying on task by section headers. Similarly, the sponsor conserves resources by streamlining administrative responsibilities such as checking page limitations and completion requirements and can focus on the intellectual merit and quality of the proposal itself.

Not all sponsors use specifically tailored electronic processing programs for proposal submissions. In developing a nonelectronic table of contents, authors should use the same sort of algorithm as encoded into the electronic processors. The goal is to develop a table of contents that follows sponsor guideline headers and sections, adheres to the proposal guideline page limitations, and presents a well-organized chronology that matches the sections of the narrative and supporting documents such as vitas or appendices. The table of contents should assist the reviewer in finding important information and simultaneously create a positive impression on the reviewer, who would then anticipate reviewing a complete, well-constructed, aesthetically pleasing, organized, and thoughtful proposal.

Whether relying on a computer software package or creative writing skills, the table of contents should follow the order of the guidelines using the same or similar sections as outlined. Subsections should be included when the proposal exceeds 10 pages, or where additional organization becomes critical in facilitating the location of required material necessary for meeting review criteria. Appendices listed on the table of contents should only be used for relevant information. Large appendices are rarely fully reviewed, so they should be selectively scant and never manipulated to circumvent any proposal page limitations.

Project Narrative

The project narrative is the core of the proposal. The narrative section includes all relevant information used for determining the importance of the proposal, what particular problem will be addressed, and which procedures will be used to solve the described problem. The narrative also includes a description of the relevant prior experience and credentials the investigator has that will enable him/her in carrying out the proposed project. In total, the narrative section provides the reviewer with a description of ambitious, yet achievable goals and objectives and a sensible management plan to complete the project within the designated timeframe. Therefore, the goals and objectives must be achievable and not so expansive as to appear overly ambitious in relationship to the timeframe allowed to accomplish the work. The investigator(s) must also bear in mind their other responsibilities and not promise more dedicated time to the project than they have available.

a. Introduction   To begin the narrative, the investigator should orient the reader with one or two introductory paragraphs as space allows to introduce the significance of the topic and to establish the credibility of the organization or individual(s) conducting the research. Since most proposals are submitted by organizations on behalf of individual investigators, introductory paragraphs can be used to provide important information about the institution and the context of the research environment. The introductory paragraphs frame an image of the existing research environment and the support structure available to assist the investigator throughout the project. Although not necessarily explicit, in essence the writer is establishing credibility of the organization. This descriptive portion of the narrative can be used to suggest that the parent organization is the perfect location for the performance of the research. Note the distinction of these paragraphs from an abstract that is used to summarize the entire proposal.

EXAMPLE

Introductory paragraphs

Here is an example of introductory paragraphs:

The XYZ University was established in 1868 as a teachers' college with a strong emphasis on physical fitness. For over 100 years, XYZ University has provided national leadership on human performance, especially in the areas of athletic training, kinesiology, and physical education. The faculty at XYZ University are selectively recruited to advance teaching, research, and service. The faculty to student ratio is 1 to 12, allowing for individualized instruction and collaborative research and practicum experiences to prepare each graduate with the skills and know how of addressing some of today's most plaguing problems confronting human performance in the twenty-first century. With the escalation and zealousness of human performance lawsuits, XYZ University has been called upon by National College Athletic Association (NCAA) to provide case law curriculum for the nation's athletic training programs. The NCAA call is intended to reach all accredited athletic training programs to serve as a guide in helping instructors navigate civil and criminal law suits creeping into each of the NCAA divisions. The curriculum will be designed to guide students in understanding and creating defendable protocols for preliminary diagnostics, treatments, and physician referrals. The protocol documentation and insurance company claims and court testimonial course sections will include the most recent case law on human performance to guide institutions in best preparing the next generation of athletic trainers confronting civil and criminal law suits.

b. Significance   The significance section of the proposal narrative educates the reader to the importance of and the urgency of the research. The significance section should also help justify funding the proposal. Through documented evidence, the writer explains the necessity of this research and stimulates the curiosity of the reviewer to further investigate how the proposed project will address a gap in the body of scientific knowledge.

By drawing from the previously described nine steps to frame a method of problem solving, the writer can provide clear and logical evidence of the proposal's merit and fundability. The author should begin by identifying the need and describing how the need developed. Supportive facts along with specific references and citations should be used, with care taken to include the most current and relevant work in the field. Once the problem is outlined and the case made for the need for a pressing and timely solution, the next step is identifying the specific question to be addressed and answered. This is the scaffolding technique described earlier. At this point, a broad picture or vision of the solution can then be described, but specifics should be addressed in the methods section. Lastly, if the research project addresses regional, state, or federal priorities, refer to those priorities in this section.

In general, the significance section should not exceed two to three pages. The majority of the proposal narrative should be focused on the method section that is described later on in this chapter. Rather, the significance section is used to educate the reader about the identified problem and its importance and further entices the reader to continue to the next section.

c. Rationale   Now that the investigator has educated the reader about the significance of the proposed research, the rationale section should then document the scientific literature covering the investigator's topic. This section typically demonstrates a gap in the body of knowledge and supports the argument that the proposed investigation will contribute significant advances to the body of scientific knowledge. Any criticisms of previous studies or methods when identifying gaps in the literature should be avoided. Instead, the rationale should be composed in a positive light, identifying alternatives that may be considered to address unanswered questions.

Given that it is quite possible that the cited references may include previous publications from the proposal's reviewers, the wise investigator will retain a positive respectful tone in addressing all prior work. Any perceived weaknesses, limitations, or inaccuracies, should be couched as interesting or provocative questions remaining to be addressed. For example, imagine a reviewer having devoted years to researching a problem, arduously pursuing alternative solutions and serving on a proposal panel with peers who have done similar work and made substantive commitments to research. The proposal being reviewed and currently under discussion in their review group references their life careers' work and provides a convincing summation that their approach is limited, misguided, and has done little to advance the understanding of the problem. The reviewer's discussion group colleagues, also considered top experts in the field, have never met the investigator who purports that an alternative strategy deviating from commonly accepted practices by the reviewers is methodologically superior and is certain they know the "right" questions and research and have a clearer vision of the solution. From this example, one might surmise that there would be a lack of enthusiasm for the proposal, even if the limitations and criticisms detailed are true.

To navigate the political minefield of proposing improvements to prior work, the writer should still cite the accepted study(s), but carefully emphasize how the strengths of the previous study piqued their interest and reinforced their commitment for further investigation. Additional research should hopefully be able to build upon the accepted work of prior experts and lead the science in a new direction. The writer can achieve the intended result of identifying the limitations of prior work but accentuate the positive while doing so. In this manner, all persons are given credit for their contributions and the review team can discuss the next phase of the research or an interesting alternative that may yield new findings rather than dwell upon the criticism of an investigator.

As previously stated, the federal government allocates over $400 billion annually for US research and development. According to the OMB, approximately 80% of that federal funding goes directly to states for managing their priorities and coordinating competitions based on joint priorities. As a result, state and federal government reports are considered credible sources of citation information and help frame the significance of the proposed research on a state or national level. Effective and timely citations may advance the reviewers' desire to fund a project to meet parallel purposes: that of their own mission along with the state's or nation's priorities.

As a general rule, the rationale and literature cited within this section should not exceed two to three pages. Although important, the rationale section is not the most important section of the proposal. The emphasis of the proposal should be directed toward the methods section as outlined below.

d. Methods Section   The methods section is the heart and soul of a proposal. This section provides readers with a step-by-step process of solving a particularly important problem. The methods section is a merger of traditional academic writing paired with business and economic writing to create a feasible plan of action that has a high probability of achieving important results. The methods section, like a business plan, is not reflective like the rationale section, but rather an active line of inquiry that articulates in great detail the investigator's plan. This section is the most lengthy in the entire proposal and requires a logical order to educate the reader. Once again using a scaffolding concept is recommended, introducing the basic concepts initially, and then increasing the complexity as the reader progresses through the text.

The methods section should be introduced by identifying the research question(s) or study objectives. The questions or objectives should be accented or highlighted using bold font, indentations, numbering, or underlines. This allows the reviewers to quickly analyze the overall goals of the project, and then permits rapid scanning of the subheaders to provide an initial impression of the general cohesiveness, organization, and feasibility of the study.

Clarity and brevity are key when writing research questions or objectives. Impractical or highly theoretical questions and goals will appear unfocused. Rather, specificity, practicality, and the use of active tense help the reviewer embrace the questions and objectives as important, valid, and timely.

EXAMPLE

Overall project goal and corresponding research questions

Here is an example of an overall project goal and corresponding research questions:

The goal of this study is to investigate the long-term implications of repeated shoulder injuries on the health and lifestyle of retired NFL football players between the ages of 55 and 60.

(continued)

The study will investigate five research questions:

1. What impact, if any, has repeated shoulder injuries had on the quality of life of retired NFL players between the ages of 55 and 60?
2. What pain treatments, if any, are these same retired NFL football players using to maintain their quality of life after having experienced repeated shoulder injuries during their NFL career?
3. What impact, if any, has self-prescribed pain treatment had on the health and physical functionality of these same retired NFL football players?
4. What impact, if any, has physician-prescribed pain treatment had on the health and physical functionality of these same retired NFL football players?
5. What impact, if any, has repeated shoulder injuries had on the psychological and social aspects of the lives of these same retired NFL football players?

Note how each successive question builds upon the previous question logically and how the overall set of questions appears manageable during a typically funded 1- to 3-year study. Also note that the questions are composed in a manner such that several answers may result, rather than a simple positive or negative response.

Research questions should be composed in an exploratory way. Many investigators mistakenly pose questions that are self-explanatory and therefore appear insignificant. For example, the question below is self-evident because common sense dictates that repeated injuries lead to long-term pain and people typically self-medicate to manage their own pain.

EXAMPLE

Poorly stated research question

Here's an example of a poorly stated research question:

1. Does repeated shoulder injuries of retired NFL football players between the ages of 55 and 60 lead to frequent use of low-dose pain medications as a self-prescribed pain treatment?

Writing a question that allows a simple yes/no response is a common misstep. When composing research questions, think carefully and pose powerful well thought out questions that not only cut through to the core of the issue, but also demonstrate the amount of time and effort that went into the thought process.

Once the research questions are identified, subsections can be created using the research questions as headers. These subheaders keep both the investigator and the reader focused. Subheaders may be included in the table of contents. Regardless, the discovery process and methodology must be detailed and described to the reviewer.

Draw upon sound scientific methods that have been confirmed as accurate, valid, and reliable in similarly structured studies. For example, if the study typically uses an experimental group and a control group, then the proposed study should reference prior studies and offer a rationale for the number of participants that will yield statistically reliable data for analysis and interpretation of the results. If a study is a longitudinal analysis of a specified group and follows up with focus group analysis, then the investigator should reference prior work of similar size and scope and alert the reader that control questions will be embedded in the overall survey to assure reliability of data. If available, the help of a statistician should be enlisted to ensure that the study size and design is powerful enough to ensure statistical significance, and that the analytical methods are properly suited for appropriate analysis of the specific type of data collected.

With all methodological procedures, be straightforward and honest about any particular methodological limitations. Reviewers appreciate knowing the limitations and may already have forecasted challenges with particular procedures before reading the entire methods section. The effort to describe any weaknesses in advance may actually illustrate to the reviewer that the investigator has anticipated other potential problems and issues ahead of time. It is essential to describe the contingencies in place for dealing with the known limitations and assurances should be made to the reviewer that these limitations do not affect the overall study integrity. One method of illustrating this concept uses parallels of prior work that included similar limitations with little impact. In this manner, the investigator can reference how other projects confronted the same issue and used alternative measures to alleviate the difficulties. Specific citations and references must be used. If the investigator is proposing a new methodology for simplifying earlier work or developing a new instrument, it is important that some pilot data and a description of preliminary work, design, or studies is provided. Pilot or preliminary data offers the reviewers some evidence that preliminary investigations are promising and that further study may yield important information.

It is important to stay focused and committed to the research plan. The methods section must describe in detail the investigator's proposed solutions to the research questions. All pertinent information supporting the described procedures and methods used must be included. For example, necessary information includes listing data encoding software packages, a description of the actual encoding procedures, the detailing of how validity scores are assigned within the method used, the expected time duration of the various subsections along with the anticipated deliverables or goals from each subsection, and the assignment of responsibilities for each subsection to various members of the team. Using a well-organized outline, ample spacing, diagrams, charts, and a well-illustrated timeline will not only greatly assist reviewers in the analysis and interpretation of the text, but will also create appeal in the attractiveness of a well thought out, well-organized, concise, and focused proposal.

Lastly, an investigator must be realistic in the self-evaluation of strengths, skills, weaknesses, and deficiencies. One's strengths must be emphasized, and one's weaknesses must be supplemented with team members or consultants possessing expertise in these weak areas. As described above, statisticians are almost always useful in designing appropriate data analysis algorithms. Other potential team members include clinicians to augment the research scientist, engineers to augment clinicians, and so on.

e. Personnel/Management Section   The personnel section, also referred to as the Management Plan Section, demonstrates the investigator's ability to provide leadership. This section provides the reviewer with a synopsis of the investigator(s) previous research activities, honors and recognition, and with insight into their dedication and commitment. It also allows for the writer to illustrate the suitability of their institution or corporation to host the research, along with a summation of the resources the institution can bring to bear upon the problem. Larger universities or corporations may provide themselves with a slight edge by demonstrating a myriad of different personnel, equipment, laboratory space, or other facilities unavailable to smaller firms or institutions. A brief but relevant synopsis of the investigator(s) credentials focused on their ability to carry the research to fruition is required, along with a description of institutional facilities and resources, and a timeline describing the projected research goals and deliverables. This section is usually brief, but full of information used by the reviewer to evaluate the skills of the individuals administering the award.

EXAMPLE

Synopsis of the investigator(s) credentials and description of institutional facilities and resources

An example of establishing an investigator's credentials follows:

> [Name of Investigator] is a Professor of Kinesiology at XYZ University and Chair of the National Association of Kinesiology Practitioners' higher education committee. The Investigator received a lifetime achievement award from the XYZ University system in recognition for her work in advancing PDQ. She has successfully administered five prior awards from the National Institutes of Health, two projects with the US Education Department, and recently completed a nationally

(continued)

recognized study on ABC funded by the Robert Wood Johnson Foundation. This long, highly successful career has prepared her well for undertaking the current proposed study. Her specific responsibilities will include oversight of the research team that is comprised of one research specialist and two graduate assistants. All administrative components of the grant (purchasing, payroll, budgeting, etc.) will be supported by a departmental secretary assigned, but not charged, to the proposed grant.

An example of describing relevant institutional resources follows:

The Investigator will have full access to the kinesiology research laboratory for performing the study. The laboratory consists of 30 × 50 foot space, gait tachometer, bipod, two treadmills, four laptop computers, and a printer for data analysis. Participants for the study will be recruited from the Kinesiology Department's undergraduate student research subject's pool where students may obtain extra credit for engaging in research studies. Under the supervision of the research specialist, the 2 graduate assistants will conduct experiments on XYZ using 100 undergraduate student volunteers. Each volunteer will receive 5 extra points in their research methods course for participation. An alternative incentive of writing a 5-page paper will be provided for those participants seeking extra credit without research volunteer experience.

f. Timeline   Timelines are effective tools to chronologically organize, order, and sequence the events and activities in a proposal. The investigator must be realistic about the time required for each activity or experiment. Many timelines include multiple headers including information such as Task, Description of Task, Date of Completion, Team Leader. Others use headers such as Goal, Objective, Activity, Timeframe, Person(s) Responsible. Use of a table format that can be created in Microsoft Word or Excel is highly desirable to easily mesh the generated timeline with the other charts or data outlined previously in the prior sections.

g. Evaluation   The evaluation section is becoming increasingly more important to sponsors. Sponsors want investigators to explain how they will confirm and validate that the methods used on project activities or interventions are functioning properly. How will the investigator know if the funded project is producing appropriate and valid results? What interim safeguards will allow the investigator to determine throughout the process that the experiments, procedures, or activities are functioning as intended? These are important questions and should be carefully considered well before the experimental design is finalized.

There are several types of evaluation methods. Typically a mixed-methodological approach is warranted. For example, researchers often employ both qualitative and quantitative measures and use formative and summative data collection and analysis procedures. Many investigators include outside evaluation consultants as part of their study personnel to assure unbiased feedback and analysis of the validity of the study design and its broader impacts. Evaluations should indicate the expected outputs and outcomes and/or deliverables so that there can be tracking measurements from the beginning to the end of a study. Outputs, outcomes, and deliverables also aid the investigator in keeping focused and on track with the main purpose and significance of the research.

h. Dissemination   The dissemination section informs the reviewer of the investigator's intent as to publication of the results. The intent is to present the results of the study to those who would benefit most from the results. This includes the research scientist who would then use the results in furthering their own research, or the clinician, who would use the results to improve their practice, or directly to the general public, who could use the results to improve their lives.

Dissemination of investigative findings is accomplished via several methods. The most traditional method of dissemination occurs through publication of articles in peer-reviewed journals, conference presentations and workshops, website information resources, and stories or reviews in newspapers or newsletters. Each of these methods offers the public access to research findings and ensure that the research benefits the greatest number of people. Authors are encouraged to accentuate dissemination strategies traditionally used within their discipline and most relevant to the project. For example, if a study investigates the impact of technology on rural school children, the dissemination strategy should include the use of electronic media for sharing information about the project and a website that lists exemplary resources and links to professional associations along with model projects that effectively demonstrate the use of this technology to improve children's learning. Conversely, should a study test the pediatric efficacy of a drug and develop recommendations for dosage levels for children, the study should be summarized and submitted to a reputable medical journal and presented at regional and national pediatric conferences. Although negative results are sometimes thought to be less publishable, these results should still be disseminated, because important negative results still add to the greater body of knowledge.

i. References   The references section identifies the sources used, quoted, and referred to throughout the proposal. If only a few references are used, they can easily be embedded within the text within parentheses. If there are a number of references, a separate section using a style format acceptable within the discipline is appropriate. Formats are readily available on the World Wide Web by using any search engine and searching the words "reference style manuals." A list of style guides and information distinguishing between citations for monographs/books and electronic material is also available. References should be listed in chronological order as they appear throughout the proposal narrative. Software such as Endnote® may be used for ease of reference manipulation and storage for future use.

PREPARING A BUDGET

Federal proposals submitted by colleges and universities must adhere to the cost principles outlined in OMB Circulars A-110, A-21, and A-133. The Federal Acquisition Regulations refer to the OMB Circulars when costing and pricing out a contract (FAR Part 33). The Circulars outline the basic cost principles for (i) the organizational systems institutions must have in place for the acceptance and management of federal funding (A-110); (ii) the determination of what constitutes an allowable and unallowable cost, and what can be budgeted as a direct cost verses and an indirect cost (A-21); and (iii) what documentation and costing analysis is required for federal compliance for audits (A-133). The term "costing" refers to the act of establishing pricing by activity or by unit of cost. State and local governments must adhere to Circular A-87 and nonprofit organizations must follow Circular A-122 for their budgeting principles. The different circulars have similarities, but also have their differences. Investigators should follow cost principles appropriate to their institution.

Given the array of regulations, cost accounting standards, and financial principles involved in federal budgeting, institutions rarely establish different procedures for budgeting for federal, state, nonprofit, or corporate proposal applications. Rather, one universal system applies to all proposals. And, because so many accounting regulations apply to budgeting within organizational contexts, sponsoring agencies require authorizing officials' approval of the budget prior to the final proposal submission.

The circulars applicable to budget preparation are A-21, A-87, and A-122. These circulars communicate three fundamental principles for budget development. First, the funds requested must be "allowable." Budgets may not include requests for gifts, alcohol, unrelated project supplies, advertising, memberships, and other costs that are not directly related to the project. Second, costs must be "reasonable." Reasonable is defined as what a prudent business person in the industry would consider a normal cost based on fair market value. This concept necessitates that investigators obtain a minimum of three quotes for equipment items over $5000 and any unusually large bulk supply purchases (i.e., laboratory cages, reference materials). Sponsors desire a "good value" for their money and it is essential to present costs that are competitive, attractive, and comparable for similar work or supplies.

The following categories are used when preparing budgets:

    a. Personnel
    b. Employee Benefits
    c. Equipment
    d. Travel
    e. Supplies and Materials
    f. Other Direct Costs
    g. Indirect Costs

Each of these sections is discussed in the following paragraphs.

a. Personnel

When presenting costs for salaries, investigators should use their own institutional base salary (current salary) as a basis for computation with an added small escalation factor for cost of living increases each year. If a position is new, the salary level should be appropriate to the position and the level of expertise (e.g., education level and experience) required for the job. Costs budgeted for personnel should be realistic and not overinflated. Some types of federal grants, such as those administered by the NIH, have salary caps, which may be determined via NIH guidelines and discussion with the grant administrator. Investigators are reminded that they cannot devote more salaried time toward a grant than allowed within the demands of any other responsibilities. For example, academic investigators may be required to devote 50% of their time toward teaching. Therefore, time available for grant work is capped at 50%, and only 50% of the investigator's salary may be drawn from grant funds. Within the culture of grant "giving" and "getting" investigators are also encouraged to contribute some of their time/effort toward the project at no charge to the sponsor.

The lead investigator on a project is called the "Principal Investigator" (PI) or "Project Director" (PD), and he/she either charges or contributes a percentage of effort reflected in the budget. The amount of time allocated to the project is a function of the PI's other commitments and the amount of involvement required. Investigators should propose a "reasonable" amount of dedicated time. What constitutes reasonable is a judgment call. If the scope of the project requires substantive time and effort, then perhaps 30% to 50% effort should be budgeted. Conversely, if there are other personnel working on the project, the PI should devote less effort to the project. Levels of effort on a project vary depending on the expertise, role, credentials, and number of additional staff on the project. Questions about the management plan and personnel for the research project should be directed to the institution's authorizing official. This individual will be able to assess the required level of staffing that will then appear competitive to a sponsor.

> **EXAMPLE**

Budgeting for PI effort

This example proposes 15% effort directly charged to the sponsor.

Dr. Jane Doe, PI: $65,000 base salary × 15% effort = $9,750 requested from the sponsor in year 1

PI: $66,950 (3% escalation of base salary) × 15% = $10,042 requested in year 2

PI: $68,959 (3% escalation of base salary) × 15% = $10,344 requested in year 3

Co-Principal Investigators (Co-PIs) are individuals who share equal responsibility for the research plan. In collaborative proposals, Co-PIs are typically individuals with expertise in specialized areas of the research that is beyond the scope of the PI's expertise and are considered essential to fulfilling the objectives. These individuals are budgeted exactly as PIs.

Other titles used in research proposals include Co-Investigator, Senior Research Associate, Statistical Analyst, Coordinator, Manager, and Graduate Research Assistant. Human Resource Officers maintain a list of titles that relate to the level of expertise required for each position within their organization. These titles should be used reflecting comparable salary ranges between like positions at other institutions and then budgeted accordingly.

EXAMPLE

Budgeting for collaborative research proposal

An example of a collaborative research proposal submitted by a higher education institution with three researchers committed to the project would look like the following:

Dr. Jane Doe, PI: $65,000 base salary × 5% effort = $3,250 requested from the sponsor in year 1

PI: $66,950 (3% escalation of base salary) × 5% = $3,348 requested in year 2

PI: $68,959 (3% escalation of base salary) × 5% = $3,448 requested in year 3

Dr. John Miller, Co-PI: $62,000 base salary × 5% effort = $3,100 requested from the sponsor in year 1

Co-PI: $63,860 (3% escalation of base salary) × 5% = $3,193 requested in year 2

Co-PI: $65,776 (3% escalation of base salary) × 5% = $3,288 requested in year 3

Senior Research Associate (SRA): $40,000 base salary × 100% = $45,000 requested in year 1

SRA: $41,200 (3% escalation of base salary) × 100% effort = $41,200 requested in year 2

SRA: $42,436 (3% escalation of base salary) × 100% effort = $42,436 requested in year 3

In the above illustration, two senior personnel are co-directing the project and plan to hire a full-time researcher to carry out the daily activities of the project. Less seasoned investigators often have less staff and devote more time to a project than a senior PI or Co-PI. Regardless of the level of experience of the various members of the research team, salary budgeting needs to be appropriate and realistic as compared to the scope of the project.

Many reviewers already have unofficially established a project cost target well before reviewing the budget. Therefore, budgets should be cost-effective. If the personnel costs are unrealistic, the proposal may be rejected.

b. Employee Benefits

In this section, investigators should use the percentage rates that are negotiated by their Human Resource Office and multiply the percentage(s) for the salary listed under personnel costs. Sometimes different benefit rates apply to different job titles or employee union classifications. Like personnel costs, the employee benefit rates typically include a small escalation factor for the cost of inflation for each additional year of the project. If an investigator works for a small organization without a Human Resource Officer, the investigator can apply a pro-rated amount for benefits that is based on the insurance plans offered within the organization for health coverage, dental, eye, or workman's compensation programs. In this circumstance, it is best to fully detail the calculation process used to determine the benefit percentage applied to the project. The description of computation and types of benefit coverage should be described in the budget narrative and must be attested by a certified accountant.

EXAMPLE

Employee benefits

In either scenario above, employee benefits consist of a percentage rate that is applied to a salary in the following manner:

Dr. Jane Doe, PI: $65,000 base salary × 15% effort = $9,750 × 35% benefits = $3,413 requested in year 1

PI: $66,950 (3% escalation of base salary) × 15% = $10,042 × 35% benefits = $3,515 requested in year 2

PI: $68,959 (3% escalation of base salary) × 15% = $10,344 × 35% benefits = $3,620 requested in year 3

c. Equipment

Equipment is defined by the federal government (and most state governments) as a cost over $5000 and a useful life of 2 years. Any purchase under a $5000 threshold is considered supplies and should be listed within the supply budget line. As stated earlier, equipment purchases require vendor quotes to assure the sponsor that they are receiving the best possible rate for equivalent merchandise.

d. Travel

Travel costs include funds needed for airfare, ground transportation, car rental, taxis, hotel, meals and general incidentals (M&IE). General incidentals are considered gratuity costs that are incurred for tipping cab drivers, baggage handlers, hotel room service providers, and dining staff. The U.S. General Services Administration (GSA) is the official federal agency that publishes the maximum lodging and per diem rates that can be charged to a federal grant or contract. The GSA website is located at http://www.gsa.gov/Portal/gsa/ep/home.do?tabId=0. The GSA rates for lodging and M&IE should be applied to all travel expenses listed in the budget.

To obtain reasonable airfare costs, the investigator should compare airline ticket prices using travel websites or by contacting a travel agent. Since most awards are received several months after a proposal's submission, investigators should use a small escalation factor for airline tickets to take into account cost increases over time.

EXAMPLE

Travel costs

An example of how to present travel costs follows:

> New York City, NY to Ocean City, MD (1 traveler) total = $978 per traveler
> - Airfare from NYC to Salisbury, MD roundtrip = $366
> - Per diem @ $149/day (per diem includes $85 lodging + $64 M&IE allowance) × 3 days = $447
> - Car rental @ $55/day for 3 days = $165

e. Supplies and Materials

Supplies and materials are those items that are necessary for the research project. Typically, laboratory glassware, chemicals, reference materials, equipment parts, software, laptops, inventories, and other associated project costs are outlined in this section. For new investigators, estimating the cost of supplies can be a challenge because every funded project changes over time and estimating the costs of unknown changes requires experience. Generally, adding a small amount of funds for unknown supplies is prudent, and the amount will vary depending on the total desired award and project scope.

f. Other Direct Costs

The other direct costs category is intended to capture all other direct costs that the above categories do not include. Here, investigators list costs for subcontracting with partnering institutions, consultants, facility costs such as hotel rent for hosting a conference outside of their institution, participant costs for human subjects, and so on. When budgeting for subcontracts, the total cost of the subcontractor should be listed in one budget line, accompanied by a note indicating that the individual budget of the subcontractor is attached. Subcontracts are used to engage collaborators who are considered "essential to the scope of work" and without whom the project could not be completed. Because subcontractors may have their own budgeting principles (based on whether they are a nonprofit, corporate, educational, or medical institution), they prepare their own budget for reviewers' analysis. In general, the PI will reach an agreement with a subcontractor during the initial phase of budget construction, and then allow the subcontractor to determine the specific financial details as long as they follow the guidelines of the sponsor.

g. Indirect Costs

Once all of the direct costs have been identified in sections a to f above, indirect costs are applied to the above. Indirect costs are also called "facilities and administrative" (F&A) costs. The F&A costs for institutions that conduct significant amounts of research are negotiated between the institution and a federal agency that specializes in reviewing cost accounting formulas for an organization's general operating costs. The general operating costs include utilities (e.g., lighting, heat, and air conditioning), snow removal, library resources, administrative and budgeting support, space, secretarial and janitorial services, computer networking, liability insurance coverage, and other logistical and physical plant services. Every 4 to 5 years F&A agreements are established between research institutions and the federal government and a percentage rate is added to the overall budgetary costs of personnel, fringe benefits, travel, equipment, supplies and materials, and other costs for contracted services. Typically, costs exceeding $25,000 of a subcontract, participant support costs that support the attendance of individuals at conferences or workshops, and the amount equivalent to tuition and fees are excluded from indirect cost calculations. Once the subcontracting costs, participant support costs, and tuition and fees have been subtracted from the total direct cost, the remainder of the costs is multiplied by the F&A rate to derive the indirect costs included in the budget. A sample budget is given in Table 20-1.

Investigators should submit a budget narrative that details the costs outlined in the budget to help reviewers understand how costs are derived and how the project will be managed to assure alignment of the project objectives with the expenditures.

CHAPTER SUMMARY

Getting funded is an honor and a privilege. Once the process is understood, the most important part of grant writing is convincing others that the proposed investigation is relevant, timely, important, and within the investigator's capabilities in

TABLE 20-1 Sample budget

RESEARCH PROJECT TITLE

PI NAME		DATES OF PROJECT		
A. PERSONNEL	**YEAR 1**	**YEAR 2**	**YEAR 3**	**TOTAL**
1. PI, J. Doe, 5% effort @ $65K base salary with 3% escalation factor	3,250	3,348	3,448	10,045
2. Co-PI, J. Miller, 5% effort @ $62K with 3% escalation factor	3,100	3,193	3,289	9,582
3. Sr. Research Associate @ 100% @ $45K	45,000	46,350	47,741	139,091
Subtotal Personnel	**51,350**	**52,891**	**54,477**	**158,718**
B. EMPLOYEE BENEFITS				
1. PI and Co-PI @ 35% of salary	2,223	2,289	2,358	6,870
2. Sr. Research Associate @ 47% of salary	21,150	21,785	22,438	65,373
Subtotal Benefits	**23,373**	**24,074**	**24,796**	**72,242**
C. EQUIPMENT				
1. Diode machine with ventilator (Quote from XYZ Laboratories)	35,000	0	0	35,000
Subtotal Equipment	**35,000**	**0**	**0**	**35,000**
D. TRAVEL				
1. NYC to Ocean City, MD, one trip per year for 3 days each trip				
a. Airfare @ $366 × 3 travelers	1,098	1,131	1,165	**3,394**
b. Per diem @ $149/day × 3 days × 3 people	1,341	1,381	1,423	**4,145**
c. Car rental @ $55/day for 3 days	165	170	175	**510**
2. National conference (3) estimated @ $1,800 each	5,400	5,562	5,729	**16,691**
Subtotal Travel	**8,004**	**8,244**	**8,491**	**24,740**
E. MATERIALS AND SUPPLIES				
1. Laboratory supplies (glassware, chemicals, cables)	1,200	1,236	1,273	**3,709**

(continued)

2. Statistical software, 3 copies of Softpro @ $500 each	1,500	0	0	**1,500**
3. Laptop for data collection and analysis for Sr. Research Assoc.	2,300	0	0	**2,300**
Subtotal Materials and Supplies	**5,000**	**1,236**	**1,273**	**7,509**
F. OTHER				
1. Subcontract to University of XYZ	54,237	55,864	57,540	**167,641**
2. Facility costs for symposia in NYC	0	10,000	0	**10,000**
3. Human participant stipends @ $15 per subject × 35 subjects each	525	525	525	**1,575**
Subtotal Other	**54,762**	**66,389**	**58,065**	**179,216**
G. TOTAL DIRECT COSTS	**177,489**	**152,833**	**147,103**	**477,425**
H. INDIRECT COSTS				
1. 47.5%—participant support costs, costs of subcontract over $25,000 and tuition and fees	**58,544**	**46,060**	**42,542**	**147,147**
I. TOTAL PROJECT COSTS (G+H)	**236,033**	**198,894**	**189,645**	**624,572**

order to advance the human, animal, and global condition. The concept of research through grant award is founded on the principle of "doing good for humanity." An investigator's ability to collaborate with sponsors through relationship building and conveying a convincing argument using sound evidence is the recipe for successfully obtaining funding. In essence, grants provide funding for leaders and visionaries who seek change. Leadership is an important responsibility that includes the widespread sharing of advances so that the greatest number of individuals can learn and benefit from work supported by federal, state, corporate, and nonprofit sponsors.

KEY POINTS

- Grant writing and the concept of research through grant award are founded on the principle of "doing good for humanity."
- Collaborating with sponsors through relationship building and conveying a convincing argument using sound evidence is the recipe for successfully obtaining funding.
- Grants provide funding for leaders and visionaries who seek change.

Critical Thinking Questions

1. Why is it important to use both library resources and sponsor databases and archives to research your subject?

2. Consider why a frequent mistake made by new investigators is assuming that the reviewers of the proposal are as knowledgeable as they are in their specific discipline.

3. What are some important considerations for finding the *right* funding source? And, why is this important?

4. Why are investigators strongly advised to contact their institutional research officer(s), if available, to help match their expertise and interests with the best-fit funding opportunities and programs?

Applying Concepts

1. Consider reasons why leadership is an important responsibility that includes the widespread sharing of advances so that the greatest number of individuals can learn and benefit from work supported by federal, state, corporate, and nonprofit sponsors.

2. Offer examples of how the concept emphasized above applies to health care and clinical practice.

3. Consider important ethical issues associated with grant writing and seeking funding from sponsors for advancement in health care and clinical practice.

4. Discuss the "culture of grants."

5. Offer examples illustrating ways to search for funding sources for a specific clinical issue of your choice.

6. Consider key points that you would need to include if you were to write a competitive grant proposal for the issue you identified above in question #5.

REFERENCES

Bauer D. *The "How to" Grants Manual: Successful Grantseeking Techniques for Obtaining Public and Private Grants.* 2nd ed. New York: Atheneum; 1984.

Britt R. Universities report stalled growth in federal R&D funding in FY 2006. *INFOBRIEF, Science Resources Statistics, NSF 07-336.* 2007.

Pallister A. *Magna Carta: The Heritage of Liberty*. London: Oxford University Press; 1971.

The Foundation Center's Statistical Information Service. [http://foundationcenter.org/findfunders/statistics/pdf/02_found_growth/03_05.pdf]. New York, NY: The Foundation Center [Producer]; 2007.

The Foundation Center's Statistical Information Service. NIH issues call for perspectives on peer review. *Federal Grants & Contracts Weekly*. 2007;3(13).

SUGGESTED READING

1. Bauer D. *How to Evaluate and Improve Your Grants Effort*. 2nd ed. Westport, CT: The American Council on Education and The Oryx Press; 2001.

2. Bauer D. *The "How to" Grants Manual: Successful Grantseeking Techniques for Obtaining Public and Private Grants*. 6th ed. Westport, CT: Praeger Publishers; 2007.

3. Bowers L. *Physical Educators' Guide to Successful Grant Writing*. Reston: National Association for Sport and Physical Education; 2005.

4. Markin K. The mysteries of budgeting for a grant. *The Chronicle of Higher Education*. 2005;May 27:C2–C4.

5. McVay BL. *Proposal that Win Federal Contracts*. Woodbridge: Panoptic Enterprises; 1989.

6. Molfese V, Cerelin J, Miller P. Demystifying the NIH proposal review process. *The Journal of Research Administration*. 2007;38:127–134.

7. Orlich D. *Designing Successful Grant Proposals*. Alexandria, VA: Association for Supervision and Curriculum Development; 1996.

8. Quinlan Publishing Group. *Writing the Winning Grant Proposal, A Quinlan Special Report*.[Report]. Boston, MA: DiMauro J [Managing Editor].

9. U.S. General Services Administration website was reviewed on February 23, 2008, available at http://www.gsa.gov/Portal/gsa/ep/home.do?tabId=0.

PART V

INTEGRATING EVIDENCE-BASED MEDICINE INTO THE EDUCATIONAL EXPERIENCE

CHAPTER 21

EVIDENCE IN LEARNING AND TEACHING

Tell me, I will forget. Show me, I may remember. Involve me and I will understand.

> —*Chinese Proverb (attributed to Confucius, 450 BC) found in Experiential Learning Cycles as quoted on wilderdom.com/ experiential/elc/ExperientialLearningCycle.htm*

CHAPTER OBJECTIVES

After reading this chapter, you will:

- Recognize the elements necessary for successful learning and teaching in an evidence-based curriculum.
- Understand that clinical research often does not provide the "black and white" answers we seek.
- Know that skill development is fostered by discussion and constructive feedback.
- Learn why making decisions about individual patients is the central focus of clinical epidemiology.
- Be able to explain why the reality of clinical practice is that most cases involve common diagnoses with patients responding to conventional interventions and natural history.
- Understand how learning and teaching from a body of evidence requires active pursuit of the best available evidence by the student.
- Know why the case analysis must not focus on the decisions of the individual care provider.
- Understand that often the evidence is insufficient to fully guide clinical practice.

KEY TERMS

active learning	credentialing exam	framework
clinical rotations	critical appraisal	outcomes
cognitive learning theory	evidence hierarchy	problem-based learning

INTRODUCTION

Learning to practice evidence-based health care requires more than classroom teaching focused on clinical epidemiology. Such a course and the contents of this book provide only a **framework** on which talented professionals-in-training will build upon in their quest to integrate the best available evidence in their practices. The next generation of practitioners-in-training must develop the ability to identify and critically appraise clinical research; and, these learning objectives should be introduced in texts as we have strived to do, and in entry-level courses. If, however, such **critical appraisal** ends with a course rather than becoming a common theme across a professional curriculum, the graduates are not likely to be well prepared to practice evidence-based health care.

The challenges of learning and teaching in a developing curriculum that embraces evidence-based practice are not trivial. To build upon the preparation in clinical epidemiology in advanced courses, time for learning and teaching clinical epidemiology must be allotted early in the curriculum. Preparation in inferential statistics may help students more readily grasp the nuances of probability, risk, odds, and likelihood that permeate discussions related to diagnostic testing, prognostication, and intervention **outcomes**. The greater challenges, however, usually lie in building upon a foundation in clinical epidemiology in clinical courses. One of the greatest challenges we have faced is the desire of students to "have the right answer" and "know how to examine, evaluate, diagnose and treat patients." Some are better than others at coping with the uncertainties uncovered after careful consideration of the myriad of decisions made daily in clinical practice. Testing strategies used to evaluate student performance that ask for the "correct" answer, while easing the burden of assessment, only add to the stresses emanating from uncertainty. Katz (2001) wrote that "the life span of medical facts is short and shortening further all of the time," certainly not comforting news to the student working hard to learn what the current facts are.

Uncertainty is a stressor on those who teach, as well as those who seek to learn. How does one approach, for example, teaching students the "best" way to learn an examination technique that they will likely be expected to perform on **clinical rotations** and perhaps be held accountable for on a **credentialing exam** when the best available evidence suggests the technique is of little use in effectively treating patients? How does the dynamic of a shared learning environment unfold when a well-informed student presents evidence that is contradictory (and stronger) to that offered as the instructor? How does an instructor assist the student caught between the best available evidence and a clinical instructor/preceptor's order to "practice like I have shown you?" Let's face it, it is easier for instructors to be authoritarian, to ask students to identify correct answers and strive to become replicas of themselves as faculty. And, many students are both accustomed to and comfortable with such an approach to learning. In this approach, however, we drift toward expert opinion, falling toward the bottom of the **evidence hierarchy**, thus failing ultimately as practitioners.

The success of a curriculum, students, and a faculty embracing evidence-based health care requires humility, a willingness to address rather than hide from conflicting conclusions and insufficient data, and the time to keep abreast of the best available evidence. Students must be prepared to appraise the clinical literature, empowered to debate the issues, and encouraged to view uncertainty as a challenge rather than a threat. Idealistic goals perhaps, but so is the goal of the universal practice of evidence-based health care optimizing the care of each patient. So the student's, the educator's, and the clinician's missions merge and it all begins in a classroom.

✔ CONCEPT CHECK

The success of a curriculum, students, and a faculty embracing evidence-based health care requires humility, a willingness to address rather than hide from conflicting conclusions and insufficient data, and the time to keep abreast of the best available evidence.

LEARNING CRITICAL APPRAISAL

*Read not to contradict and confute, not to believe and take
for granted, not to find talk and discourse, but to weigh
and consider*

*Sir Francis Bacon (from http://www.quotationspage.com/
quote/29246.html, accessed February 12, 2010)*

These words of wisdom are perhaps more applicable today than ever before as the volume of and accessibility to the clinical literature continues to expand. Contradictory findings are common, as is the need to make decisions as to whether the results of clinical research can or should be applied to decisions about the care of individual patients. In other words, the clinical research often does not provide the "black and white" answers we seek, thus adding to the sense of uncertainty experienced by students, faculty, and clinicians. How is it possible that two groups of investigators can study the same question, yet reach a different conclusion? Perhaps one study was substantially larger allowing for greater statistical power, or the research method of one was considerably stronger. Perhaps the methods of data analysis differed. The knowledgeable research consumer is able to consider these and other issues in a critical appraisal of the reports they read. The foundation for critical appraisal is found in this and other texts and related coursework. Critical appraisal, however, is a skill that is developed with practice over time.

✔ CONCEPT CHECK

Clinical research often does not provide the "black and white" answers we seek, thus adding to the sense of uncertainty experienced by students, faculty, and clinicians.

Skill development is fostered by discussion and constructive feedback. We have found that students working in small groups to address a clinically relevant question often find themselves in a dynamic discussion regarding the strength of the clinical literature. When the groups report out further discussion ensues allowing a large number of students to learn and develop their skills. Such a process is often messy and requires faculty to empower students and guide rather than direct the activities of the class. It is natural for students to feel doubtful and tentative when first involving themselves in this dynamic process of learning and teaching.

The mechanics of locating, identifying, and critically appraising the literature is reviewed in Chapters 6 and 7, and the issues of research design and data analysis are presented in Chapters 8 to 18 and thus not reintroduced in this chapter.

There are a couple of approaches to beginning the process of helping students acquire critical appraisal skills. Students can be provided with specific papers to read, appraise, and discuss, be provided a specific topic and directed to particular databases, or be given very lose guidelines where they select the clinical question, choose the databases to search, and report the results of their work. Students may be provided guidelines on which to base their critical appraisal or may be asked to base their appraisal on criteria of their choosing. Decisions as to how best to proceed depend on the level of preparation of the students across a spectrum of skills including experience searching databases, level of clinical preparation, level of preparation in research design and statistics, and the time available to complete the work. We have found that lesser prepared students do best with more guidance while those with greater preparation enjoy the freedom and challenges in seeking out answers to questions that are of particular interest to a working group.

> ✔ **CONCEPT CHECK**
>
> Students working in small groups to address a clinically relevant question often result in dynamic discussion regarding the strength of the clinical literature. When the groups report out further discussion ensues allowing a large number of students to learn and develop their skills. Such a process is often messy and requires faculty to empower students and guide rather than direct the activities of the class.

LEARNING AND TEACHING FROM A BODY OF EVIDENCE

The only people we know who think effective teaching is easy have never taught a course in their lives. Courses with content directed at clinical care present an additional challenge as the clinical research evolves more rapidly than ever. Staying current across the spectrum of even a single course requires a commitment of time to identify, read, appraise, and integrate new research. For faculty committed to their own research and teaching multiple courses, the task of staying current in all areas of instructional responsibility is an impossible mission: Success in staying as current as possible and teaching from a body of evidence may depend more on perspective and strategy than effort. Teachers are often viewed and view themselves as conveyors of knowledge and truth. Students become recipients rather than active participants. Learning and teaching from a body of evidence requires active pursuit of the best available evidence by the students who, while becoming a labor force, gain the experience necessary to support a lifetime of independent learning. Take, for example, a course in therapeutic modalities. While the elements of such a course and the textbooks used to support the course are fairly universal, currency in the available clinical research across all modality applications for a multitude of medical conditions is a tall task. Groups of students, however, assigned to identify and appraise the literature on specific topics can provide the latest information to the group and thus inform teaching and clinical practice. The quality of these contributions is largely dependent on the foundation developed through a course in clinical epidemiology. When the foundation is lacking, elements of information retrieval and critical appraisal must be integrated into the course, which while good for students diminishes the time available to devote to specific course elements. It can be difficult to strike a balance between developing the topic-specific knowledge base and a skill set to support critical appraisal and lifelong learning. Recognition of the skill set as an important component of the curriculum is, however, often an important step in building a curriculum that promotes evidence-based clinical practice.

> ✔ **CONCEPT CHECK**
>
> Learning and teaching from a body of evidence requires active pursuit of the best available evidence by the students who, while becoming a labor force, gain the experience necessary to support a lifetime of independent learning.

PROBLEM-BASED LEARNING

Making decisions about individual patients is the central focus of clinical epidemiology and is really the vehicle that permits the integration of the best available research with clinician experience and patient values in the hospital and clinic environment. Thus, once students have developed the basic skills of information retrieval and critical appraisal, learning through case analysis provides a powerful means of integrating evidence-based practice into a curriculum. Case- or **problem-based learning** (PBL), sometimes referred to as situation-based learning, also effectively integrates the continuum of the patient care process into the learning process.

EXAMPLE

Learning through case analysis

The case: A 17-year-old female volleyball player presenting with an acutely injured knee sustained while landing awkwardly from a jump.

Elements of discussion: The athlete's gender, activity, and age put her at risk for injury to the anterior cruciate ligament. The risk increase related to these factors, as well as discussion of risk reduction strategies, introduces elements important to clinical practice.

Certainly, differential diagnosis of acutely injured knees offers numerous opportunities to explore issues related to physical examination and imaging. Prognosis and treatment outcomes are issues that also warrant critical review of the clinical literature. The elements of such a case could constitute a large project for an individual student or be assigned to multiple individuals or groups. It is also possible to investigate only selected components, physical examination procedures for the knee for example, of a case. While such a process limits the integration of curriculum components, the use of case analyses serves to ground the discussion in the realities of clinical practice.

✔ CONCEPT CHECK

Making decisions about individual patients is the central focus of clinical epidemiology and is really the vehicle that permits the integration of the best available research with clinician experience and patient values in the hospital and clinic environment. Thus, once students have developed the basic skills of information retrieval and critical appraisal, learning through case analysis provides a powerful means of integrating evidence-based practice into a curriculum.

Case analysis also offers the opportunity to integrate classroom and clinical experiences. The use of information regarding patients receiving care or those recently discharged raises concerns regarding confidentiality as well as opening the door for criticism of care providers known to students and faculty. Obtaining permission to use personal information in case analyses is essential when it is possible that the information may identify the individual patient. Potentially identifying information can take many forms. Unique diagnoses and injuries sustained in particular incidents may identify a patient as can their profession, position on a team, or role in the community. The point is that it is best to secure permission to discuss a case rather than assuming the steps taken to secure confidentiality will be sufficient. This is especially true when the care was provided in the local community.

Cases are analyzed to help students learn to make clinical decisions based on the best available evidence. The reality is that often the evidence is insufficient to fully guide clinical practice and the case analysis is completed outside of the influence of clinical experience, patient preferences, and other factors influencing care. Thus the case analysis must not focus on the decisions of the individual care provider but rather focus on how the research literature can inform practice when similar cases are encountered. Moreover, the process is best not confined behind the closed doors of a classroom open only to faculty and students but rather be inclusive of those participating in the case when possible.

One final consideration regarding problem and case-based teaching and learning that seems to perplex students relates to the nature of the case or problem of interest. Since most cases presented in the literature are rather unique, often in the form of a fairly rare diagnosis, students often assume that the cases and problems they investigate must also be unique. The reality of clinical practice is that most cases involve common diagnoses with patients responding to conventional interventions and natural history. Common cases offer as many or more opportunities for critical appraisal of the related clinical research than those cases that warrant presentation in peer-reviewed settings. While every clinician strives to identify those patients who warrant additional evaluations to rule out potentially serious but uncommon conditions, it is the critical review of routine practices that will have the greatest impact on the broadest spectrum of patients. Consider the once common use of superficial heat, ultrasound, and massage to treat nonspecific low back pain. Certainly, the diagnosis and the interventions are very common and not worthy of a published case report. However, the review of a case involving a patient with nonspecific low back pain is ripe for analysis from perspectives including risk factors and prevention, diagnostic considerations, and intervention effectiveness. Students exploring such a case might gain a wealth of understanding of the challenges faced by clinicians in some settings, very frequently.

✔ **CONCEPT CHECK**

While every clinician strives to identify those patients who warrant additional evaluations to rule out potentially serious but uncommon conditions, it is the critical review of routine practices that will have the greatest impact on the broadest spectrum of patients.

✔ **CONCEPT CHECK**

The reality is that often the evidence is insufficient to fully guide clinical practice and the case analysis is completed outside of the influence of clinical experience, patient preferences, and other factors influencing care. Thus the case analysis must not focus on the decisions of the individual care provider but rather focus on how the research literature can inform practice when similar cases are encountered.

PROMOTING LEARNING AND ASSESSING OUTCOMES

Clinical epidemiology has been described as a unique body of knowledge that enables critical appraisal of the clinic research and the integration of the best available evidence into clinical practice. The goal of developing an understanding of clinical epidemiology in our students is to foster individual preparation, and ultimately cultivate a culture prepared to practice evidence-based health care.

Since clinical epidemiology and evidence-based practice cannot be separated into unique entities, it is really not possible to separate preparation in clinical epidemiology from the development of a talented clinician. The connections between clinical epidemiology and evidence-based practice must be appreciated when developing instructional strategies and assessment instruments. Instruction and assessment must occur along a continuum that begins with a general understanding of clinical epidemiology and the paradigm of evidence-based practice, continues into information retrieval and critical appraisal, and ends when students demonstrate the integration of the best available research into their patient management decisions.

Assessment related to the mechanical issues of data retrieval, methodologic quality appraisal, and data analysis is relatively straightforward. Students and clinicians must also value and strive to practice evidence-based care, which while refining skills also promotes expansion of the paradigm. Successful integration of clinical epidemiology and evidence-based care can only be assessed once students are completing clinical experiences or have graduated and begin practice. Thus, assessment of the student regarding application of the principles developed in the classroom must continue into their clinical experiences. Such assessment requires a planned communication between faculty, clinical instructors, coordinators of clinical education, and students. Such "additional" assessment may be viewed as adding to the burden on clinical instructors already stretched to provide patient care and quality instruction.

In the big picture evidence-based practice is a new paradigm that many current clinical instructors were not exposed to during their training. Over time more clinical instructors will enter this role with expectations that students will integrate clinical research into their patient care recommendations. This demographic shift will permit greater on-site assessment of how effectively students function in an evidence-based practice model. In the current environment, however, some creativity is required to assess students attempting to adapt to "treating patients in the real world" and integrating research evidence into their developing practice patterns. We have found that case reports and postclinical affiliation debriefings permit a level of assessment and remediation when necessary to develop skills within the context of the overall academic mission. The truest test of success comes from the assessment of practicing alumni. Assessment of alumni can be a tall challenge due to geographic dispersion and often low return rates on alumni surveys. Including items related to the value for and practice of evidence-based health care on such surveys, however, provides data related to how effectively an academic curriculum impacted upon practice. Recurring assessment from the classroom to clinical experiences to postgraduation practice also conveys the measure of importance a faculty and an academic unit place on evidence-based health care.

CHAPTER SUMMARY

The goal of this chapter was to encourage the use of evidence in the classroom as we strive to prepare our students with the research skills that are necessary for clinicians in this new millennium of evidence-based medicine (EBM). As American medical schools and professional curriculum are moving from "providing instruction" toward "promoting learning" education is shifting towards modes of learning that require students to apply concepts, follow procedures, solve problems, and make predictions (Amato, Konin, & Brader, 2002; Clark & Harrelson, 2002). These methods of learning have evolved from recent developments in the science of learning and from constructivist theory (Brooks & Brooks, 2001; National Research Council, 2001/2002). In contrast to traditional approaches to learning based on rote memory and recall, these contemporary theories of learning emphasize the way knowledge is represented, organized, and processed. Thus, we are faced with the challenge of introducing research methods as a framework for evidence-based clinical practice. Part of this challenge is to prepare our students with the necessary skills for accessing, synthesizing, interpreting, and applying empirical research findings to determine the best clinical practices when they have not yet become practicing clinicians.

Research skills must be learned, and to do so, they must be taught and practiced (Wingspread Group, 1993). These skills include written and oral communication, information gathering, critical analysis, interpersonal competence, and the ability to use data and make informed judgments following an evidence-based best practice model. Spence (2001) states that we will not meet the needs for a more and better higher education until professors shift to designers of learning experiences and not teachers. The focus in the classroom must shift from "how will I teach this information" toward "how will my students learn this information."

As instructors of preservice students of physical therapy and athletic training, we have realized the need to model the use of high-quality learning experiences. Under this premise, we have delved into PBL, situation-based and case-based learning to help foster the skills of critical analysis and integration and application of research findings following hierarchies of evidence (in EBM) among our students. We have found that PBL, if done well, can improve learning by promoting "enduring understanding" (Wiggins & McTighe, 1998) and help connect the classroom to authentic learning experiences that increase the transfer of key concepts to other contexts outside of the classroom.

What has become clearer to us over the past few years is that "process is content." Stated more specifically, our teaching philosophies have matured and developed around the belief that the *learning process* is as equally important as the subject discipline content. For that reason, when we teach research methods courses there is a strong focus on process skills in addition to traditional research method content. As part of the evolution from "professional lecturer" to "facilitator" of learning, we try to overtly model the following process skills throughout the course: teamwork, assessment, written and oral communication, technology integration, critical thinking, and problem solving (SCANS, 1993; NASPE/NCATE, 2001). We also try to have our students think and write about their performance of these skills in the context of the physical therapy and athletic training disciplines. These skills are more obviously important to the next generation of educators; however, it is important that future certified athletic trainers and physical therapists be able to peer teach, communicate effectively with the health care system and parents, locate available community-based resources for patients involved with substance abuse or other psychosocial issues, demonstrate technology use, interpret professional literature, and make effective presentations (Knight, 2001).

Cognitive learning theory and its constructivist approach to knowledge suggest that we should not look for what students can repeat or mimic, but for what they can generate, demonstrate, and exhibit (Brooks & Brooks, 1999). As constructivists and instructors of future clinical practitioners (e.g., physical therapists and certified athletic trainers), we've found PBL to be a logical and refreshing instructional practice for us to follow when teaching research methods as a framework for evidence-based clinical practice.

PBL is an **active learning strategy**. Active learning suggests that students demonstrate what they know and are able to do. Rather than emphasizing discrete, isolated skills, PBL emphasizes the application and use of knowledge in research methods and EBM. In order for PBL and EBM to be effective, we believe both PBL and EBM must be done well, and that comes with practice by the instructor and students alike.

KEY POINTS

- One of the greatest classroom challenges is the desire of students to "have the right answer" and "know how to examine, evaluate, diagnose and treat patients."
- Contradictory findings are common.
- Critical appraisal is a skill that is developed with practice over time.
- Skill development is fostered by discussion and constructive feedback.
- Staying current requires a commitment of time to identify, read, appraise, and integrate new research.
- Students often assume that the cases and problems they investigate must also be unique.
- Obtaining permission to use personal information in case analyses is essential when it is possible that the information may identify the individual patient.
- The connections between clinical epidemiology and evidence-based practice must be appreciated when developing instructional strategies and assessment instruments.
- Instruction and assessment must occur along a continuum.
- Assessment requires a planned communication between faculty, clinical instructors, coordinators of clinical education, and students.

Critical Thinking Questions

1. Discuss some approaches to beginning the process of helping students acquire critical appraisal skills.
2. Consider problem-based learning as an active learning strategy. What does that mean for the use of evidence in the classroom?
3. Discuss the types of skills that should be learned and practiced as research skills.
4. What is the goal of developing an understanding of clinical epidemiology?
5. Discuss how problem-based learning, if done well, can improve student learning.

Applying Concepts

1. Consider cognitive learning theory and its constructivist approach to knowledge. Choose a course (i.e., epidemiology, therapeutic modalities, etc.) and suggest ways that students can generate, demonstrate, and apply their understanding of course content through case studies and other problem-based learning strategies.
2. Offer examples of how to efficiently and effectively assess students' basic skills of information retrieval and critical appraisal learning through case analysis.

REFERENCES

Amato H, Konin, JG, Brader H. A model for learning over time: the big picture. *J Athl Train.* 2002; 37(4 Suppl): S236–S240.

Brooks JG, Brooks MG. *In Search of Understanding: The Case for Constructivist Classrooms.* Alexandria, VA: Association for Supervision and Curriculum Development; 1999.

Clark R, Harrelson G. Designing instruction that supports cognitive learning processes. *J Athl Train.* 2002;37(4 Suppl): S152–S159.

Katz DL. *Clinical Epidemiology & Evidence-based Practice.* Thousand Oaks, CA: Sage Publications; 2001:xvii.

Knight K. *Assessing Clinical Proficiencies in Athletic Training: A Modular Approach.* Champaign, IL: Human Kinetics; 2001.

National Association for Sport and Physical Education/National Council for the Accreditation of Teacher Education (NASPE/NCATE). *Guidelines for Initial Physical Education Program Reports: NASPE/NCATE 2001 Initial Physical Education Standards.* 3rd ed. Reston, VA: NASPE; 2001.

National Research Council. How people learn: brain, mind, experience, and school. Committee on developments in the science of learning and committee on learning research and educational practice. In: Bransford JD, Brown AL, and Cocking RR, (eds). *Commission on Behavioral and Social Sciences and Education.* Washington, DC: National Academy Press; 2002.

National Research Council. Knowing what students know: the science and design of educational assessment. Committee on the foundations of assessment. In: Pelligrino J, Chudowsky N, and Glaser R, (eds). *Board on Testing and Assessment, Center for Education.* Division of Behavioral and Social Sciences and Education. Washington, DC: National Academy Press; 2001.

Secretary's Commission on Achieving Necessary Skills (SCANS). *What Work Requires of Schools: A SCANS Report for America 2000.* Washington, DC: US Department of Labor; 1991.

Spence L. The case against teaching. *Change Magazine.* 2001; 33 (6):10–19.

Wiggins G, McTighe J. *Understanding by Design.* Alexandria, VA: Association for Supervision and Curriculum Development; 1998.

Wingspread Group on Higher Education. *An American Imperative: Higher Expectations for Higher Education.* Johnson Foundation; 1993, pp. 1, 13.

CHAPTER 22

THE CLINICAL EXPERIENCE

It is a miracle that curiosity survives formal education.

—Albert Einstein (1879–1955), as quoted in
Albert Einstein Quotes on ThinkExist.com
Quotations (http://www.thinkexist.com)

CHAPTER OBJECTIVES

After reading this chapter, you will:

- Understand the importance of evidence-based medicine (EBM) in the classroom.
- Be able to discuss the role of clinical education in student learning.
- Understand the similarities and differences between didactic education and clinical education.
- Be able to describe the concept and practice of grand rounds in clinical education.
- Understand the differences between case reports and case studies.
- Recognize the three parts of a case study.
- Be able to discuss the benefits of case-based learning in clinical education.
- Understand strategies to integrate evidence-based medicine into classroom experiences.
- Appreciate the continued preparation of clinicians in the practice of evidence-based medicine.
- Understand how patients, students, and the public can be educated through grand rounds.

KEY TERMS

case reports	evaluation	interventions
case-based learning	evidence-based medicine	outcomes
critical review	grand rounds	
didactic lecture	informed consent	

INTRODUCTION

Chapter 21 discussed strategies to help students and instructors integrate **evidence-based medicine** into classroom experiences. These experiences build an important foundation for students. It is through clinical education, however, that students apply what has been learned, demonstrate professional behaviors, and often come to appreciate that the "real world" of health care practice differs from the comfort of the classroom where greater certainty often exists and mistakes don't affect real patients. Classroom or didactic education and clinical education are not two unrelated parts of an educational experience. In fact, it is likely that the more these experiences can be integrated, the richer the educational program will be. Thus, this chapter serves as extension of Chapter 21 and focuses on the continued preparation of clinicians in the practice of evidence-based medicine once they have progressed into clinical education. The timing of clinical experiences for students in the health care professions varies widely between disciplines and academic program. Thus, there is not a single strategy. We have chosen to focus on two common assignments required of student–clinicians, **case reports** and **grand rounds** but also identify other opportunities to apply many of the principles found in this text during clinical education.

CASE REPORTS

Case reports, also referred to as case studies, have appeared in many clinical journals and are frequently required of students in the health care professions. There is continuing debate as to the values of case reports in today's clinical literature, although some are valuable additions to the knowledge base. Our purpose is not to debate the extent to which case reports should be included in the literature but rather to focus on those student-generated reports that rarely warrant publication. In this context the case report really becomes a form of **case-based learning**. In many instances students are seeing what they have learned being applied to the care of a real patient.

Case reports may be retrospective or prospective and when prepared by students either a description of what was observed or what the student did. As the clinical education experience progresses, the student assumes more responsibility and thus can prepare a case report prospectively based on their actions. This type of case report generally requires the student to acquire and review a detailed medical history, complete and describe a thorough examination, review findings of additional testing and imaging, and consider the diagnostic possibilities. The student is then faced with the challenge of developing a plan of care that is agreeable to the patient. Lastly, the outcome of the case must be described. Regardless of the student's role in the case these reports are usually presented in written form, sometimes followed by oral presentation.

> ✔ **CONCEPT CHECK**
>
> Case reports may be retrospective or prospective and when prepared by students either a description of what was observed or what the student did.

Case reports serve to guide professional development, enhance writing skills, and require a review of pertinent literature. The literature review component of case reports is a critical juncture in the integration, or lack thereof, of evidence-based medicine in the academic experience. Each of the authors of this book has prepared case reports and identified literature that was supportive of our positions and conclusions. In these cases the literature search was often incomplete while the papers retrieved received only limited **critical review**.

The practice of evidence-based medicine requires consideration of the best available evidence rather than the identification of evidence that supports or refutes a particular position. When one considers a case, including all of the interactions with a patient and each of the decisions made, there are multiple opportunities for critical inquiry. Perhaps it is the number of opportunities that pose the greatest barrier to maximizing instruction in the practice of evidence-based medicine.

EXAMPLE

Multiple opportunities for critical inquiry

Consider a case involving an acutely injured knee. A typical case report might begin with a description of the patient, their presentation, and initial findings. There is then a rapid transition to the physical examination that extends into the results from imaging. While convention suggests moving on to **interventions** and a description of the outcome of treatment, it may be time to slam on the breaks and consider what has occurred. What does or should the student know based on the patient's presentation and response to the initial interview questions? Assuming the knee injury was traumatic, what structures may be involved and how should one proceed to narrow the diagnostic possibilities. For example, based on the Ottawa knee rules is imaging indicated? How does the student propose to proceed with the physical examination? How likely are the proposed examination procedures to result in false findings, or stated differently, how confident should one be when an examination procedure result is positive or negative?

In posing the questions in the above example, the student and their learning, rather than an external audience, becomes the focus of the case study. Ending the case study at the **evaluation** stage paints an incomplete picture, but is it necessary for the student to go further? The answer will depend on where the student is in their training and the context in which the case study is completed. A case study that serves as a culminating experience likely needs to be further developed to address interventions and **outcomes**. For the student early in their academic preparation focusing on the evaluation of patients the purpose of the case study has been served and the process ended. We suggest that purpose-specific case studies are valuable in teaching student to practice evidence-based health care. By breaking cases into evaluation, intervention, and outcome assessment across an academic program permits sufficient attention to the issues related to diagnostic accuracy, efficacy, and effectiveness of interventions and the properties of the outcomes measurement instruments to truly identify and apply the best available evidence.

Before leaving the subject of case studies we would like to share additional observations. The first is that cases that are sufficiently unique to be of interest to an external audience are relatively uncommon. Those in academia that have been subjected to culminating case reports can likely attest to the state of boredom that sets in somewhere in the grading process and the jubilation that accompanies completion. However, when one asks students to examine the components of a case and address diagnosis, intervention, or outcomes, the common cases we encounter daily provide sufficient fodder because it is not the case but the appraisal and application of the literature that draws the reader's attention. The second observation is that detailed, well-prepared case studies require a good bit of effort. Our collective observation is that when a student prepares a case report they often lose the forest through the trees, therefore losing the opportunity to critically evaluate the management of the case and thus clinical practice in general. There is not a single or simple solution to this dilemma; however, failure to appreciate the time required to acquire and carefully appraise the salient literature will sentence the instructor to the continued reading of case reports that are neither interesting nor generally informative.

✔ CONCEPT CHECK

The practice of evidence-based medicine requires consideration of the best available evidence rather than the identification of evidence that supports or refutes a particular position.

GRAND ROUNDS

In using the term "grand rounds" we are borrowing from the long-standing practice of hospitals and other health care facilities of scheduling regular plenary sessions for providers (or subgroups of providers) in the organization. In their original form grand rounds involved live patient evaluations and interactive discussion of the diagnostic process and plan of care. The format of grand rounds has changed markedly over the past few decades and now the presence of patients is uncommon (Herbert & Wright, 2003). Often grand rounds that were intended to spark debate and discussion resemble a typical classroom lecture. The most common format is now a **didactic lecture** (Mueller et al., 2006). A single speaker completes a presentation and provides, hopefully, time for questions and, more importantly, discussion. Moreover, the didactic format tends to lead the audience through a case rather than engaging in an effort to identify the best course.

We chose to use the term grand rounds in the context of integrating evidence-based health care into the educational experience because the critical analysis of cases often does not occur in typical courses. Moreover, active student participation in such classes is often limited. We also wish to distinguish what we have labeled grand rounds from presentations made by students in a classroom as a component of an academic course. It is not our intention to judge the values of such presentations but simply point out that most are delivered in front of one or a few faculty rather than a community of clinicians. In fact, it is the community of clinicians sharing their knowledge and debating the issues that best distinguishes events as grand rounds. While the presence of patients is uncommon at grand rounds today, returning to this format has some attraction especially for students early in their training with limited patient contact. We also do not believe that grand rounds be limited to being led by a recognized expert. In fact, we would encourage some sessions be led by students. Siri et al. (2007) described the experiences of surgical residents charged with reviewing components of a case involving the death of a patient. While we hope that our readers will not face this challenge in the context of the preparation as health care providers, cases with unsatisfactory outcomes often provide the best opportunities to learn. Regardless of the outcome of the case, grand rounds create a format where the case defines the direction of the learning rather than a syllabus or an instructor. Often a clinician attending grand rounds is quite familiar with the various diagnostic and treatment procedures discussed. However, the pearls of wisdom that enhance our abilities are frequently found at grand rounds. These may be in the form of the consideration of a diagnosis that had not crossed our mind, a better technique for treatment, and a better means of assessing treatment outcomes. Filling in the gaps in what we know is at the core of lifelong learning and grand rounds can be a wonderful forum for our professional development.

> ✔ **CONCEPT CHECK**
>
> We chose to use the term grand rounds in the context of integrating evidence-based health care into the educational experience because the critical analysis of cases often does not occur in typical courses.

Requirements

Clinician Support

The first piece to developing a system of regularly scheduled grand rounds that will impact student learning is the support of clinicians associated with the academic program and/or the community. Certainly, faculty members are welcome but unless the faculty member sees patients on a regular basis, they will not bring fresh cases to the table.

Willing Participation of Students

The second piece is the willing participation of students. Grand rounds can foster the development of professional behaviors partially because participants are taking responsibility for their continuing education rather than being compelled to participate in order to receive a grade or meet a requirement imposed by an employer. Garnering the enthusiastic participation in grand rounds is not a slam dunk if one considers some of recent reports. The group, however, does not need to be large. Representation of practicing clinicians is essential while the active and hopefully enthusiastic participation by students can be sustaining.

The Cases

The next pieces to grand rounds are the cases. Circumstances will influence whether patients are present for all or a portion of the session or whether someone will be charged with presenting the case. In all circumstances steps must be taken to protect the confidentiality of medical information. Patients should be informed of the process if they are to appear and provide **informed consent** for their information to be discussed. The participants in the grand rounds should hold the information they have about the patient with the same rigor as that of a patient seen during routine clinical care. If a case is presented by a clinician, permission to discuss the case should also be sought. While it is possible to present a case without revealing the identity of the patient, the more unique the case and the smaller the practice community, the more likely confidentiality will be breached. It is also likely that efforts to maintain anonymity will lead to some failure to present information germane to the case. Thus, we recommend obtaining informed consent from the patient that is the subject of the case regardless of whether they will be present.

CONCEPT CHECK

The participants in the grand rounds should hold the information they have about the patient with the same rigor as that of a patient seen during routine clinical care.

Critical Review and Debate of Relevant Literature

The final piece to grand rounds and the one that is really related to teaching the practice of evidence-based health care is critical review and debate. Each participant possesses a unique set of experiences and a unique understanding, or lack thereof, of the relevant literature. Each case should provide or, even better, stimulate a quest for the best available evidence. Students should be included when participants are asked to cite the literature supporting a particular view and participate in the critical review of relevant literature. Much like a good research paper, the value of grand rounds often is found in the pursuit of what is left unanswered rather than in the answers provided through the event. It is certainly possible that one case may span more than one meeting as time may be required to gather and appraise the literature regarding elements of a particular case.

Other Considerations

Professionalism, mutual respect, and the quest for knowledge that defines practice are more critical to the success of grand rounds than rules and structure. The focus is on learning rather than teaching and while senior clinicians often guide those with lesser experience and expertise, every effort should be made to avoid top-down presentation of information characteristic of many classrooms found in health care education programs.

Case-based learning is not a new concept. The quest for the best available evidence, however, is not always evident especially when cases are recycled in course materials. Case reports and grand rounds foster the pursuit of the best available evidence and help students identify what they don't know as opposed to a structured course where efforts are made to help them learn what the faculty believes they should know. As educators strive to prepare students to practice evidence-based health care and apply the contents of this text, these educational strategies can prove quite useful.

✔ CONCEPT CHECK

Case reports and grand rounds foster the pursuit of the best available evidence and help students identify what they don't know as opposed to a structured course where efforts are made to help them learn what the faculty believes they should know.

CHAPTER SUMMARY

Grand rounds are a ritual of medical education, consisting of presenting the medical problems and treatment of a particular patient to an audience consisting of doctors, residents, and medical students. The patient is usually present for the presentation and may answer questions. Grand rounds have evolved considerably over the years, with most current sessions rarely having a patient present and being more akin to lectures.

KEY POINTS

- The practice of evidence-based medicine requires consideration of the best available evidence rather than the identification of evidence that supports or refutes a particular position.
- Case reports may be retrospective or prospective and when prepared by students either a description of what was observed or what the student did.
- The literature review component of case reports is a critical juncture in the integration, or lack thereof, of evidence-based medicine in the academic experience.
- The format of grand rounds has changed markedly over the past few decades and now the presence of patients is uncommon.
- Grand rounds create a format where the case defines the direction of the learning rather than a syllabus or an instructor.
- Grand rounds can foster the development of professional behaviors partially because participants are taking responsibility for their continuing education rather than being compelled to participate in order to receive a grade or meet a requirement imposed by an employer.
- In all circumstances steps must be taken to protect the confidentiality of medical information.
- Each case should provide or stimulate a quest for the best available evidence.
- Much like a good research paper, the value of grand rounds often is found in the pursuit of what is left unanswered rather than in the answers provided through the event.
- Case reports and grand rounds foster the pursuit of the best available evidence and help students identify what they don't know as opposed to a structured course where efforts are made to help them learn what the faculty believes they should know.

Critical Thinking Questions

1. What are the benefits of case reports in evidence-based medicine?
2. How are case studies used in education today?
3. What are the three parts of a case study?
4. Case reports serve as guides to the development of what three key elements?
5. What is the historical significance of grand rounds in medical education?

Applying Concepts

1. Consider various clinical and health care situations in which steps must be taken to protect the confidentiality of medical information. Discuss potential challenges and ethical considerations for the responsible conduct in clinical practice (refer to Chapter 5, if necessary).
2. Discuss the educational and medical significance of grand rounds in teaching and learning from an evidence-based practice perspective.

REFERENCES

Herbert RS, Wright SM. Re-examining the value of medical grand rounds. *Acad. Med.* 2003;78:1248–1252.

Mueller PS, Segovis CM, Litin SC, et al. Current status of medical grand rounds in departments of medicine at US medical schools. *Mayo Clin Proc.* 2006;81:313–321.

Siri J, Reed AI, Flynn TC, et al. A multidisciplinary systems-based practice learning experience and its impact on surgical residency education. *J Surg Educ.* 2007;64:328–332.

GLOSSARY

Note: The more basic key terms found in the chapters are not defined in this glossary. For these definitions, please consult Merriam-Webster's online dictionary (http://www.merriam-webster.com/dictionary/).

A

active learning suggests that students demonstrate what they know and are able to do

analysis of covariance (ANCOVA) a special case of ANOVA where a variable is introduced for the purpose of accounting for unexplained variance. ANCOVA increases statistical power (chance of rejecting the null hypothesis)

a priori power analysis estimation of an appropriate sample size for a study is done before the study takes place

B

Belmont Report is a written report that originated from the Department of Health, Education and Welfare (HEW) which concentrates on and lays down the guidelines for the protection of human subjects used in research

bench research is often thought of as being conducted in a laboratory environment under tightly controlled conditions. Also known as basic science

beneficence is the ability of the practitioner to secure and stabilize the condition or well being of the client while they are receiving treatments or involved in a research project. It can also be understood as acts of kindness, charity, or comfort to the individual client that go beyond their normal obligation to the client

benefit versus risk a written document that states the benefits and the risks of a potential activity. The benefits must outweigh the risks to be useful

biomedical research a vast and diverse field where questions related to the functions of the body, disease, responses to medications, injury mechanisms, and disease and injury patterns are addressed

blinding is a technique where the subjects, members of the experimental team, or clinicians are not fully aware of a certain component of a study. An example is if an individual is a control or part of experiment

Boolean search is a search based on the notion of logical relationships among search terms. Specifically, from a computer programming perspective, the operator terms of "OR," "AND," and "NOT" effect strict logically collated outcome or search results. Stated differently, each of the operator terms (i.e., or, and, not) used to combine search terms instructs a different operation or set of search directions for the computer to follow

C

call for abstracts in order to present research findings at a professional meeting the investigators must respond to a call for abstracts from the organization sponsoring the meeting and submit an abstract for review

case reports "a detailed report of the diagnosis, treatment, and follow-up of an individual patient. Case reports also contain some demographic information about the patient (for example, age, gender, ethnic origin)" (1)

case-based learning case reports and grand rounds foster the pursuit of the best available evidence and help students identify what they don't know as opposed to a structured course where efforts are made to help them learn what the faculty believes they should know

CINAHL electronic database

clinical epidemiology what can be done to help prevent or treat a patient's condition (disease/injury) in a clinic or office

clinical practice guidelines systematically developed statements to assist practitioner and patient decisions about appropriate health care for specific clinical circumstances

clinical prediction guides also known as clinical prediction rules. Prefer the term clinical practice guide, as opposed to rule, since the true purpose of these reports is to guide, rather than dictate, clinical decisions

clinical prediction rules developed from a cluster of exam findings or characteristics and may assist in the evaluative or treatment phase of patient care

clinical research "research that either directly involves a particular person or group of people or uses materials from humans, such as their behavior or samples of their tissue, that can be linked to a particular living person" (2)

clinical rotations "a period in which a medical student in the clinical part of his/her education passes through various 'working' services" (3)

Cochrane collaboration "an international not-for-profit and independent organization, dedicated to making up-to-date, accurate information about the effects of health care readily available worldwide. It produces and disseminates systematic reviews of health care interventions and promotes the search for evidence in the form of clinical trials and other studies of interventions" (4)

cognitive learning theory suggests that we not look for what students can repeat or mimic, but for what they can generate, demonstrate, and exhibit

conceptual framework "a group of concepts that are broadly defined and systematically organized to provide a focus, a rationale, and a tool for the integration and interpretation of information" (5)

control biases methods of studies of prevention, treatment and diagnostic procedures, and steps that minimize investigational bias

correlations between variables the methods and statistical analysis of research into relationship

credentialing exam examination required prior to receiving professional certification

credibility also known as validity in qualitative research. Credibility is based on a set of standards by which honesty, accuracy, and dependability of the data can be judged. The intensive, first-hand presence of the researcher is the strongest support for the validity or credibility of the data collected through qualitative inquiry

criterion variable "in regression analysis (such as linear regression) the criterion variable is the variable being predicted. In general, the criterion variable is the dependent variable" (6)

critical appraisal to assess and regard the significance of efficiently accessing and effectively determining the applicability, reliability, and validity of published research in order to distinguish best clinical practices

critical review the practice of evidence-based medicine requires consideration of the best available evidence rather than the identification of evidence that supports or refutes a particular position

cultural codes codes, or the unwritten rules, that make ones culture

D

data information collected through observation and/or experimentation, and later scrutinized through a series of statistical analyses to determine results.

database electronic libraries of indexed journals, books, and nonjournal bibliographic literature and documents that are overseen, managed, and updated on a regular basis

dependability in research is associated with a judgment of the repeatability of research findings. If findings are repeatable, then they are considered to be reliable. In qualitative research, the notion of reliability is referred to as dependability. Also associated with consistency

dependent variable something that is measured by the researcher

diagnosis "the determination of the nature of a disease, injury, or congenital defect" (7)

diagnostic continuum the differences between research into diagnostic testing and prevention or treatment strategies

didactic lecture a single speaker completes a presentation and provides hopefully, time for questions and more importantly, discussion

disablement model "an evaluation and treatment model based on specific impairment, functional loss, and attainable quality of life rather than a medical diagnosis" (8)

disease-oriented measures measures that provide insight into the physiology of illness or injury. DOE measures provide information about a patient's pathology and are of most interest to health care providers, as opposed to being important to patients

E

empirical research a methodological approach to problem solving in which decisions are based upon findings and conclusions established as a result of analyzing collected data about variables and the relationships that connect them. A process or set of ideas used for asking and answering questions

epidemiology the study of why disease and injury occur in a population

estimates of sensitivity and specificity the ability of a test to identify those with and without a condition and are needed to calculate likelihood ratios

ethical issues the contrast of appropriate and inappropriate behaviors, and are based on personal, moral, professional (i.e., cultural), and societal views of accepted, principled criteria, and guidelines for responsible conduct

ethnography focuses on the study of the group and their culture. Closely associated with the fields of anthropology and sociology. The studying of cultural or cultural groups, but it is not limited to this inquiry and includes topics of investigation such as office settings/corporate culture, youth sport groups, cults, community-based groups, feminism/sexism in communities or institutions, policy application and delivery, and racism

evidence hierarchy rank reviews based on the strength of the argument made and the evidence given

evidence-based medicine (EBM) "the process of applying relevant information derived from peer-reviewed medical literature to address a specific clinical problem; the application of simple rules of science and common sense to determine the validity of the information; and the application of the information to the clinical problem" (7)

evidence-based practice the process by which decisions about clinical practice are guided from evidence in research based on scientific models and theoretical paradigms

external validity relates to how generalizable the results of a study are to the real world

F

false negative results test results may fail to detect pathology when it is present

false positive results test results may suggest pathology is present when it is not

G

generalizability of research findings the reader must assess whether the investigators used research methods that minimized potential bias and maximized data validity

global and region-specific measures survey instruments used to assess global health status typically focus on quality of life and disability. These often are multidimensional scales and include questions that specifically address both physical health and emotional well-being

grand rounds live patient evaluations and interactive discussion of the diagnostic process and plan of care

grounded theory is a method of qualitative inquiry that results in the generation of a theory. The theory can be thought of as a by-product of the data because it develops and perhaps even changes during the qualitative inquiry process. The resultant theory evolves and is derived from the data, thus the theory is considered anchored or "grounded" in the research

H

human participants a individual who partakes in a activity

I

independent variable something that is manipulated by the researcher

Injury Rate refers to the number of new injuries per unit of exposure time

internal culture standards, values, philosophy and professional guidelines shared by a societal ethos

internal validity refers to the validity of a study's experimental design. For example, most experiments are designed to show a causal relationship between an independent variable and a dependent variable. If an experiment can conclusively demonstrate that the independent variable has a definite effect on the dependent variable, the study is internally valid. If, however, other factors may influence the dependent variable and these factors are not controlled for in the experimental design, the study's internal validity may be questioned

interpretivism also known as qualitative inquiry. To understand the meaning of an experience for particular participants, one must understand the phenomena being studied in the context of the setting for the participants of interest

intervention the magnitude of change on one or more measures or as a probability of a favorable or adverse outcome

intervention outcomes results attributed to treatment

invisible web areas of the Internet that are inaccessible to search engines

L

levels of evidence following the CEBM classification of levels of evidence, the highest level of evidence is Level 1 evidence that comes from randomized controlled trials (RCT), which are the gold standard for clinical trials methodology

likelihood ratios "the likelihood ratio, often denoted by Λ (the capital GREEK LETTER LAMBDA), is the ratio of the maximum PROBABILITY of a RESULT under two different hypotheses" (8)

limits of agreement (LOA) the absolute differences between two measurement techniques are compared to each other and specifically looks for systematic error. To perform this analysis, data must be on a continuous scale and both techniques must produce the same units of measurement

M
methodologic flaws threaten the validity of data reported in studies
methodologic quality in research Whiting et al. developed a 14-item assessment tool to assist consumers in evaluating the methodological quality of research into diagnostic tests. Scores of 10 or more are considered to reflect sound research methods

N
nonclinical research research and development of new diagnostic technologies. However, not until a diagnostic test is studied in the population it is intended to benefit can the true magnitude of benefit and risk be elucidated

O
outcome measures the data analysis conducted in preparation of a guide can also generate likelihood ratios that translate the probability of a successful outcome with an intervention when a patient presents with a group of characteristics derived from investigations where outcomes are dichotomous
outcomes instruments instruments designed to address functional limitations and disabilities that are often associated with patients who have the specific injury or illness

P
paradigm shift "an adjustment in thinking that comes about as the result of new discoveries, inventions, or real-world experiences" (8)
parametric and nonparametric statistics nonparametric statistical methods of comparison are used to analyze nominal data. Parametric statistics analyze the (distribution of) variance and are appropriate to analyze interval and ratio data under most circumstances
pathology "the medical science, and specialty practice, concerned with all aspects of disease but with special reference to the essential nature, causes, and development of abnormal conditions, as well as the structural and functional changes that result from the disease processes" (7)
patient-important outcomes consideration of patient values serves as a reminder that clinicians should not get carried away interpreting numbers and forget that the patient is the focus of attention

patient-oriented measures measures that are of direct interest to patients rather than clinicians. POE often involves information that is subjectively self-reported by patients as opposed to objective clinical or laboratory measures that are taken by health care providers or researchers

patient values principles, morals, ethics, standards fundamental to the individual person

phenomenology refers to how people describe things and how they experience them via their senses and the role of the researcher(s) is to then study and describe these experienced situations

point estimates of association "when a parameter is being estimated, the estimate can be either a single number or it can be a range of numbers such as in a CONFIDENCE INTERVAL. When the estimate is a single number, the estimate is called a "point estimate" (9)

position statements synthesize the best available evidence and provide concise recommendations for patient care

positive and negative prediction values a positive likelihood (+LR) ratio is indicative of the impact of a positive examination finding on the probability that the target condition exists. A negative likelihood ratio addresses the impact of a negative examination on the probability that the condition in question is present

predictor variables "a variable that can be used to predict the value of another variable (as in statistical regression)" (10)

prevalence the proportion of a sample which has a given injury or illness at a single time point

prevalence ratio the ratio of the injury prevalence estimates between two groups

probability estimates provided in association with point estimates of association

problem-based learning integrates the continuum of the patient care process into the learning process

procurement principles the protection of due process, equal access to opportunities, and the receipt of funding for research to benefit society are codified in statutes governing the procurement process

publication guidelines provides guidelines regarding the length and style of the abstract and publishes submission deadlines

PubMed a journals database provided as a service of the U.S. National Library of Medicine and the National Institutes of Health. The database contains journal abstracts and citations and includes links to full text articles and other related resources

P-values an indication that the differences observed when studying a sample are reflective of true population differences

R

randomized clinical trials "clinical trials that involve at least one test treatment and one control treatment, concurrent enrollment and follow-up of the test- and control-treated groups, and in which the treatments to be administered are selected by a random process" (11)

randomized trials require that each patient enrolled in a study receive all intervention for prescribed periods of time in randomized order

receiver operator characteristic curves provides a clinicians information about tests that generate measures on a continuous scale such as blood pressure, range of motion, and serum enzyme levels

regression analysis "a technique used for the modeling and analysis of numerical data consisting of values of a dependent variable (response variable) and of one or more independent variables (explanatory variables)" (8)

relative risk provides a proportion of injury incidence between two groups and is identical to the calculation of risk ratio

relevant literature information that is related to the topic of discussion, it is most important in the introduction of the paper

research hypothesis predicts the answer to the question (also see Chapter 1)

S

scientific method a systematic process where the creation of a research hypothesis that is based on existing knowledge and unconfirmed observations. Experiments are then designed and conducted to the test these hypotheses in an unbiased manner. The scientific method requires that data be collected via observation or, in the health sciences, often via instrumented devices in a controlled manner

scientific paper conveying and discussing the results of an investigation

scientific writing writings exhibiting the methods and principles of science

selection bias characteristics that subjects have before they enroll in a study may ultimately influence the results of the study. These may include things like age, maturation, sex, medical history, injury or illness severity, and motivation, among many others

special tests patient interviews and the performance of physical examination procedures

standard error of measurement (SEM) "a test based on error with regard to reliability. The difference between the obtained test result and the hypothetical true result" (7)

statistical power chance of rejecting the null hypothesis. Statistical power increases the likelihood of finding "statistically significant" differences or in other words rejecting the null hypothesis

strength of evidence can vary between and even within a clinical practice guideline depending upon the quality and quantity of research available

systematic review a research process where the investigators identify previous studies that address a particular question, summarize findings, and when possible collapse data for meta-analysis, a process where statistical analysis is performed on data combined from multiple studies

T

theoretical model a strict statement of relations that can be put into equation (e.g., Theory of Relativity). Used to represent a type of physical analogy (e.g., the brain is like a computer)

theoretical research hypothesis describes how expected changes in the dependent variable depend on the independent variable as a result of the study

theory a tentative explanation for the facts and findings that evolve from the research process

therapeutic intervention the clinician needs to know what is wrong before it can be made right

translational research a more recent term that is used to describe investigations that apply the results from basic science to the care of patients. Sometimes referred to as "bench-to-bedside," translational research seeks to speed the development of more effective patient care strategies

translational research consists of expert opinion and disease-oriented evidence

treatment outcomes "evaluation undertaken to assess the results or consequences of management and procedures used in combating disease in order to determine the efficacy, effectiveness, safety, practicability, etc., of these interventions in individual cases or series" (11)

Type I and II errors Type I errors occur when a null is rejected and in fact population differences do not exist. Type II error occurs when a null is not rejected yet a study of the population would reveal differences between groups

V

variables the things or stuff being questioned or measured in the study. Must have two or more categories of distinguishing qualities or distinctive characteristics, a range of values, parameters, or quantifiers

REFERENCES

1. National Cancer Institute. Retrieved March 08, 2010, from http://www.cancer.gov/dictionary/?CdrID=44007
2. Clinical Research & Clinical Trials. (2009, July 23). Retrieved March 8, 2010, from http://www.nichd.nih.gov/health/clinicalresearch/
3. McGraw-Hill Concise Dictionary of Modern Medicine. (2002). Retrieved March 4, 2010, from http://medical-dictionary.thefreedictionary.com/

4. The Cochrane Collaboration website: About Us section. http://www.cochrane.org/docs/descrip.htm
5. Mosby's Medical Dictionary, 8th edition. (2009). Retrieved February 20, 2010, from http://medical-dictionary.thefreedictionary.com/
6. Online Statistics: An Interactive Multimedia Course of Study. Retrieved March 08, 2010, from http://onlinestatbook.com/glossary/index.html
7. Stedman's Medical Dictionary for the Health Professions and Nursing, 6th ed. Baltimore, Maryland: Lippincott Williams and Wilkins; 2008.
8. The Free Dictionary by Farlex. Retrieved March 7, 2010, from http://www.thefreedictionary.com
9. Online Statistics: An Interactive Multimedia Course of Study. Retrieved March 08, 2010, from http://onlinestatbook.com/glossary/
10. WordNet® 3.0. Retrieved March 08, 2010, from http://dictionary.reference.com/
11. Medical Dictionary online. Retrieved March 7, 2010, from http://www.online-medical-dictionary.org/

Page numbers followed by *f*, *t* and *b* indicate figures, tables, and boxes, respectively.